A Manual of

ORTHOPAEDIC TERMINOLOGY

A Manual of
ORTHOPAEDIC TERMINOLOGY

CAROLYN TALIAFERRO BLAUVELT

Writer/Editor, Medical-Dental Publications;
Midatlantic Chapter, American Medical Writers' Association,
Bethesda, Maryland

FRED R.T. NELSON, MD, FACS, FAAOS

Clinical Assistant Professor of Surgery,
Visiting Assistant Professor, Human Performance Laboratory,
Uniformed Services University of the Health Sciences, Bethesda, Maryland;
Adjunct Assistant Professor of Health Sciences,
George Washington University, Washington, D.C.

FOURTH EDITION

with 94 illustrations

The C. V. Mosby Company

ST. LOUIS · BALTIMORE · PHILADELPHIA · TORONTO   1990

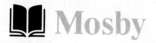

Editor: Eugenia A. Klein
Developmental editor: Kathryn Falk
Assistant Editor: Jo Salway
Production/editing: Editing, Design, & Production, Inc.
Design: Gail Morey Hudson

The opinions or assertions contained herein are the private ones
of the authors and are not to be construed as official or as reflecting
the views of the Uniformed Services University of the Health Sciences
or the Department of Defense.

FOURTH EDITION

The C.V. Mosby Company
11830 Westline Industrial Drive, St. Louis, Missouri 63146

Library of Congress Cataloging in Publication Data

Blauvelt, Carolyn Taliaferro, 1933-
  A manual of orthopaedic terminology/Carolyn Taliaferro Blauvelt,
Fred R. T. Nelson.—4th ed.
    p.   cm.
  Includes bibliographical references.
  ISBN 0-8016-0157-6
  1. Orthopedics—Terminology.   I.   Nelson, Fred R. T., 1941-
II.   Title.
    [DNLM: 1.   Orthopedics—terminology.   WE 15 B645m]
RD731.B63   1990
617.3'0014—dc20
DNLM/DLC
for Library of Congress   89-13189
                                                      CIP

GW/D/D 9 8 7 6 5 4 3 2

The Fourth Edition
is dedicated to all

ORTHOPAEDIC NURSES AND TECHNICIANS

in recognition of their professional skills,
loyalty, and dedication within the orthopaedic community.
Their support to physicians and patients
is gratefully appreciated.

Foreword to third edition

Since its publication as a first edition in 1977, *A Manual of Orthopaedic Terminology* has been a valuable reference to provide quick access to lucid definitions of the extensive and specialized terminology used by orthopaedic surgeons and others concerned with the musculoskeletal system.

Musculoskeletal structures represent a major system of the human body, encompassing those anatomic elements of structural support vital to dynamic and static biophysical function of the body as a whole. Effective function of this system in relation to the whole depends on normal and abnormal reactions of the various tissues comprising the musculoskeletal system. Proper understanding of the morphology and functions of the musculoskeletal system in health or disease states demands a multidisciplinary interest in the anatomy, physiology, biochemistry, and biomechanics of bones, cartilage, muscles, tendons, nerves, and ligamentous and synovial tissues.

Maintenance of function requires effective application of new information to disease prevention and investigation, preservation, restoration, and development of the form and function of the entire musculoskeletal system.

The authors recognize that the terminology generated by orthopaedic surgeons, neurosurgeons, physiatrists, other specialists, and researchers working with the musculoskeletal system is as extensive as the system itself. Therefore the primary purpose of this condensed reference is to make learning that terminology an easier task for the newcomer to the field.

Although the terms used in the practice of orthopaedic surgery are frequently complex words or word groups, some are better known by acronyms. Acronyms, which may have a narrow origin or geographic significance, appear frequently, making communication difficult in some instances. A secondary purpose of this text is its intended use as a repository of acronyms in common usage today. Some of these have been determined to be obsolete and have been deleted from this edition.

The authors have updated and expanded the text to include the newest and most recent terms in the field. The section on research terminology has been revised. The chapter on prosthetic and orthotic terminology has been modified. Joint replacement, electric stimulation of fracture healing, scanners, and other new technologic terms have been added in the revision to reflect current usage.

A Manual of Orthopaedic Terminology satisfies the purpose intended by the authors. It is an invaluable resource for nurses, secretaries, technicians, and physicians who must identify words or acronyms. This is particularly true for the newcomer to orthopaedics.

As an orthopaedic surgeon, I wish to express appreciation to the authors for a most valuable contribution to the educational armamentarium available to all of us in the field. Better understanding and communication are the likely benefits for the user of this text. Each will contribute to improved quality of medical care for all patients.

Charles V. Heck, M.D.

Consultant to the Executive Director, American Academy of Orthopaedic Surgeons

Preface

Since the inception of *A Manual of Orthopaedic Terminology* in 1977, the manual has continued to grow in keeping with the many changes taking place in the orthopaedic specialty. With the third edition, the manual experienced a Japanese translation (1986). As we present this fourth edition, the purpose and objectives remain the same: to describe with brevity and clarity the language of orthopaedics and, hopefully, contribute to the understanding of this specialty. We have attempted to find a convenient way of sorting out, rearranging, and distributing the many terms in their proper category to assist both the professional and the layman.

Usually one must refer to many textbooks to obtain specific meanings of terminology within the specialty. This compendium of terms will enable the reader to deal with the language of orthopaedics more effectively. The manual was designed to assist nurses, orthopaedic residents, technicians, office assistants, researchers, librarians, allied health professionals, and others who interface with or are a part of the orthopaedic community.

How does one use this manual? Unlike a standard dictionary, the chapters are defined according to areas of orthopaedic specialty. A reader interested in a certain type of x-ray examination, disease process, or surgical procedure refers to that chapter. Each chapter introduction presents a format divided into sections to give greater coherence to related terms. The expanded index lists and cross-references all key words and their appropriate pages. However, with increasing familiarity and knowledge of orthopaedics, the user will recognize the terms and their place in a certain chapter.

Proper names (eponyms) are listed in alphabetic order and grouped together in context within a chapter. This will readily assist those looking for a specific name that is related to a disease process or surgical procedure.

The interlude between the third and fourth editions produced a significant amount of new material, and the fourth edition reflects these changes. We have updated, expanded, and revised the chapters where constant revision is necessary in keeping with the rapid growth in the field. Fundamentals may not change, but materials, methods, and techniques do.

The last decade of the twentieth century will see a tremendous surge in the application of biochemical and biophysical knowledge in clinical orthopaedics. This will include applications in electrobiology, diagnostics, oncology, and immunology. Changes in pharmacology and nonsurgical modalities will have a wide influence in orthopaedic practice. Chapters updated for this edition include the following:

The *classification of fractures by region of bone and degree of injury* has more recently appeared in the literature. These classification systems by types and grades are presented in this edition.

Certain diseases have been recognized *as distinct entities*. Terms for some disorders have changed as the understanding of the biology or mechanism of the disorder is better understood. Included are some classification systems that have gained general acceptance.

The use of *magnetic resonance imaging* in orthopaedics has expanded markedly in the last 5 years. Terms related to this technology and some advancements in radiology have been added.

In the area of *tests, signs, and maneuvers,* physical examination reports are more frequently including eponyms. One area of considerable confusion has been the knee examination, and a table has been added to clarify this examination.

As the quality and spectrum of *laboratory testing* improved, so did the approach to the terminology. Normal values are no longer listed, and reference is made to the local testing facility for those values. This important chapter has meticulously been updated.

The establishment of trauma centers has lead to greater use of *orthopaedic first aid appliances.* These and other treatment methods have been added to Chapter 6.

The area of frequent change is in *orthotics and prosthetics.* However, the material changes in prosthetics and new orthotics fabricated for specific purposes did not alter the devices still being used and current with this edition.

Reconstructive joint surgery continues to produce the most material and latest concepts. Materials, past and present, are included to show the tremendous strides made in operative orthopaedics as well as other surgical fields. Replantation surgery with microvascular techniques has produced terminology similar to general surgical terms. Numerous figure illustrations have been added to complement this chapter.

The hand and the foot are subspecialties of orthopaedics intricate enough to be set apart individually. The anatomy, diseases, and surgical procedures are covered in Chapters 9 and 10 with an updated vocabulary.

Professionals in the field of orthopaedics work closely with members of their allied health specialties in patient care—*occupational therapy* and *physical therapy.* For that reason terms from those associated areas are included, and their importance to orthopaedics is noted. The current trends and services of the specialties of occupational therapy and physical therapy have been brought up to date with complete revisions in both areas.

Musculoskeletal research within orthopaedics is rapidly expanding. Research terminology is unique

and unlike that which is used in a clinical setting. It includes the language of biochemistry, biomechanics, immunology, physics, engineering, and prosthetics. The introduction to Chapter 12 outlines the various stages of research, from the idea to the written protocol, the research in progress, and the end results and findings. Advances in technology are presented, incorporating clinical and biomedical research. A conscious effort was made to keep the chapter relatively brief. Terms that might overflow into applied orthopaedics are maintained, but a complete reference was not appropriate for this edition.

No one can write a book on all areas of orthopaedics and keep it current without the help of many competent people. This manual is no exception. We have chosen contributors whose background and experience make them well qualified to assist in updating material for each edition and who work directly or indirectly in this specialty. These people have generously given of their time, in view of other professional commitments, to improve the correctness and accuracy of information, provide an update, and give constructive criticism. We can share in the success of this manual with them, and we wish to express our appreciation and thanks to the following individuals and/or organizations who participated in the revisions of the fourth edition:

The American Occupational Therapy Association, Division of Professional Practice, Rockville, Maryland.

The American Physical Therapy Association, Department of Practice, Alexandria, Virginia.

Robert W. Chambers, MD, Chairman, Department of Pathology, Suburban Hospital, Bethesda, Maryland. *Laboratory.*

Gary E. Friedlaender, MD, Professor and Chairman, Department of Orthopaedics and Rehabilitation, Yale University School of Medicine, New Haven, Connecticut. *Tissue banking and bone grafts.*

John J. Gartland, MD, James Edwards Professor Emeritus of Orthopaedic Surgery; Director, Office of Departmental Review, Jefferson Medical College, Philadelphia, Pennsylvania. *Musculoskeletal diseases.*

Joshua Gerbert, DPM, MS, Dean for Academic Affairs, Professor of Podiatric Surgery, California College of Podiatric Medicine, San Francisco, California. *Podiatry terminology, The Foot.*

Donald P. Jenkins, PhD, Associate Professor of Surgery, Georgetown University, Washington, DC; Visiting Associate Professor of Anatomy, Uniformed Services University of the Health Sciences, Bethesda, Maryland; Anatomy Consultant to the CIBA Collection. *Anatomy.*

David M. Lichtman, MD, FACS, Rear Admiral, Medical Corps, U.S. Navy; Commander, Naval Medical Command, Northwest Region, Oakland, California; Professor of Surgery, Uniformed Services University of the Health Sciences, Bethesda, Maryland. *The Hand.*

James M. Salander, MD, FACS, Colonel, Medical Corps, U. S. Army; Chief, Peripheral Vascular Surgery Service, Walter Reed Army Medical Center, Washington D.C.; Associate Professor of Surgery, Uniformed Services University of the Health Sciences, Bethesda, Maryland; Director, Military Region, American College of Surgeons Committee on Trauma. *Vascular.*

For past contributors of the first, second, and third editions, we would like to acknowledge Wilton H. Bunch, MD, PhD; John F. Burkart, MD; Helen F. Delaney, OT; J.M. Dennis, DPM; Stephen F. Gunther, MD, FAAOS; Carole Hays, MA, OTR, FAOTA; Donald L. Hiltz, PT; Steve Kramer, CPO; David M. Lichtman, MD, FAAOS; Donna M. Mathisen, GPT; W. Patrick Monaghan, PhD; Francesca C. Music, MS, MT (ASCP); James M. Salander, MD, FACS; Barton K. Slemmons, MD, FAAOS; J. Craig Stevens, MD; Myron D. Tremaine, MD, FAAOS; and David Q. Wilson, MD, FAAOS.

We are especially indebted to the late Charles V. Heck, MD, the former executive director of the American Academy of Orthopaedic Surgeons. It was through his support and encouragement that the book became a reality.

The success of the first three editions proved the need for a reference of this kind for this specialty. It is with pleasure that we present this fourth edition with many, many thanks not only to our contributors but also to the editorial staff and those "behind the scenes" at The C.V. Mosby Company, whose continued guidance, support, and publication skills have contributed much to the book's success.

Carolyn Taliaferro Blauvelt
Fred R.T. Nelson

Contents

Introduction to the orthopaedic specialty

Or"tho-pae'dic. Orthopaedic means correction or prevention of bony deformities (formerly, especially in children). The word comes from the Greek *orthos*, meaning straight, upright, right, or true—hence, also correct or regular—and from the Greek *pais*, meaning child.

The scope of orthopaedic surgery includes the treatment, management, and rehabilitation of patients with musculoskeletal conditions affecting bones, muscles, joints, tendons, ligaments, cartilage, blood vessels, nerves, and related tissues through surgical, nonsurgical, and other medical measures. The nature of these conditions may involve congenital abnormalities, metabolic disease processes, metastatic (tumor) pathology, or traumatic injuries (fractures), to name a few conditions requiring the expertise of the orthopaedic specialty. When surgery is indicated, postoperative rehabilitation is equally important in the continued care and treatment of musculoskeletal conditions.

The orthopaedic surgeon is a specialist on the musculoskeletal system as applied to adult and childrens' orthopaedics and the management of trauma. In addition, he or she possesses a working knowledge of neurology, cardiopulmonary physiology, and bioengineering in the care of the orthopaedic patient. This expertise has expanded in recent years to include computerized tomography, electrical and magnetic bone stimulation, microsurgery, and knowledge of the advances in internal and external fixation devices. Orthopaedic medicine is continually changing, and the orthopaedic surgeon is challenged with the responsibility of keeping informed of new techniques through continuing education in the field.

The orthopaedic surgeon develops many skills in the practice of this specialty. Nonoperative measures include the artful application of casts for immobilization and management of fractures or scoliosis, to the treatment of diseases and disabilities through conservative management. In the operating room, the orthopaedist is skilled in the repair and reconstruction of major skeletal defects, which include replacing diseased joints with plastic implants, inserting metallic rods and other devices for stability, or performing fusions, revisions, or amputations. Of a more delicate nature, he or she performs surgery that applies arthroscopic and microvascular techniques that encompass skin grafts, finger transplants, nerve repairs, and similar difficult procedures.

From a team approach, the orthopaedic specialty depends on many other disciplines in the management of patients. The immediate team members are the professional nurses who provide and participate in the primary care of patients and who are assisted by the invaluable services of the orthopaedic technicians, both in the clinic and hospital setting. The second group of team members includes the allied health professionals, the physiatrist, physical therapist, and occupational therapist. These individuals are directly involved in, and may be consulted for, the development of a treatment plan in a patient's rehabilitation. The next group of team members providing assistance includes the prosthetists (artificial limbs) and orthotists (braces), who measure, fit, design, and fabricate devices for the orthopaedic patient. Indirectly, the manufacturer of orthopaedic appliances plays an important role, as does the researcher who tests the biocompatibility of materials used in the musculoskeletal system.

All of these specialties are an important and integral part of the orthopaedic team, providing a combination of skills that benefits thousands of patients with musculoskeletal problems. Other disciplines that interface with orthopaedics include bioengineering, electrobiology, transplantation, diagnostic imaging, oncology, biochemistry, and similar areas.

Orthopaedic medicine has become so diverse that specialization within the specialty is becoming an accepted practice. In addition to general orthopaedics, a physician may specialize in diseases and surgery of the spine, soft tissues, the hand, the foot, major joints, trauma, sports medicine, or the fascinating, ever-changing area of orthopaedic research. Many physicians are exposed to orthopaedic surgery during their training years, but only a select group actually pursues this difficult and diverse field to the point of certification.

The qualifications for certification by the American Board of Orthopaedic Surgery (ABOS) are 4 or 5 years of graduate education following medical school, and an additional year of practice in which his or her ethical conduct is monitored. The physician must complete all requirements to become "board certified" and a diplomate of the Board. Following completion of the certification requirements, an orthopaedic surgeon becomes eligible for fellowship in the American Academy of Orthopaedic Surgeons (AAOS), the national organization of the specialty. The admission to fellowship in the Academy is based on a 2-year practice period beyond certification and certain other specific requirements. The Academy fellowship at present represents about 81% of the orthopaedic surgeons in the United States.

The national organization of the specialty, the American Academy of Orthopaedic Surgeons, developed the accepted definition of orthopaedics in 1952:

Orthopaedic Surgery is the medical specialty that includes the investigation, preservation, restoration, and development of the form and function of the extremities, spine, and associated structures by medical, surgical, and physical methods.

1

Classifications of fractures, dislocations, and sports-related injuries

---

The musculoskeletal reaction to trauma can result in a variety of bone, muscle, and ligamentous disruptions; sometimes fracture and ligamentous injuries occur concurrently. The general types of musculoskeletal trauma are fractures, dislocations, subluxations, sprains, strains, and diastases.

This chapter defines the classification system of fractures and dislocations in two parts: the first is a general description that can be easily understood by the nonspecialist, and the second part gives a more complicated grading system used within the orthopaedic specialty. Most patients with musculoskeletal injuries present to an emergency room in an acute stage and are treated by the emergency room physician until it is determined an orthopaedic specialist may be required. Good communication is essential, and it is beneficial to the nonspecialist to understand the language of orthopaedics in relating the assessment of acute injuries. This understanding is also useful in situations involving telephone consultations between physicians' assistants at the scene of an accident and the emergency room physician. A brief and accurate description is vital to the evaluation and treatment of the injured, and familiarity with the six-step classification system that follows will help in understanding the significance of accurate communication. The second part, a system of grades, types, and mechanisms, is not new, but is included to supplement the existing information on musculoskeletal trauma.

Familiarity with the correct terms will enable one to identify a fracture immediately. For example, "open, midshaft, femur, comminuted fracture" is a brief description, but relates a lot. To achieve this degree of accuracy, learning the classifications is necessary. They are:

1. Open versus closed
2. Portion of bone involved and general appearance
3. Position and alignment of fragments
4. Classic and descriptive names
5. Contributing factors
6. Degree and nature of healing

Interestingly, fractures have specific terminology that varies from time of occurrence to healing. Fractures may be given anatomic names, or those of a person, a place, or the method by which they occurred; they are further defined in terms of how they occurred, reason for the break, and degree; and, as fractures begin to heal, the degree and nature of healing is described. Also in need of clarification is the management of fractures. *Closed* management (or reduction) means surgery was not indicated and that treatment was in the form of a manipulation, cast, splint or traction application, or some combination of the three. *Open* management (or reduction) means that surgical reduction and incision with or without metallic fixation were required.

There have been many new advances in the treatment of fractures, and a recent trend is from casting to bracing or the combination of both in fracture management. The term *cast brace* has been applied to the form of treatment in which brace design is often incorporated into temporary standard cast materials. This method allows for limited motion in braces during the early healing stage with "controlled" fracture movement. Its use has shown greater callus weld around the fracture site, improved ligamentous healing, and earlier recovery of joint mobility and muscle control.

Another method of fracture management employs electrical devices called *surface electrodes* externally applied to a fracture site. For certain types of fractures, this method has diminished the need for braces.

The mainstay of traumatic fracture management has been in external fixation devices and frames, also known as "fixateurs." External fixation is a diverse system for managing loss of skeletal stability with various components placed in bone.

Treatment methods and external skeletal fixation devices are discussed in Chapters 6 and 7.

General and specific types of dislocations, subluxations, sprains, strains by anatomic location, and sports-related soft-tissue injuries are also given.

Classification for trauma registry

Some research on outcome of fracture management requires the coordination of many treatment centers. To facilitate the comparison of specific types of fractures, the Orthopaedic Trauma Association has approved a specific classification for use in the Trauma Registry. The classification system uses many of the terms that follow in this chapter. However, it is highly specific as to location and nature of associated injuries. Anyone working in this area should refer to Gustilo, RB: The classification of fractures and dislocations, Chicago, Year Book Medical Publishers (in press).

TERMINOLOGY OF FRACTURES AND DISLOCATIONS

fracture (L., *fractura*): structural break in the continuity of a bone, epiphyseal plate, or cartilaginous joint surface, usually traumatic with disruption of osseous tissue.

fracture-dislocation: fracture of a bone that is also dislocated from its normal position in a joint.

dislocation (L., *luxatio*): the complete displacement of bone from its normal position at the joint surface, disrupting the articulation of two or three bones at that junction and altering the alignment. This displacement affects the joint capsule and surrounding tissues (muscles, ligaments). Dislocation (*luxation*) may be traumatic (direct blow or injury), congenital (development defect), or pathologic (as in muscle imbalance, ligamentous tearing, rheumatoid arthritis, or infection).

subluxation: incomplete or partial dislocation in that one bone forming a joint is displaced only partially from its normal position; also, a chronic tendency of a bone to become partially dislocated, in contrast to an outright dislocation, for example, shoulder, patella, and, in infants, hip.

diastasis: may be one of two types: (1) a disjointing of two bones that are parallel to one another, for example, radius and ulna, tibia and fibula complex, or (2) the rupture of any "solid" joint, as in a diastasis of the symphysis pubis. Such injuries tend to occur in association with other fractures and are then called "fracture-diastases."

sprain—ligament rupture (L., *luxatio imperfecta*): the stretching or tearing of ligaments (fibrous bands that bind bones together at a joint) varying in degrees from being partially torn (stretched) to being completely torn (ruptured), with the continuity of the ligament remaining intact. Following a sprain the joint may become inflamed, swollen, discolored, and extremely painful. Rest, elevation, and a restrictive bandage, splint, or cast are methods of treating these injuries until properly healed. When a ligament or tendon has been torn completely, dislocation may also occur. Surgical repair may be required in some cases.

strain: stretching or tearing of a muscle or its tendon (fibrous cord that attaches the muscle to the bone it moves) resulting in sore, painful, and sometimes stiff muscles. With rest, strains will subside in 2 to 3 days, but symptoms may persist for months.

CLASSIFICATIONS OF FRACTURES
Open versus closed (Fig. 1-1)

closed f.: fracture that does not produce an open wound of the skin but does result in loss of continuity of bone subcutaneously. Formerly called simple f.

open f.: fracture in which one of the fragments has broken through the skin and in which there is loss of continuity of bone internally. Formerly called compound f.

Portion of bone involved

To denote the portion of bone involved or the point of reference of a fracture, the distal third may be expressed as D/3 or distal/3, the middle third as M/3 or middle/3, and the proximal third as P/3 or proximal/3. Middle/3 fractures are commonly known as midshaft fractures. (The abbreviations are acceptable for clinical notes but should be spelled out in formal correspondence.) For highly specified anatomic locations, the following terms are commonly used.

apophyseal f.: avulsion fracture of an apophysis (bony prominence) where there is strong tendinous attachment.

articular f.: fracture involving a joint surface. Also called joint f. and intraarticular f.

cleavage f.: fracture involving shelling off of cartilage with avulsion of small fragment of capitellum humeri. Also called Kocher f.

condylar f.: fracture of any round end of a hinge joint; see Femoral and distal humeral fractures.

cortical f.: fracture involving cortex of bone.

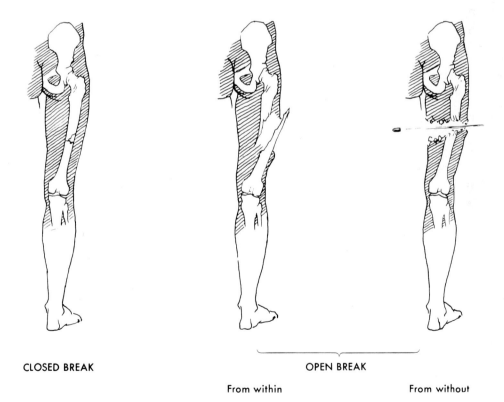

CLOSED BREAK   OPEN BREAK

From within   From without

Fig. 1-1. Closed versus open fracture. (From Schneider FR: Handbook for the orthopaedic assistant, ed 2, St Louis, 1976, The CV Mosby Co.)

diacondylar f.: transcondylar fracture (line across the condyle).

direct f.: fracture resulting at specific point of injury and due to the injury itself.

extracapsular f.: fracture that occurs near, but outside, the capsule of a joint, especially the hip.

intracapsular f.: fracture within the capsule of a joint.

periarticular f.: fracture near but not involving a joint.

transcondylar f.: fracture occurring transversely between the condyles of the elbow. This term is also used in fractures of the femur and bones with condyles. Also called diacondylar f.

tuft f.: fracture of the distal phalanx (tuft) of any digit. Also called bursting f.

General appearance (Fig. 1-2)

avulsion f.: tearing away of a part; a fragmentation of bone where the pull of a strong ligamentous or tendinous attachment tends to forcibly pull the fragment away from the rest of the bone. The fragment is usually at the articular surface.

bursting f.: multiple fragments, usually at the end of a bone; classically, f. of the first cervical vertebra.

butterfly f.: a bony *fragment* shaped like a butterfly and part of a comminuted f. Usually involves high energy force delivered to the bone.

chip f.: a small fragment, usually at the articular margin of a condyle.

comminuted f.: fracture with more than two fragments; lines of fracture that may be transverse,

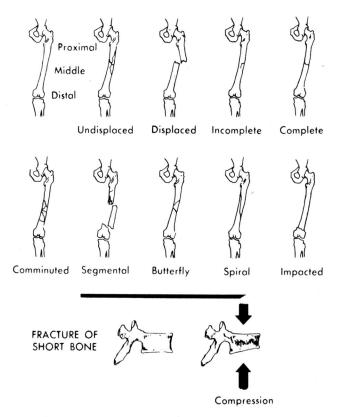

Fig. 1-2. Fracture terminology, general appearance. (From Schneider FR: Handbook for the orthopaedic assistant, ed 2, St Louis, 1976, The CV Mosby Co.)

oblique, spiral, or T or Y shaped. Also called splintered f. Locations of fractures most likely to be comminuted are:

supracondylar f. of humerus: immediately above humeral condyle.

supracondylar f. of femur: immediately above femoral condyle.

intertrochanteric f. of femur: line of fracture extending between lesser and greater trochanters.

bimalleolar f.: of inner or outer malleoli of ankle.

long bone f.: of the proximal, middle, and/or distal third of shaft.

complete f.: the bone is completely broken through both cortices.

compression f.: crumbling or smashing of cancellous bone by forces acting parallel to the long axis of bone; applied particularly to vertebral body fractures.

depressed f.: usually used to describe skull or articular surface fractures where the fragment is displaced below the overall level of the skull or articular surface.

displaced f.: fragments are moved away from each other.

double f.: segmental fracture of a bone in two places.

epiphyseal f.: involves the cartilaginous growth plate of a bone. Also referred to as epiphyseal slip f., Salter f., and Salter-Harris f.

fissure f.: crack in one cortex (surface) only of a long bone.

greenstick f.: in children, incomplete, angulated fracture with a partial break. Also called incomplete f., interperiosteal f., hickory-stick f., and willow f.

hairline f.: a nondisplaced fracture line (crack) in the cortex of bone.

impacted f.: fracture in which fragments are compressed by force of original injury, driving one fragment of bone into adjacent bone.

incomplete f.: cortices of bone are buckled or cracked but continuity is not destroyed; the cortex is broken on one side and only bent on the other. Microscopically, the fracture is present on bent side and resorption and callus will occur on this side as well. Types are greenstick f., torus f.

infraction f.: small radiolucent line seen in pathologic fractures, most commonly resulting from metabolic problems.

leadpipe f.: in children, a forearm fracture in the cortex of long bone shaft where one of the cortices is compressed and bulging at point of impact on one side, with a linear fracture on opposite side.

linear f.: lengthwise fracture of bone; implies that there is no displacement.

multiple f.: two or more separate lines of fracture in the same bone.

oblique f.: slanted fracture of the shaft on long axis of bone.

occult f.: hidden fracture (undetected by radiograph), generally occurring in areas of the ribs, tibia, metatarsals, and navicula.

plastic bowing f.: curved deformity of a tubular bone without gross fracture.

Salter-Harris f.: epiphyseal fractures in children involving epiphyseal growth plate (types I through V), the seriousness of which could arrest growth or cause deformity. The Aitken classification types I, II and III are the same as Salter-Harris types II, III, and IV, respectively. Epiphyseal fractures are also described anatomically (Fig. 1-3).

secondary f.: pathologic fracture of bone weakened by disease.

segmental f.: several large fractures in the same bony shaft.

spiral f.: one in which fracture line is spiral shaped, usually on shaft of long bones. Also called torsion f.

stellate f.: fracture with central point of injury, from which radiate numerous fissures.

subperiosteal f.: a fracture in which the bone but not its periosteal tube is broken; uncommon, usually the result of a direct blow.

torsion f.: see Spiral f.

torus f.: usually noted in children; a stable, often incomplete fracture in which one distal cortical surface appears to be wrinkled by compression

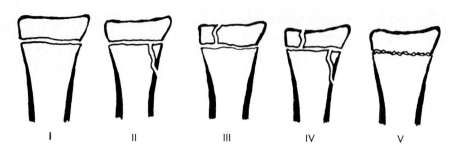

Fig. 1-3. Epiphyseal fracture types classified by the Salter method.

forces and the opposite cortex may or may not be infracted by tension forces.

transverse f.: line of fracture across the shaft at right angles to the long axis of bone.

Position and alignment of fragments
(Fig. 1-4)

The position of a fragment refers to any displacement of one bony fragment in reference to the next. Displacement, should it exist, can be in any plane.

Alignment refers to rotatory and/or angular deviation of the distal fragment in relation to the proximal fragment. For example:

posterior bow: in a completely displaced midshaft femoral fracture with a 3 cm overriding and 20 degree anterior angulation, the bone ends are not in apposition; there is a 3 cm shortening, and the distal end is angulated in an anterior direction.

bayonet position: when the fragments touch and overlap, but with good alignment.

Internal and external rotation can also be stated in degrees.

Classic and descriptive names

The following fracture types are listed according to anatomic location.

Shoulder fractures (proximal humerus and scapula)

anatomic neck f.: fracture in the area of tendinous attachments, the true neck of humeral metaphysis.

Hill-Sachs (Hermodsson) f.: A moderate com-

pression fracture of the humeral head usually seen after an anterior dislocation of the shoulder.

surgical neck f.: fracture in area below the anatomic neck of the humerus.

Arm and elbow fractures

boxer's elbow: a chip fracture at the tip of the olecranon caused by a fast extension of the elbow in a missed jab (punch).

condylar f.: fracture of the medial or lateral articular process of the humerus at the elbow.

epicondylar f.: fracture through one of the two epicondyles, medial or lateral.

Kocher f.: semilunar chipped fracture of capitellum with displacement into joint.

supracondylar f.: fracture through the distal metaphysis of the humerus.

T f.: intercondylar fracture shaped like a T.

Y f.: intercondylar fracture shaped like a Y.

Forearm and wrist fractures

Barton f.: dorsal dislocation of carpus on radius with associated fracture of the dorsal articular surface of radius; deformity similar to Colles f.

chauffeur's f.: fracture of the radial styloid caused by a twisting or snapping type of injury. Also called backfire f., lorry driver's f.

chisel f.: incomplete, medial head of radius with fracture line extending distally about ½ inch.

Colles f.: through the distal radius within ½ to 1 inch of the articular surface with dorsal displacement of the distal fragment, producing a *silver-fork deformity;* generally associated with a fracture of the ulnar styloid.

de Quervain f.: combination of a wrist scaphoid

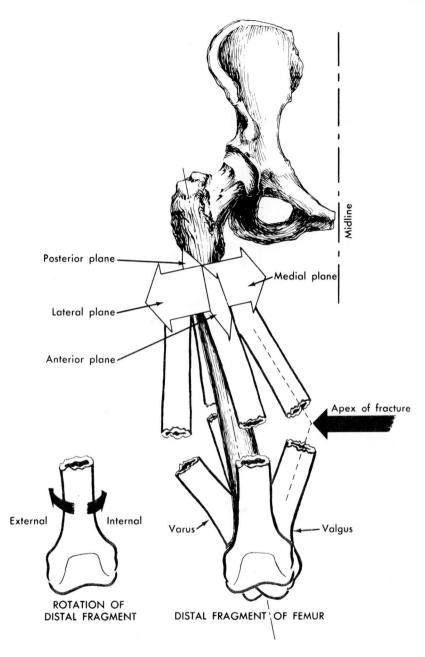

Fig. 1-4. Description of fracture deformity. (From Schneider FR: Handbook for the orthopaedic assistant, ed 2, St Louis, 1976, The CV Mosby Co.)

fracture with volar dislocation of scaphoid fragment and lunate.

Essex-Lopresti f.: comminuted head of radius with distal radioulnar dislocation.

Galeazzi f.: fracture of the distal radius, with disruption of the distal radioulnar articulation. (Also called Dupuytren f., Darrach-Hughston-Milch f.)

Monteggia f.: isolated fracture of proximal third of ulna, with either posterior or anterior dislocation of radial head allowing angulation and overriding of ulnar fragments.

Moore f.: like a Colles f., but specifically fracture of distal radius with dorsal displacement of ulnar styloid with impingement on annular ligament.

nightstick f.: an undisplaced fracture of the ulnar shaft caused by a direct blow.

Piedmont f.: oblique fracture, usually at the proximal portion of distal third of the radius; obliquity runs from proximal ulnar aspect to distal radial aspect, allowing distal fragments to be pulled into the ulna by the pronator quadratus muscle. *Fracture of necessity* requiring operative management.

radial head f.: fracture of the most proximal part of the radius, a dish-shaped portion of bone called the radial head.

reverse Barton f.: volar displacement of carpus on radius, with associated fracture of volar articular surface of radius.

Skillern's f.: open fracture of distal radius associated with greenstick f. of distal ulna.

Smith f., reverse Colles f.: with distal fragment displaced volarly.

Hand fractures

Bennett f.: dorsal subluxation or dislocation of thumb metacarpal on greater multangular with associated avulsion fracture of the volar articular surface of the metacarpal.

boxer's f.: volarly displaced impacted fracture of the neck of the fifth and/or fourth metacarpal, caused by striking close-fisted hand on hard object.

mallet f.: avulsion fracture of the dorsal base of the distal phalanx of any digit that includes insertion of extensor apparatus, thus allowing distal segment to "drop" into flexion. Also called baseball finger.

Rolando f.: T-shaped intraarticular fracture at the base of the first metacarpal.

Spine fractures

Chance f.: of vertebra, with horizontal splitting of spinous process and neural arch with disruption through vertebral body; an unstable fracture.

clay shoveler's f.: of spinous process(es) C-6, C-7, T-1, T-2, or T-3.

hangman's f.: posterior element (pedicles) fracture with anterior subluxation of the cervical neck of C-2 on C-3.

Jefferson f.: bursting fracture of the ring of the first cervical vertebra (atlas).

posterior element f.: broad term used to describe any fracture of the spinous process, lamina, facets, pars interarticularis, or pedicle.

teardrop f.: avulsion fracture, in the shape of a teardrop, of the anterior lip of a cervical vertebral body.

vertebra plana f.: wafer-thin compression fracture of a vertebral body resulting from intrinsic bony pathologic condition.

wedge f.: anterior compression fracture of any vertebra; most common in the dorsal spine.

Pelvis, hip, and proximal femur fractures

basal neck f.: fracture at base of femoral neck at junction of trochanteric region.

central f.: acetabular fracture, centrally displacing through inner wall of pelvis.

dashboard f.: posterior lip of acetabulum chips when femoral head is driven against it; often caused by a sudden jolt when knee hits dashboard.

dome f.: acetabular fracture involving weight-bearing surface of the acetabulum.

Duverney f.: fracture of the ilium just below the anterosuperior spine.

extracapsular f.: fracture outside of joint capsule of humerus or femur.

femoral neck f.: transcervical fracture through midportion of femoral neck.

intertrochanteric f.: fracture along a line joining the greater and lesser trochanters.

Malgaigne f.: fracture through wing of the ilium or sacrum with associated fractures through the ipsilateral pubic rami, allowing upward displacement of hemipelvis. Often associated with internal injuries.

pertrochanteric f.: fracture of proximal femur where the fracture line passes through both the lesser and greater trochanters.

ring f.: fracture involving at least two parts of pelvic circumference.

shaft f.: fracture between subtrochanteric and supracondylar area.

sprinter's f.: fracture of anterosuperior or antero-inferior spine of ilium, with a fragment of bone being pulled forcibly by sudden muscular pull.

straddle f.: double fracture or dislocation of the pubis usually caused by a straddling mechanism, for example, falling onto a rail with the point of contact being between the legs.

subcapital f.: femoral fracture at head-neck junction.

subtrochanteric f.: transverse fracture of femur just below lesser trochanter.

Femur, knee, tibia, and fibula fractures

bumper f.: fracture of the tibia or femur caused by a direct blow in area of the tibial tuberosity; commonly caused by a car bumper accident and may be bilateral.

Gosselin f.: fracture of the distal tibia shaped like a V, with apex of V extending into ankle joint.

patellar f.: fracture of kneecap.

pillion f.: T-shaped fracture of distal femur with displacement of the condyles posteriorly to femoral shaft, caused by severe blow to knee.

Segond f.: an avulsion of tibial attachment of iliotibial band.

Steida f.: fracture of internal condyle of femur.

supracondylar f.: fracture involving distal shaft of bone above condyles of humerus.

tibial plateau f.: fracture involving proximal tibial articular surface.

wagon wheel f.: of distal femoral epiphysis in children. Also called cartwheel f.

Y and T f.: combined supracondylar and intercondylar fractures of the distal femur.

Ankle and foot fractures

ankle mortise diastasis: separation of tibia and fibula at ankle; often associated with a fracture or dislocation.

aviator's astragalus: denotes a wide variety of talar fractures caused by sudden impaction of foot into ankle; may be associated with other fractures about the foot and ankle.

boot-top f.: fracture of transverse, distal-third of tibia, occurring at boot top. Also called skier's injury.

Bosworth f.: fracture-dislocation of the ankle, with oblique fracture of the distal fibula and displacement of the proximal fibular fragment out of fibular groove to a place posterior and medial to the posterolateral ridge of the tibia.

Conrad-Bugg trapping: incarceration of soft tissue, usually the posterior tibial tendon, between fragments of an ankle fracture. This produces an injury that must be reduced by open methods.

Cotton f.: partial forward dislocation of the tibia to produce a fracture of the posterior inferior margin of the tibia, sometimes called the posterior malleolus. This is most commonly associated with a fibular fracture.

Dupuytren f.: a spiral fracture of the distal end of fibula; associated with ankle diastasis.

Gosselin f.: V-shaped fracture of the distal tibia into the tibiotalar joint.

Jones f.: fracture at base of fifth metatarsal at diaphyseal/metaphyseal junction resulting from athletic injury; unlike a styloid f., it does not heal readily.

Lisfranc f.: usually a fracture-dislocation, with displacement of the proximal metatarsals.

Maisonneuve f.: spiral fracture of proximal end of fibula, near the neck, associated with a tear of the anterior tibiofibular ligament and the potential for ankle diastasis.

march f.: stress fracture of metatarsal caused by excessive marching. Also called fatigue f.

Montercaux f.: fracture of fibular neck associated with diastasis of ankle mortise.

paratrooper f.: fracture of posterior articular margin of tibia and/or malleolus.

Pott f.: spiral oblique fracture of distal fibula with associated rupture of the deltoid ligament; avulsion of the medial malleolus and lateral displacement of foot on tibia.

plafond f.: any fracture that involves the surface of the tibia that comes into contact with the dome of the talus.

Shepherd f.: of posterior talus shearing off piece of bone and in some instances, actually a separate piece of bone (os trigonum).

Tillaux Kleiger f.: fracture of distal lateral tibia, vertically extending into the joint; sometimes associated with diastasis and other fractures about the ankle.

triplane f.: a fracture of the ankle in three planes: coronally through the posterior tibial metaphysis, transversely through the growth plate, and sagittally through the distal tibial epiphysis.

Wagstaffe f. (Le fort f.): separation of a distal anterior fragment of the fibula, that is, the portion of attachment of the anterior tibiofibular ligament.

Volkmann f.: fracture of a triangular portion of the posterior lateral tibia into the joint, leaving a triangular bony fragment sometimes called *Volkmann's triangle.*

Contributing factors

Aside from a single obvious traumatic event, there are other factors contributing to fractures.

dyscrasic f.: fracture resulting from weakening of bone by a disease process; endocrine f.

fatigue f.: a spontaneous fracture in "normal" bone resulting from fatigue or stress produced by excessive physical activity in a short period of time; seen in fibulas/tibias of young long-distance runners, the hips and heels of young military recruits, and in the metatarsals. Also called stress f., march f.

inflammatory f.: fracture that occurs in association with inflammation secondary to an infection, such as syphilis.

insufficiency f.: a stress fracture that occurs in

bone because of its diminished volume (that is, osteopenia).

neoplastic f.: a form of pathologic fracture. Presence of a tumor in bone, whether originating in the bone or metastatic from elsewhere, causes sufficient weakening to allow it to fracture spontaneously or with less trauma than it would normally take to break a healthy bone.

pathologic f.: fracture that occurs with or without trauma where bone has been weakened by a local or systemic process. The most common causes are a tumor (benign or malignant), local infection, or bone cyst. This term is less widely applied to congenital disorders such as osteogenesis imperfecta, osteopetrosis, and neurofibromatosis. The term is applied more to congenital or acquired disorders such as osteomalacia, rickets, Paget disease, scurvy, and osteoporosis.

stress f.: crack in bone from overexertion placed on bone structure of limb or metatarsals and from pull of muscle on bone. Not noticeable initially on x-ray examination, but on later films when callus formation has taken place at the site. A bone scan will show the fracture. Also called march f.

Degree and nature of healing

The quality of bone healing is stated in terms of the solidarity of adhesiveness of the bone fragments. As most fractures heal, a surrounding "sleeve" of bone, or *callus*, is formed. This new bone formation is composed of cartilage, bone, blood vessels, and fibrous tissue and is often referred to in discussing bone healing. If the bone is completely healed, the term *healed* is used. Anything less is considered a *state of healing*, unless there is *a failure of progression of healing with expectation of no further healing*. This is then considered a *nonunion.*

The absence of complete union is called *ununited*, but this term by some users implies an expectation of failure to unite. In *delayed union* the speed of callus formation (fracture healing) is slower than anticipated, but this does not imply expectancy of either total healing or nonunion. A *pseudoarthrosis* is the formation of a jointlike structure at the old fracture site and is a type of nonunion. It consists of fibrocartilaginous tissue and a synovial fluid sac. If a bone unites but in abnormal position and/or alignment, the term *malunion* is used. If two bones parallel to one another unite by osseous tissue, such as the tibia/fibula or ulna/radius complex, the result is a *crossunion*, or synostosis. For example, in a simple fracture of the midshaft of the radius and ulna, assume that the radius adheres to the ulna at the distal fracture site and that the radius does not heal because of angulated healing of the ulna. Such a situation can be described as a *malunited fracture* of the *midshaft* of the ulna with a nonunion of the radius and crossunion of the distal radius and ulna. When the diagnoses are listed, they might be given as (1) malunion, fracture, closed, midshaft, ulna, right, or (2) nonunion, fracture, closed, midshaft, radius, right, associated with crossunion.

Secondary union is a term that has multiple meanings. It implies delayed healing either by the eventual adhesion of granulating surfaces of bony fragments or surgical intervention late in the course of fracture healing to promote union.

Nutritional support is important in bone healing to augment medical and surgical care. Bones need mineral and protein to heal, providing another consideration in treatment.

By grades, types, and mechanisms

Fractures in specific anatomic areas have been classified by the relative position of the fragments, angles of fracture lines, or some other systematic grading method. Following are some of those systems.

Anderson and D'Alonzo

This system is for grading odontoid fractures.
type I: oblique fracture through the upper part of the odontoid process.
type II: fracture at the junction of the odontoid process with the body of the second cervical vertebra.
type III: fracture extending downward into the cancellous portion of the axis, the fracture line progressing inferiorly to the anterior vertebral body.

Ashhurst

The Ashhurst system is for classifying ankle fractures and sprains, classed by direction or mechanism of force.

External rotation injuries

first degree: transsyndesmotic fracture of the fibula.
    alternate first degree: rupture of anterior tibiofibular ligament with or without spiral fracture of the proximal fibula
second degree: rupture of the deltoid ligament.
    alternate second degree: avulsion of the medial malleolus.
third degree: fracture of the entire lower end of the tibia and fibula with external rotation deformity.

Abduction injuries

first degree: transverse fracture of the fibular malleolus with fracture line at or below its base with no displacement.
second degree: rupture of the deltoid ligament or fracture of the medial malleolus followed by fracture of the distal fibula.
third degree: fractures of both lower ends of the tibia and fibula with lateral displacement.

Adduction injuries

first degree: avulsion of the fibular malleolus at or below its base.
second degree: avulsion of the fibular malleolus at or below its base with a shear (vertical into tibial shaft) fracture of the medial malleolus.
third degree: supramalleolar fracture of both tibia and fibula with medial displacement.

Fracture by compression in long axis of leg

first degree: isolated marginal fracture of the distal bearing plate of the tibia.

second degree: comminution of the tibial plafond.

third degree: T or Y fractures.

ASIF

ASIF is a classification system for ankle fractures based on the level of fracture in reference to the tibiotalar joint space.

A: fractures below level of tibiofibular syndesmosis (surgery not required).

B: fracture across the tibiofibular syndesmosis.

C: fracture above syndesmosis.

Boyd and Griffin

This system is for trochanteric fractures of the femur.

type I: fractures extending along the intertrochanteric line from the lesser to greater trochanter.

type II: comminuted fracture with the main fracture being in the intertrochanteric line.

type III: basically subtrochanteric fracture with at least one fracture line passing a point just distal to or at the lesser trochanter.

type IV: fracture of the trochanteric area and proximal shaft with fracture lines in at least two planes.

Bucholtz

The Bucholtz system is for the classification of pelvic fractures.

type I: nondisplaced, such as pubic fracture.

type II: diastasis pubis, but no superior displacement.

type III: total ring disruption with or without superior migration of segment.

Cemented prostheses

A grading system for fractures of the femur around cemented hip prostheses has been developed.

type 1: "explosion" type with comminution around the stem.

type 2: oblique around the stem of the implant.

type 3: transverse at the level of the tip of the implant.

type 4: fracture distal to the implant.

Evans

The Evans system is for grading intertrochanteric femoral fractures.

type I: fracture line extends upward and outward from the lesser trochanter. These may be undisplaced and stable, displaced but stable on reduction, displaced and unstable with no apposition on attempted reduction, and comminuted with no apposition and instability on attempted reduction.

type II: the obliquity of the major fracture line is outward and downward from the lesser trochanter. These are not stable in reduction.

Fielding

The Fielding system is for grading subtrochanteric fractures of the femur.

type I: at level of the lesser trochanter.

type II: between 2.5 and 5.0 cm below level of lesser trochanter.

type III: between 5.0 and 7.5 cm below level of lesser trochanter.

Frykman

The Frykman system is for grading distal radial and ulnar fractures.

Radial involvement	Without fracture of ulnar styloid	With fracture of ulnar styloid
extraarticular only radiocarpal joint	type I	type II
only	type III	type IV
distal radioulnar joint only	type V	type VI
both radiocarpal and distal radioulnar joint	type VII	type VIII

Garden

The Garden system is for grading femoral neck fractures. The angles of the primary trabeculae are taken into account to define displacement and degree of reduction. This is 160 degrees on an AP x-ray and 180 degrees on the lateral x-ray.

grade I: fracture is incomplete with head tilted in

a posterolateral direction. This is an impacted fracture.

grade II: complete but undisplaced fracture.

grade III: complete but partially displaced, the two fragments remain in contact with each other.

grade IV: fracture fragments are completely displaced.

Hawkins

The Hawkins system is used for classifying fractures of the talus.

type I: nondisplaced vertical fracture of the talar neck

type II: displaced fracture of the talar neck with subluxation or dislocation of the talar joint (ankle joint remains aligned)

type III: displaced fracture of the talar neck with dislocation of the body of the talus from both the subtalar and ankle joints

Herbert and Fisher

The Herbert and Fisher system is for classifying scaphoid fractures.

type A1: nondisplaced tubercle hairline fracture.

type A2: nondisplaced hairline waist fracture.

type B1: oblique fracture of distal-third.

type B2: displaced of mobile fracture of waist.

type B3: proximal pole fracture.

type B4: fracture dislocations of carpus.

type B5: comminuted fractures.

type C: delayed unions.

type D1: fibrous nonunion.

type D2: sclerotic nonunion (pseudarthrosis)

Hohl

The Hohl system classifies tibial condylar (plateau) fractures. This classification system does not use numbers or letters, but is the named nature of the fracture.

undisplaced
local compression
split compression
total condylar compression
split
comminuted

Kyle

The Kyle classification system is for intertrochanteric fractures.

type III: intertrochanteric fracture with varus deformity, as well as fracture fragments of the posteromedial part of the cortex and greater trochanter.

Lauge-Hansen

The Lauge-Hansen system is based on five possible positions of the foot at the time of injury.

Supination-adduction

first stage: tear of fibular collateral ligament or fractured fibula.

second stage: stage one plus shear (vertical) fracture of medial malleolus.

Supination-eversion

first stage: rupture of tibiofibular ligament.

second stage: first stage plus fracture of fibula.

third stage: second stage plus fracture of posterior tubercle of the tibia or rupture posterior of tibiofibular ligament.

fourth stage: third stage with rupture of the deltoid ligament or fracture of the medial malleolus.

Pronation-eversion

first stage: tear of the deltoid ligament or fracture of the medial malleolus.

second stage: first stage with rupture of the anterior tibiofibular ligament with or without fracture of the anterolateral column.

third stage: second stage with spiral fracture of the distal fibula.

Pronation-abduction

first stage: deltoid ligament torn or fracture of medial malleolus.

second stage: first stage with rupture of anterior and posterior tibiofibular ligaments with or without fractures of the tubercles.

third stage: second stage plus fracture of fibular distal shaft.

Pronation-dorsiflexion

first stage: vertical fracture of the medial malleolus.

second stage: first stage with fracture through anterior weight-bearing plate of the distal tibia.

third stage: second stage with fracture of the fibula.

fourth stage: comminuted fracture of the distal tibia.

Mason

The Mason classification system is for radial head fractures.

type I: nondisplaced.

type II: displacement of segment of radial head.

type III: severely comminuted.

Milch

The Milch classification system is for humeral condylar fractures.

type I: the lateral trochlear ridge remains with the intact segment leading to a stable medial to lateral elbow stability.

type II: the lateral trochlear ridge is a part of the fracture that may allow the radius and ulna to translocate.

Muller

The Muller classification system is for fracture of the distal humerus.

type A1: medial epicondyle.

type A2: transverse supracondylar.

type A3: comminuted supracondylar.

type B1: trochlear-epicondylar fragment.

type B2: capitellar lateral epicondylar fragment.

type B3: capitellar dome only.

type C1: Y condylar through trochlea.

type C2: Y condylar through trochlea with comminution of supracondylar area.

type C3: comminuted intraarticular fracture.

Navicular

The navicular system is based on the location of the fracture in the bone.

proximal pole fracture
waist fracture
distal body fracture
tuberosital fracture
distal articular osteochondral fracture

Neer

The Neer classification system is for femoral supracondylar and intercondylar fractures.

type I: minimal displacement.

type IIA: medial displacement of condyles in reference to the femoral shaft.

type IIB: lateral displacement of condyles in reference to the femoral shaft.

type III: conjoined supracondylar and shaft fractures.

The Neer is also applicable to humeral head and neck fractures with or without dislocation. The system categorizes (without numbers or letters) and describes the fracture on two aspects—the number of parts (2, 3, or 4) and the location (anatomic neck, surgical neck, greater tuberosity, and lesser tuberosity) and fracture dislocation in a posterior or anterior direction). There is the additional category of articular surface involvement.

Neer and Horowitz

The Neer and Horowitz classification system is for shoulder (proximal humeral) fractures in children based on degree of separation of the epiphysis from the shaft.

grade I: 0% to 25% slip.

grade II: 25% to 50% slip.

grade III: 50% to 75% slip.

grade IV: 75% or more slip.

Ogden

The Ogden classification system is for epiphyseal fractures based on subclassifications.

type IA: distraction pure epiphyseal fracture.

type IB: shear pure epiphyseal fracture.

type IC: regionally impacted pure epiphyseal fracture.

type IIA: shear epiphyseal fracture with attached piece of metaphysis.

type IIB: shear epiphyseal fracture with attached piece of metaphysis and detached metaphyseal fragment.

type IIC: shear metaphyseal fracture.

type IID: impaction fracture with attached metaphyseal fragment.

type IIIA: shear fracture separating an epiphyseal fragment.

type IIIB: distraction fracture separating an epiphyseal fragment.

type IIIC: impaction fracture involving a separated epiphyseal fragment.

type IIID: apophyseal fracture.

type IVA: shear fracture crossing growth plate with no epiphyseal separation.

type IVB: shear fracture crossing growth plate with separation of epiphyseal fragment.

type IVC: fracture across an apophyseal/epiphyseal complex as in a cervical fracture of the femur.

type V: impaction fracture of growth plate with destruction of a portion of the growth plate.

type VI: small chip fracture across growth plate

type VII: small chip fracture of epiphysis, not entering growth plate

Olecranon fractures (no eponym)

type I: involves only proximal-third of articular surface, or no articular surface.

type II: involves middle-third of articular surface.

type III: may occur in conjunction with anterior displacement of radius.

Open fracture grading system

type I: a less than 1 cm clean wound that communicates to fracture site.

type II: a more than 1 cm communicating laceration associated with fracture site but no extensive soft tissue damage, flaps, or avulsions.

type IIIA: extensive lacerations or flaps but adequate coverage of fracture by soft tissue, or high-energy trauma irrespective of the size of the wound.

type IIIB: extensive injury to the soft tissue with stripping of the periosteum and exposure of the bone, usually associated with massive contamination.

type IIIC: open fracture associated with arterial damage requiring repair.

Pauwels

The Pauwels classification sytem is for femoral neck fractures.

type I: angle of fracture line is 30 degrees from the horizontal.

type II: angle of fracture line is 50 degrees from the horizontal.

type III: angle of fracture line is 70 degrees from the horizontal.

Pipkin

The Pipkin grading system is for fractures of the femoral head associated with posterior dislocation of the hip.

type I: fracture of the femoral head caudad to the fovea centralis.

type II: fracture of the femoral head cephalad to the fovea centralis.

type III: fracture of the femoral head and neck.

type IV: fractures of the femoral head and acetabular rim.

Poland

The Poland is an epiphyseal classification system with types I-III the same as Salter-Harris and type IV being an epiphyseal fracture with separation of both epiphyseal fragments.

Radial head (Mason)

type I: undisplaced segmental (marginal).

type II: displaced segmental.

type III: comminuted.

type IV: comminuted with posterior dislocation of elbow.

Riseborough and Radin

The Riseborough and Radin system is for classification of intercondylar fractures of the distal humerus. As a common element these all have a transverse supracondylar component with a vertical fracture into the joint.

type I: intercondylar fracture without displacement.

type II: T-shaped intercondylar fracture with the trochlear and capitellar fragments separated but not rotated.

type III: same as type II, but with rotation of the fragments.

type IV: T-shaped intercondylar fracture with severe comminution of the articular surface and wide separation and rotation of the humeral condyles.

Schatzker

The Schatzker system is for tibial condylar (plateau) fractures.

type I: pure cleavage, an uncomminuted wedge is split off laterally and distally.

type II: cleavage combined with depression, a lateral wedge is split off and some articular surface is pushed down.

type III: pure central depression, the articular surface is driven into the plateau but the lateral cortex is intact.

type IV: fracture of the medial condyle, either as a single piece or comminuted; the tibial spines may be involved.

type V: bicondylar fracture; both tibial plateaus are split off.

type VI: plateau fracture with dissociation of metaphysis and diaphysis.

Seinsheimer

The Seinsheimer system describes five types of subtrochanteric fractures.

type I: undisplaced fracture.

type IIA: single-line transverse subtrochanteric fracture.

type IIB: oblique fracture with lesser trochanter attached to the proximal fragment.

type IIC: oblique fracture with lesser trochanter attached to distal fragment.

type IIIA: three-part fracture with a posteromedial fragment that includes the lesser trochanter.

type IIIB: three-part fracture with the third fragment being a lateral butterfly fragment.

type IV: comminuted fracture with four or more fragments.

type V: subtrochanteric-intertrochanteric fractures that include an extension into the greater trochanter.

Steward and Milford

The Steward and Milford system classifies fracture-dislocations of the hip.

grade I: simple dislocation without acetabular fracture.

grade II: dislocation with one or more large acetabular rim fragments but stability after reduction.

grade III: explosive or blast fracture with disintegration of the acetabular rim and gross instability of the hip.

grade IV: dislocation with a fracture of the head or neck of the femur.

Stress injury to bone

A grading system based on clinical and radiologic information to grade stress injuries to bone.

grade 0: positive bone scan in an asymptomatic subject with negative x-rays. Seen only in experimental surveys.

grade I: local symptoms associated with a positive scan and negative x-rays.

grade II: local symptoms with a positive bone scan and minimal changes on x-ray.

grade III: local symptoms with a positive bone scan and clear evidence of bone resorption on x-ray.

grade IV: local symptoms with positive bone scan and an actual bone fracture on x-ray.

Thompson and Epstein (Epstein)

The Thompson and Epstein system is for fractures associated with dislocation of the hip.

type I: dislocation with or without minor fracture.

type II: large single fracture of posterior acetabular rim.

type III: comminution of posterior acetabular rim with or without a major fragment.

type IV: with fracture of the acetabular floor.

type V: with fracture of the femoral head.

Tronzo

The Tronzo system classifies intertrochanteric fractures of the femur, based on reduction potential.

type 1: incomplete trochanteric fracture, reduced anatomically with traction.

type 2: uncomminuted fracture of both trochanters, with or without displacement, reduced with traction, anatomic reduction usually achieved.

type 3: comminuted fracture with large lesser trochanteric fragment, posterior wall exploded, beak of inferior femoral neck, unstable.

type 4: comminuted and unstable disengaged trochanteric fractures with explosion of posterior wall and medial displacement of femoral neck spike.

type 5: trochanteric fracture with reverse obliquity (downward from a medial to lateral direction).

Trunkey

The Trunkey system is used to classify pelvic fractures.

type I: fractures of individual bones with a break in the continuity of the pelvic ring.

type IA: avulsion fractures.
1. anterior superior iliac spine.
2. anterior inferior iliac spine.
3. ischial tuberosity.

type IB: fracture of pubis or ischium.

type IC: fracture of the wing of the ilium.

type ID: fracture of the sacrum.

type IE: fracture or dislocation of the coccyx.

type II: single break in the pelvic ring.

type IIA: fracture of two ipsilateral rami.

type IIB: fracture near, or subluxation of the symphysis pubis.

type IIC: fracture near, or subluxation of the sacroiliac joint.

type III: double breaks in the pelvic ring.

type IIIA: double verticle fractures or dislocations of the pubis.

type IIIB: double vertical fractures or dislocations of the pelvis.

type IIIC: severe multiple fractures.

type IV: fractures of the acetabulum.

type IVA: undisplaced.

type IVB: displaced.

Watson-Jones

The Watson-Jones system is used to grade tibial spine fractures.

grade I: a hinged fragment that can be managed without surgery.

grade II: retraction of the fragment, needs surgical replacement.

grade III: complete disruption of the articular surface.

Weber

The Weber classification of epiphyseal fractures adds intraarticular and extraarticular designations to Salter-Harris epiphyseal classification system.

Zickle

The Zickle classification system is for femoral subtrochanteric fractures.

type 1A: short oblique fracture from above lesser trochanter to lower lateral shaft.

type IB: long oblique fracture from above lesser trochanter to lower lateral shaft; comminution may be present.

type IC: transverse fracture just below lesser trochanter to a point near the isthmus.

CLASSIFICATION OF DISLOCATIONS

Dislocations are divided into two parts: a general list of terms applied to all joints; and a list by specific anatomic location. Posttraumatic arthritis, recurrent dislocation, limitation of joint motion, joint mice, instability, and/or avascular necrosis may accompany various dislocation types.

General dislocations

closed d.: one in which the skin is not broken. Formerly called simple d.

complete d.: one that completely separates the joint surfaces.

complicated d.: associated with surrounding tissue injuries.

congenital d.: one that exists at birth.

consecutive d.: one in which the luxated bone has changed its position since its first displacement.

frank d.: a complete dislocation in any area.

habitual d.: one that repeatedly recurs; usually congenital.

incomplete d.: subluxation with only slight displacement.

old d.: one in which inflammatory changes have occurred.

open d.: one in which the skin is broken. Formerly called compound d.

partial d.: incomplete dislocation.

pathologic d.: results from paralysis or disease in the joint or surrounding area.

primitive d.: bones remain as originally displaced.

recent d.: one in which there is no complicating inflammation.

recurrent d.: repetitive dislocation with or without adequate trauma.

traumatic d.: caused by serious injury.

Specific dislocations (anatomic)
Cervical (neck) dislocation

Bell-Dally d.: nontraumatic dislocation of the first cervical vertebra (atlas).

Shoulder dislocations

A/C joint separation: acromioclavicular joint disruption and separation.

anterior shoulder d.: dislocation of the glenohumeral joint with the humeral head displaced anteriorly and inferiorly; may be associated with one of the following:

Bankart lesion: seen surgically as detachment of the glenoid labrum and sometimes a bony fragment from the glenoid.

Hill-Sach lesion: seen radiographically as an indentation of the posteromedial humeral head, which occurred at the time of the dislocation. Also called hatchet head deformity.

luxatio erecta: dislocation of shoulder so that the arm stands straight up above the head.

posterior shoulder d.: of the glenohumeral joint with the humeral head displaced posteriorly.

sternoclavicular joint separation: disruption of the sternoclavicular joint.

subcoracoid d.: glenohumeral dislocation with the humeral head displaced medially.

subglenoid d.: glenohumeral dislocation with the humeral head displaced inferiorly.

Elbow dislocations

direct injury d.: posterior displacement of the olecranon.

divergent d.: one in which the ulna and radius are dislocated separately.

milkmaid's d.: of radial head superiorly and anteriorly. Also called superior radial head dislocation, milkmaid's elbow.

Monteggia f.-d.: fracture of the ulna with a radial head dislocation.

Wrist dislocations

Desault d.: at the radiocarpal joint with dorsal displacement of carpus and ulnar styloid process.

lunate d.: volar semilunar dislocation in the wrist; a type of dislocation often not recognized.

perilunate d.: a dislocation of all carpals, which are shifted posteriorly, leaving the lunate in proper position; may be associated with a scaphoid fracture, in which case it is termed a *transscaphoid perilunate dislocation*. Rarely do other carpi dislocate singularly or in association with fractures about the wrist. Wrist instabilities may be associated with fractures, but specifically relate to ligamentous instabilities of the carpal bones.

DISI: dorsiflexed intercalated segment instability is associated with a capitolunate angle greater than 20 degrees and a scapholunate angle greater than 70 degrees when the wrist is held in a neutral posture.

VISI: volarflexed intercalated segment instability has an average reduced scapholunate angle of 35 degrees, and the capitate is tilted dorsally when the wrist is held in a neutral posture.

Hand dislocations

Dislocation can occur at all the small joints of the hand. Dislocations at the carpometacarpal (CMC) and metaphalangeal (MP) joints generally occur in a dorsal direction. Dislocations at the MP joints can sometimes be irreducible without surgery. Dislocations in the hand are often associated with intraarticular fractures. Fracture-dislocations often require surgical reduction and fixation to realign joint surfaces.

Bennett d.: lateral or dorsal displacement of the first carpometacarpal joint.

boutonniere deformity: flexion contracture of the

proximal interphalangeal (PIP) joint that may progress to subluxation. Associated with hyperextension contracture of the distal interphalangeal (DIP) joint. Deformity begins with rupture of the extensor tendon insertion of the PIP joint and later becomes a fixed deformity.

carpal instability: partial or complete dislocations between individual wrist bones, causing a click-clunk with wrist movement. Most often occurs at the scapholunate joint, but can occur at the triquetrolunate, midcarpal, and even the radiocarpal joint.

gamekeeper's thumb: partial subluxation and instability of the thumb metaphalangeal joint due to rupture of the ulnar collateral ligament. Originally described as due to twisting neck of geese, and now commonly due to a ski-pole strap injury.

Kienböck d.: of semilunar bone. Also called isolated d.

Spine dislocations

spondylolisthesis: not a true dislocation, since it rarely occurs as a result of trauma or muscle imbalance, but is a forward displacement of one vertebral body over another; usually occurs as a result of a defect in the pars interarticularis.

spondylolysis: acute (traumatic) dissociation of pars interarticularis or posterior elements (lamina) with or without spondylolisthesis.

unilateral facet subluxation: dislocation of one of the two facets at any given level; most common in the cervical region.

Hip dislocations

anterior d.: dislocation of the femoral head anteriorly.

central d.: one in which the femur jams into the acetabulum. Also called bursting dislocation.

luxatio coxae congenita: congenital dislocation of the hip (CDH).

luxatio perinealis: dislocation of femoral head into the perineum.

Monteggia d.: dislocation of femoral head to near the anterosuperior spine of the ilium; hip joint dislocation.

Otto pelvis: gradual central displacement of the femur by unknown causes.

posterior d.: one in which the femoral head slips posteriorly; more common than anterior d.

posterior f.-d.: chip fracture of the acetabulum with a posterior dislocation of the femoral head.

Patella (dislocation versus subluxation)

One of the most common dislocations is a patellar dislocation, erroneously called a dislocated knee. The dislocated patella simply goes out of the femoral groove. A subluxation is a tendency for the patella to move partially out of the groove.

knee d.: slippage of the femur off the tibia. Commonly called a true knee dislocation to distinguish it from a dislocated patella.

Ankle dislocations

Chopart d.: navicula and cuboid dislocate across talus and calcaneus (Chopart joint).

fracture-dislocation of ankle: any combination of tibial and fibular fractures resulting in a displaced talus.

Lisfranc d.: a tarsometatarsal dislocation; not to be confused with a frank dislocation, which denotes a complete dislocation in any area.

metatarsophalangeal joint d.: dislocation at the base of the toe.

Nélaton d.: dislocation of the ankle in which the talus is forced between the end of the tibia and fibula.

Smith d.: upward and backward dislocation of the metatarsals and medial cuneiform bone.

subastragalar d.: separation of the calcaneus and navicular bone from the talus.

tarsal d.: usually an ankle dislocation associated with a fracture of the neck of the talus; commonly an open injury. This term may also denote other tarsal bone dislocations such as of the cuneiform and cuboid.

DISLOCATIONS BY TYPES

Dislocations are generally classified by degree of separation or by nature of the associated injuries.

Acromioclavicular

Classifying by the acromioclavicular system deals with degree of separation and complicating configuration of clavicular separation at the joint.

type I: sprain of the ligament with no significant fiber disruption and no separation.

type II: partial separation of the joint but with some intact ligament. The joint does not separate by one bone width or more at the joint, and the coracoclavicular interspace is essentially normal.

type III: complete separation of the joint with 25% to 100% separation at coracoclavicular space.

type IV: like type III with clavicle displaced into trapezius muscle.

type V: the displacement of the clavicle is more severe with the coracoclavicular space 100% to 300% or normal.

type VI: clavicle is incarcerated under the acromion, whereas the deltoid muscle, torn in types III to V, is only partially torn in this case.

Epstein

The Epstein classification system is for anterior dislocations of the hip.

type I: superior dislocation (includes pubic and subspinous dislocations).

type IA: no associated fracture.

type IB: associated fracture of head of femur.

type IC: associated fracture of the acetabulum.

type II: inferior (includes obturator, thyroid, and peroneal dislocations).

type IIA: no associated fracture.

type IIB: associated fracture of head of femur.

type IIC: associated fracture of acetabulum.

Rowe and Lowell

The Rowe and Lowell classification system is for central acetabular fracture-dislocations.

type 1: undisplaced (single line or stellate).

type 2: inner wall fractures.

type 2A: femoral head reduced under acetabular dome initially.

type 2B: femoral head not reduced under acetabular dome initially.

type 3: superior dome fractures.

type 3A: acetabulum generally congruous with femoral head.

type 3B: acetabulum incongruous with femoral head.

type 4: bursting fracture (all elements of acetabulum involved).

type 4A: fractures with congruity between femoral head and acetabular dome.

type 4B: fractures with incongruity between femoral head and acetabular dome.

SUBLUXATIONS

Subluxations are categorized by anatomic location as there are no eponymic terms.

facet s.: malalignment of opposing facet, allowing one cervical vertebral body to rotate around another.

radioulnar s.: subluxation of the distal ulnar radial joint.

sacroiliac s.: subluxation of the sacroiliac joint usually associated with a pelvic fracture and other dissociations of the pelvic ring.

shoulder s.: subluxation of the glenohumeral joint (as opposed to the acromioclavicular joint).

wrist s.: subluxation of proximal carpal bones on the radius and ulna.

SPRAINS

Sprains and ruptures of ligaments most commonly occur in the knee and ankle and sometimes in the shoulder.

Shoulder sprain

acromioclavicular s.: stretching of the ligaments of the acromioclavicular (A/C) joint but without any disruption. Often the term *shoulder sprain* implies this specific condition, as opposed to an affection of the glenohumeral joint.

Knee sprains

anterior cruciate s.: sprain commonly associated with a medial collateral ligament tear, dislocated patella, or torn meniscus; may occur as an isolated injury.

lateral collateral s.: sprain of the knee; commonly an isolated injury; may be associated with rupture of the biceps femoris tendon, anterior and/ or posterior cruciate, and iliotibial tract.

medial collateral s.: sprain occurring as a result of a clipping injury; may be associated with a cruciate ligament tear, patellar dislocation, or torn medial meniscus.

posterior cruciate s.: sprain allowing the tibia to slide backward on the femur; often seen alone.

posterior oblique s.: part of the medial collateral ligament sprain or rupture complex.

Ankle sprains

deltoid s.: sprain commonly occurring with a fibular fracture; rarely an isolated rupture.

fibular collateral s.: sprain or rupture commonly occurring as an isolated injury.

tibiofibular s.: sprain in which, without rupture, there is no spreading of the tibia and fibula; with rupture, a diastasis occurs.

SPORTS-RELATED INJURIES

Injuries from vocational and avocational sports activities has greatly increased over the past 2 decades. In the United States more than 2 million sports-related injuries occur annually. Much time and effort have been devoted to the more immediate identification and treatment of these athletic injuries, which has led to the advent of sports medicine.

Sports medicine has also had an effect on the activities themselves. Exercise as a science has opened new dimensions in health care. Improved sports equipment and design have undergone a rapid development, thanks to the combined efforts of engineers and medical support personnel. In addition, rule changes are often made in consideration of the safety of the players.

Many sports injuries are a result of muscle and tendon overuse rather than a specific sprain or strain. Some of these conditions are so common in certain sports that they are named after the sport, for example, baseball elbow.

This terminology applies to the nonathletic population, as well, who experience similar conditions. This may be the result of an increase in activity from a previously sedentary, nonactive lifestyle, or other factors such as degenerative joint

disease. The classic example is that of tennis elbow. Many people with this problem cannot attribute it to a change in activity, such as painting or tennis, but have a condition of the cervical spine that causes the muscle of the forearm to tighten, resulting in overuse of the tendon.

The following terms are related to athletic injuries of the soft tissues. The fracture-related sports injuries are listed in the preceding section.

apprehension shoulder: subluxation at the glenohumeral joint. Occurs in forced abduction and external rotation resulting in reluctance on the part of the athlete to make that motion.

backpack palsy: similar to Erb's palsy, a brachial plexus overpull caused by a heavy pack with shoulder straps, resulting in palsy of the fifth and sixth cervical nerve muscle distribution.

baseball elbow: condition of baseball pitchers where overstress on the medial side of the elbow causes medial collateral ligament bone spurs, myositis, ulnar nerve injuries, or posterior compartment loose bodies. Also referred to as javelin thrower's elbow.

black-dot heel: small dark spot on the heel fatpad caused by blood under the skin on the lateral side where there is repeated trauma to heel in athletic activity or shear stress in running. Also called black heel syndrome.

bowler's thumb: irritation of the flexor tendon of the thumb with increased nerve sensation on the lateral side caused by the repeated grasp of a large bowling ball.

breaststroker's knee: irritation of the medial capsule of the knee, tibial collateral ligament, or patellar cartilage caused by repeated thrusts of the limbs in a breaststroke swimmer.

charley horse: a sudden cramp in a muscle usually during athletic activities. Occurs often in athletes because of overuse of an undertrained muscle or inadequate salt or water intake during hot weather.

flexor origin syndrome: tendonitis of the origin of the flexor wad of five at the medial elbow. Also called medial epicondylitis, reverse tennis elbow.

football finger.: avulsion of the deep flexor tendon

of the distal phalanx of the ring finger. Often occurs when trying to tackle an opponent by hooking the finger over the pants belt line.

golfer's elbow: inflammation at the origin of the wrist and finger flexor muscles of the inner elbow. Also called thrower's elbow, medial epicondylitis, and reverse tennis elbow.

handlebar palsy: palsy of the muscles of the hand innervated by the ulnar nerve, caused by pressure against bicycle handlebar.

heel spur: an area of inflammation at the proximal attachment of the plantar fascia, usually involving the median tubercle of the plantar surface of the calcaneus, often seen in runners and commonly the result of excessive joint pronation. Anything that causes stress on the plantar fascia (weakened feet, structural deformity, or excessive pronation of the subtalar joint) will encourage the development of a heel spur.

hip pointer: a very painful irritation of the insertion of abdominal muscles along the superior iliac crest. Pain localizing here can also represent the pull of a thigh muscle from that region.

jumper's knee: infrapatellar tendonitis, often seen in athletes who jump as part of that sport, for example, in basketball and volleyball.

linebacker's arm: (tackler's arm) a myositis ossificans reaction in the lateral brachialis muscle, usually seen in the mid-arm of tacklers.

Little Leaguer's elbow: in children, a traction injury of the elbow on the medial epicondyle caused by prolonged pitching or throwing. Serious in that it may lead to fragmentation of the bone and disturbance of growth.

Little Leaguer's shoulder: a traction injury to the shoulder in the growth plate of the proximal humerus that may lead to a painful shoulder and can lead to deformity if throwing is continued.

ring man shoulder: bony resorption or sclerosis at the insertion of the pectoralis major muscle of upper arm. Seen in gymnasts who use rings.

rotator cuff injury: inflammation or rupture of one or more of the tendons that lie deep in the shoulder and bridge the glenohumeral joint. This type of injury is inhibiting in pitchers and tennis players, in particular, and can be caused by excessive use, direct blow, or stretch injury.

runner's bump: prominence of the posterior heel at the point of insertion of the Achilles tendon; associated with distance running.

runner's knee: tight and tense condition of quadriceps of thigh that directs pain to knee.

shin splints: pain in the shin usually following repeated stress such as running or walking long distances without conditioning. Describes a painful condition rather than a specific anatomic lesion. The most common causes are posterior tibial tendinitis, stress fracture of tibia, and anterior tibial compartment syndrome with the inability of blood to reach the muscle (ischemia) because of compartmental swelling during increased activity.

shoulder pointer: a tearing of the anterior deltoid muscle leading to a distinct point of discomfort at the origin (immediate vicinity of the acromioclavicular joint) of the deltoid muscle.

tennis elbow: inflammation of the wrist and finger extensor muscles at outer elbow. Also called lateral epicondylitis.

tennis leg: tear of one of the heads of the gastrocnemius or plantaris muscle, often seen in tennis players.

tennis toe: (marathoner's toe) subungual hematoma causing a black toenail. Usually painless and requires no treatment.

trigger points: this term has several different meanings. In general these are specific points of muscle or muscle attachment that are very tender and related to muscle spasm. Pressure on these points may cause pain referred distal to those points. These point areas may be the result of chronic spinal disorders or caused by overuse of specific muscle groups.

2

Musculoskeletal diseases and related terms

The musculoskeletal reaction to bone and soft tissue lesions, whether localized or referred, can be due to many factors: bones can fracture or dislocate; joints become arthritic; bursa sacs around joint areas become inflamed; muscles, ligaments, and tendons become strained, stretched, or weakened; muscles may spasm or atrophy; cartilage may degenerate; disks become compressed; vascular and metabolic changes may occur, affecting both bone and soft tissue. All of these areas of the locomotor system can be affected temporarily or permanently.

Bone disorders can be diagnosed easily by radiographs, but soft tissue lesions are harder to diagnose and symptoms can be deceptive. On examination, assessment can be made by the size, nature, position, and stage of progress of soft tissue lesions. The word *lesion* describes a wound, injury, or pathologic change in tissue. A gross lesion is that visible to the naked eye.

The terms *disease* and *syndrome* may be used interchangeably but have precisely different meanings. Diseases are a specific result of a bodily process, causing discomfort or dysfunction for the patient. Syndromes are composed of a set of symptoms that have been recognized as the hallmark of a specific disease process.

Many diseases of the musculoskeletal system overlap into other specialty areas such as neurology, neurosurgery, and vascular surgery, and the patient's symptoms often present as an orthopaedic problem; therefore terminology of other specialties as related to orthopaedics is included.

Soft tissue lesions of the locomotor system are generally associated with *referred* pain, meaning pain that is felt distant to its source of origin. For example, sciatic nerve pain in the leg is referred pain from the lumbar spine region (origin). Any pressure on nerves can cause dermatome distribution of pain in the limbs. *Localized* pain refers to lesions in a specific concentrated area. The distance a pain can travel from its source is dependent on the size of the dermatome, but pain does not necessarily follow a nerve.

It can be a real challenge to obtain an accurate diagnosis of the source of pain within the locomotor system because of the many tissue types involved. The ultimate goal in the treatment of musculoskeletal lesions is to help the patient become functional and productive as quickly as possible through a conservative approach, manipulation, surgery, or other measures.

Musculoskeletal diseases are classified here according to tissue types and by anatomic areas.

TISSUE DISEASES
Bone diseases

Osteo-, the Greek root for bone, can be used in various combinations that include more than one root, for example, osteochondral (bone and cartilage), or in terms in which *osteo-* is preceded by other terms, for example, polyostotic fibrous dysplasia.

Bone disease types are grouped together for purposes of identifying similar or related processes by anatomic name and by eponymic terms.

However, eponyms that are used more frequently than the common (Greek or Latin) term are listed separately. The bone diseases are divided as follows: (1) *osteo-* root diseases, (2) infectious bone diseases, (3) tumors of bone, (4) affections of bony alignment, (5) miscellaneous Latin and English terms, and (6) eponymic bone diseases.

Osteo- root diseases

ostealgia: pain within bone.

osteitis: inflammation of bone with enlargement, tenderness, dull aching; many varieties.

osteitis deformans: disease of unknown origin resulting in bowing of long bones and deformation of flat bones. Also called Paget disease.

osteitis fibrosa cystica: bone disease caused by hyperfunction of parathyroid gland. Also called osteoplastica.

ostemia: abnormal congestion of blood in bone.

ostempyesis: suppuration (pus) within bone.

osteoaneurysm: aneurysm in bone.

osteoarthritis: chronic disorder of a joint with excessive erosion of the cartilage surface associated with excess bone formation at the margins of the joint and gradual loss of function because of pain and stiffness. This may be the outcome of abnormal mechanical forces, such as prior injury, a systemic disorder, or part of a generalized osteoarthritic process.

osteoarthropathy: a condition of increased bone formation at the joints; sometimes used to refer to osteoarthritis. Variations of osteoarthropathy are hypertrophic, hypertrophic pulmonary, pulmonary trophic, and secondary hypertrophic.

osteoarthrosis: chronic arthritis, usually mechanical, not caused by inflammatory process. May be used as a synonym for osteoarthritis.

osteoarticular: pertaining to or affecting bones and joints.

osteocachexia: chronic disease of bone resulting in cachexia (malnutrition).

osteochondritis: inflammation of both bone and cartilage. Various types are o. deformans juvenilis, o. ischiopubica, o. juvenilis, juvenile deforming metatarsophalangeal, and o. necroticans.

osteochondrofibroma: tumor containing elements of osteoma, chondroma, and fibroma.

osteochondrolysis: osteochondritis dissecans.

osteochondroma: a benign bone tumor arising from surface of bone consisting of a bone projection topped by a cartilage cap and covered by periosteum.

osteochondromatosis: Transformation of synovial villi into bone and cartilage masses, causing loose bodies in the joint. This condition occurs in joints affected by trauma or other degenerative diseases. A condition specifically called synovial osteochondromatosis and *Henderson-Jones chondromatosis*.

osteochondropathy: condition affecting bone and cartilage, marked by abnormal enchondral ossification.

osteochondrophyte: an archaic term synonymous with osteochondroma.

osteochondrosarcoma: bone and cartilage sarcomatous tumors.

osteochondroses: diseases of children in which one or more growth ossification centers degenerate or become necrosed or inactive, followed by regeneration and usually deformity. Entities include osteochondritis dissecans, Blount's disease, Osgood-Schlatter disease, and Scheuermann's disease. Other entitites involved avulsion fractures, tertiary or irregular epiphyseal growth centers, traumatic chondral separation with secondary infarction, and intraosseous herniation of disk material.

osteochondrosis dissecans: the formation of a separate center of bone and cartilage formation on an epiphyseal surface. The osteochondral fragment may remain in place, be absorbed and replaced slowly, break loose and become a loose body. Mutliple etiologies probably exist. This was originally believed to be an inflammatory lesion, but there is no clear evidence for this, hence the change of the term from osteochondritis to osteochondrosis. Another probable etiology is a demarcation of an area of avascular necrosis. Formerly called osteochondritis dissecans.

osteoclasia: breaking down and absorption of bony tissue.

osteocope: syphilitic bone disease with severe pain within bone.

osteocystoma: cystic tumor in bone.

osteodiastasis: abnormal separation of bones.

osteodynia: pain in bones.

osteodystrophy: defective bone formation.

osteoenchondroma: benign bone and cartilage tumor confined within bones.

osteofibrochondrosarcoma: malignant tumor containing bony, fibrous, cartilaginous tissue.

osteofibroma: tumor containing both osseous and fibrous elements.

osteofibromatosis: multiple osteofibroma formation.

osteogenesis imperfecta: condition in which bones are abnormally brittle and subject to fractures; inherited and may be a function of abnormal collagen. Also called osteitis fragilitans, fragilitas ossium congenita, osteopsathyrosis idiopathica, and brittle bones.

osteohalisteresis: loss or deficiency of mineral elements of bones, producing softening.

osteolipochondroma: cartilage tumor with bone and fatty elements.

osteolipoma: fatty tumor containing osseous elements.

osteolysis: dissolution of bone.

osteoma: hard tumor of bonelike structure developing on bone: benign tumor of spongy bone as seen in young people.

osteomalacia: the adult form is rickets, a reduction of physical strength of bone caused by decreased mineralization of osteoid; may result from vitamin D, calcium, or phosphorous deficiency with or without renal disease. Osteomalacia in the child is associated with the growth deformities of rickets.

osteomesopyknosis: autosomal dominant disorder characterized by osteosclerosis similar to that in pyknodysostosis, but localized to the axial spine, pelvis, and proximal part of the long bones.

osteomyelitis: inflammation of bone marrow, cortex, tissue, and periosteum; can be caused by any organism, but usually bacteria. See next section for a more complete list of causes.

osteomyelodysplasia: thinning of osseous tissue of bone with increase in size of marrow cavities, attended by leukopenia (low white blood cell count) and fever.

osteonecrosis: death of bone tissue, usually of vascular origin.

osteoneuralgia: nerve pain in bone.

osteopathia striata: affection of bone giving distinct striped appearance on x-ray examinations; lesions characterized by multiple condensation of cancellous bone tissue, sometimes said to be in association with osteopetrosis. Also called Voorhoeve disease.

osteopathy: any disease process of bone.

osteopenia: any state in which bone mass is reduced below normal. This would include conditions of osteoporosis and osteomalacia.

osteoperiostitis: inflammation of bone and periosteum.

osteopetrosis: hereditary disease of bone, with areas of chalky condensed bone within bone. Also called Albers-Schönberg disease, osteosclerosis, osteosclerosis fragilis.

osteophyte: bony excrescence or osseous outgrowth, usually found around the joint area of bone.

osteoplastica: cystic fibrosis with bone inflammation.

osteopoikilosis: presence of multiple sclerotic foci in ends of long bones and scattered stippling in round and flat bones; usually without symptoms but noted on x-ray examinations.

osteoporosis: diminution of both the mineral and matrix components of bone such that the remaining bone is normal in composition but reduced in total bone mass. The secondary cause of osteoporosis is most commonly immobilization, such as casting. Primary osteoporosis is an age-related disorder characterized by decreased bone mass and by increased susceptibility to fractures in the absence of other recognizable causes of bone loss.

osteopsathyrosis: osteogenesis imperfecta.

osteoradionecrosis: necrosis (death) of bone following irradiation.

osteosarcoma: sarcoma containing osseous tissue.

osteosclerosis: hardening or abnormal denseness of bone. Also called eburnation, osteitis ossificans.

osteosis: formation of bony tissue with in-filtration of connective tissue within bone.

osteospongioma: spongy tumor of bone.

osteosynovitis: inflammation of synovial membranes and neighboring bones.

osteotabes: condition in which bone marrow cells are destroyed and marrow disappears; usually in infants.

osteotelangiectasia: sarcoma of bone containing dilated capillaries.

osteothrombophlebitis: inflammation through intact bone by progressive thrombophlebitis of small venules.

osteothrombosis: blood clots or plugging of veins of bone.

Infectious bone diseases

Osteomyelitis may be caused by bacteria, fungi, and perhaps even viruses.

1. A variety of bacteria may be associated with osteomyelitis
   Staphylococcus aureus
   Streptococcus organisms
   Escherichia coli
   Pseudomonas organisms
   Klebsiella organisms
   Salmonella organisms
   Neisseria gonorrhoeae
   Mycobacterium tuberculosis
2. Fungal types (rare)
   Actinomycosis
   Blastomycosis
   Histoplasmosis
3. Viral types—suggested, not proven

Terms related to osteomyelitis (bone infection)

acute o.: possibly up to 6 weeks, x-rays may be negative for first 2 weeks.

chronic o.: over 6 weeks; may last for years.

chronic sclerosing o. of Garre: minimally symptomatic long-term osteomyelitis associated with x-ray findings of densely scarred bone but not the usual abscess formation.

cloacae: in osteomyelitis, these are the openings in the infected sequestra of bone.

cystic o.: the x-ray appearance of an aborted osteomyelitis where a fluid-filled cystic cavity remains in the bone.

iatrogenic o.: an infection brought about by surgery or other treatment.

involucrum: bone formation around infected cortical bone.

nonsuppurative o.: term applied to tuberculosis of bone.

sequestrum: detached piece of dead bone.

sinus: a drainage tract extending from an area of infected bone to skin.

suppurative o.: infection of bone with active production of pus; may be acute or chronic.

Tumors of bone

Until recently the term *osteogenic sarcoma* has been used to define all the bone sarcomas, for example, osteosarcoma, chondrosarcoma, and fibrosarcoma. Currently, more specific terms are preferred.

Bone cell tumors

osteoblastoma: tumor composed mostly of osteoblasts, some giant cells, and new bone; usually benign, but may become quite large.

osteochondroma: a cartilage-capped benign growth that may be on a stalk on the surface of bone.

osteoid osteoma: benign osteoblastic tumor composed of osteoid tissue and atypical bone. Also called Jaffe disease.

osteoma: specifically benign bone-forming tumor.

osteosarcoma: sarcoma in which cancer cells are making bone.

parosteal osteosarcoma: a bone-forming tumor that is usually low grade and develops on the surface of bone and does not involve the medullary canal.

periosteal osteosarcoma: a group of sessile subperiosteal tumors that is separated (by some authors) from the parosteal group.

Cartilage tumors (affecting bone)

chondroblastoma (Codman tumor): generally benign tumor composed of early chondroblasts and some giant cells; occurs in the epiphysis of bone.

chondroma: cartilage tumor.

chondromyxoid fibroma: combination of cartilage, myxomatous cells, and fibroblasts; usually benign, oblong tumor, eccentric in shaft.

chondrosarcoma: sarcoma in which cancer cells are making cartilage.

enchondromatosis: proliferation of cartilage cells within metaphysis of several bones, causing thinning of overlying cortices and distortion of length in growth. Also called Ollier disease.

epiphyseal osteochondroma: development of intraosseous chondromas within the epiphysis with occasional extension beyond epiphyseal margins. May occur from infancy to adulthood. Formerly called *osteomatosis, ephiphyseal exostosis, intraarticular osteochondromas, epiarticular osteochondromas, dysplasia epiphysealis hemimelica,* and *epiarticular osteochondromatous dysplasia.*

parosteal chondrosarcoma: tumor composed of cartilage cells and arising from the surface of bone.

Round cell tumors

eosinophilic granuloma: a tumorlike process in bone composed of masses of histiocytes, cholesterol, and eosinophilic cells. Believed caused by a metabolic defect in lipid metabolism of the reticuloendothelial system of bone, one of several abnormal conditions of this system. Others are Gaucher's disease, Hand-Schuller-Christian disease, and Letterer-Siwe disease.

Ewing tumor: malignant tumor of bone seen in children; composed of small round cells.

Hodgkin tumor: generally a bony manifestation of a low-grade systemic process affecting the lymphatic system.

multiple myeloma: multiple plasma cell tumors in bone, usually malignant.

myeloblastoma: marrow tumor of bone.

plasma cell myeloma: usually a discrete collection of plasma cells; may develop into multiple myeloma. Also called myeloma, myelocytoma.

primary lymphoma: term used to distinguish a lymphoma arising in bone. Similar to a Ewing's sarcoma, it is a slower-growing tumor seen in adults.

reticulum cell sarcoma: a slow-growing malignant marrow tumor believed to represent an isolated focus of lymphoma.

Other tumors

desmoplastic fibroma of bone: a lytic lesion of bone containing fibroblasts separated by dense bands of collagenous tissue (benign tumor).

epithelioid sarcoma: tumor composed of a nest of epithelial-like cells but with sarcomatous activity.

fibrosarcoma: malignant tumor composed of fibroblastic-like cells and dilated vessels. May occur as a soft tissue malignancy or as a primary tumor bone.

giant cell tumor (osteoclastoma): a lesion of osteoclasts originating in the metaphysis of bone and developing eccentrically. It has a characteristic bubble pattern on x-ray and microscopically contains giant cells and stromal cells with varying amounts of vascularity. These tumors are usually benign but can be malignant.

malignant fibrous histiocytoma: bony tumor characterized by fibrous and histiocytic proliferation with the absence of osteoid and chondroid elements.

Miscellaneous Latin and English terms

aneurysmal bone cyst: single or multiple benign blood-filled cysts of bone.

apophysitis: inflammation of an apophysis. Depending on the location, specific types may be referred to as:

Osgood-Schlatter disease: tibial apophysis at the insertion of the patellar tendon.

Sever disease: apophysitis of the heel bone at the insertion of the Achilles tendon.

Scheuermann disease: osteochondrosis of the vertebral epiphysis in juveniles.

aseptic necrosis: osteonecrosis (bone death) caused by vascular insult, usually at the end of a bone. In adults the most common symptom-producing aseptic necrosis occurs in the femoral head (avascular necrosis); in children, it is called epiphyseal ischemic necrosis or epiphyseal aseptic necrosis. The precise pathology of these diseases is debatable; therefore the term is used here in reference to osteochondrosis or epiphyseal osteochondritis, and by area:

Freiberg disease: of the second metatarsal head.

Kienböck disease: of the lunate bone of wrist.

Köhler disease: of the tarsonavicular; sometimes of the patella.

Legg-Calvé-Perthes disease: of the femoral head. Also called Legg-Perthes disease, Perthes disease, coxa plana.

Panner disease: of the capitellum of the humerus.

Thiemann disease: of the proximal phalanges.

bone infarct: area of bone where blood supply is interrupted.

bone island: small areas of compact but microscopically normal bone that appear as 0.5- to 1-cm areas on x-ray film.

bone spur: the ossification of ligamentous or muscular attachment to bone. Generally applied to any bony excrescence seen on x-ray, but specifically refers to a portion of ligament or tendon that has turned to bone at the attachment to bone. The most common areas include the heel, patella, humeral epicondyles, and vertebral body margins.

brown tumor: a brown-appearing lesion in bone secondary to hyperparathyroidism. Also called osteoclastoma.

caisson disease: avascular necrosis of bone (and soft tissue) caused by sudden increase and release in air pressure causing infarct. Also called diver's disease.

condensing osteitis of the clavicle: a rare and benign disorder of unknown origin affecting the medial clavicle, characteristically in women of late child-bearing age. The level of discomfort varies, and x-rays reveal a slight expansion of the medial one third of the clavicle.

cortical fibrous dysplasia (ossifying fibroma of long bone, intracortical fibrous dysplasia): a benign anomaly of bone cortex, usually found in children and characterized by a cystic-appearing lesion on x-ray. Microscopically, this lesion is characterized by a fibrous replacement of cortex with some trabecular bone.

exostosis: excess bone formation, usually near a joint.

hypertrophic e.: sometimes used to describe excess bone formation in osteoarthritis.

hereditary multiple e.: multiple bony excrescences, growing from cortical surfaces, forming tubular extensions roughly transverse to the long axis of bone involved. Also called Jaffe disease.

familial expansile osteolysis: an autosomal dominant bone dysplasia with general and focal skeletal changes occurring in the second decade of life. There is usually pain, osteoclastic resorption, bowing, and a tendency toward pathologic fracture. Deafness and early loss of teeth may also occur.

giant cell reparative granuloma: common, benign lesion of jaw characterized by a fibrous background within which there are scattered multinucleated giant cells. A multicentric form is seen in the small bones of the hands and feet.

infantile cortical hyperostosis: painful hyperostosis with involvement of long bones and the mandible. This usually occurs in infants 5 months of age and younger and is associated with irritability, fever and soft tissue.

malacoplakia: a disease that usually involves the gut and has a probable infectious cause. Histiocytes respond with the formation of Michaelis-Gutmann bodies. Bone lesions are rare and can be destructive.

melorheostosis: a form of osteosclerosis or hyperostosis (dense bone); linear longitudinal thickenings of the shaft of long bones, very rare, resulting in a candle wax appearance (dripping) of the bone.

milk-alkali disease: excess calcium in tissue resulting from heavy ingestion of milk and certain antacids.

myelofibrosis: replacement of bone marrow by fibrous tissue.

nonossifying fibroma (fibroxanthoma, fibrous cortical defect, subcortical defect): an anomaly of bone that appears in youngsters as a sharply circumscribed, eccentrically located lesion in the metaphysis of long bones. Microscopically this lesion is characterized by whorl patterns of spindle cells, fibrous tissue, numerous xanthoma cells, and occasionally giant cells.

ochronosis: hereditary error of protein metabolism marked by accumulation of homogentisic acid resulting in degenerative arthritis and a characteristic blackening of cartilage.

periostitis: inflammation of bone covering (periosteum); usually the result of an infection such as syphilis.

progressive diaphyseal dysplasia: neuromuscular dystrophy associated with general wasting; abnormally formed shafts of long bones. Also called Engelmann disease.

pyknodysostosis: condition marked by patchy areas of thickening of the cortex of bone.

rickets: failure of deposition of bone salts within the organic matrix of cartilage and bone associated with stunting of growth and bone deformities.

skeletal amyloidosis: the deposition of amyloid (glycogen) material in bone producing bubbly-appearing lesions on x-ray. Condition is associated with plasma cell dyscrasias, primary systemic amyloidosis, focal amyloidosis, and patients undergoing hemodialysis for chronic renal insufficiency.

slipped capital femoral epiphysis: a gradual or sudden movement of the femoral head toward a posterior and medial direction; usually occurs in preteenage children. Also called Frohlich adiposogenital dystrophy.

uncommitted metaphyseal lesion: benign but radiologically-aggressive appearing lesion seen in the proximal metaphysis of children, microscopically characterized by whorls of fibrous tissue, new bone, giant cells, and vascular components.

unicameral bone cyst: a benign bone anomaly where there is a fluid-filled cavity seen in the metaphysis of a long bone of a child. Microscopically the cavity is lined with fibrous stroma, curlicues of trabecular bone similar to fibrous dysplasia, and cholesterol clefts.

weaver's bottom: ischial gluteal bursitis seen often in patients with a sedentary occupation.

Eponymic bone diseases

Albers-Schönberg disease: osteopetrosis affecting the ends of bone. Also called chalk bones, thick bones, marble bones.

Albright syndrome: precocious puberty associated with bone deformities resulting from fibrous dysplasia. Also called polyostotic fibrous dysplasia, Albright-McCune-Sternberg syndrome, and McCune-Albright syndrome.

Apert disease: hereditary disease resulting in multiple deformities and mental retardation. Also called acrocephalosyndactylism.

Blount disease: lesion of the medial proximal tibial epiphysis causing valgus (bowing laterally) deformity of the tibia. Also called osteochondrosis deformans tibia, tibia vara.

Boeck sarcoid: condition usually affecting small bones of hands and feet with granulomatous inflammatory reaction in lymph nodes, spleen, lungs, and liver.

Bouchard nodes: cartilaginous and bony enlargement of the proximal interphalangeal joints of fingers in degenerative joint disease.

Brodie abscess: chronic infection of bone resulting in a characteristic coin-sized sclerotic lesion with a lucent center.

Caffey disease: subperiosteal cortical defect; infantile cortical hyperostosis; self-limited process of excess bone formation seen in newborns to 2-year-olds.

Engelmann disease: osteosclerosis (thickened bones) affecting diaphysis. Also called progressive diaphyseal dysplasia.

Freiberg disease: aseptic (avascular) necrosis of the second metatarsal head.

Fröhlich adiposogenital dystrophy: slipped capital femoral epiphysis. Also called Babinski-Fröhlich syndrome.

Gaucher disease (cerobroside reticulocystosis): bone disorder resulting from lipid storage disease that is due to an absence of glucocerebrosidase. Excessive production of histiocytes with interference of marrow function and destruction of bone occurs.

Gorham disease (massive osteolysis): a progressive, extensive, spontaneous loss of bone tissue associated with an increase in small blood and lymph vessels.

Hand-Schüller-Christian disease: one of the so-called histiocytosis X group of diseases; a complex of bony tumors caused by either accumulation of cholesterol, metabolic error, or neoplasm; characterized by eosinophilic granuloma, exophthalmos, and diabetes.

Heberden nodes: cartilaginous and bony enlargement of the distal interphalangeal joints in osteoarthritis.

Jaffe disease: osteoid osteoma; hereditary multiple exostosis.

Kienböck disease: aseptic necrosis affecting lunate or ilium.

Köhler disease: aseptic necrosis of tarsonavicular (scaphoiditis) and sometimes patella.

König disease: osteochondrosis dissecans of the knee; a separate formation of bone and cartilage segment at the joint surface.

Legg-Calvé-Perthes disease: aseptic epiphyseal ischemic necrosis of the capital femoral epiphysis in children. Also called coxa plana; Perthes disease; Legg-Perthes disease.

Letterer-Siwe disease: histiocyte tumor of bone, usually fatal in infants and small children. Also called eosinophilic granuloma.

Marie-Bamberger disease: hypertrophied joints resulting from lung disease.

Milkman syndrome: bone disease in which multiple transparent stripes are seen on radiograph.

Niemann-Pick disease: fatal fat storage disease marked by absence of sphingomyelinase affecting bone marrow in infancy.

Ollier disease: enchondromatosis.

Osgood-Schlatter disease: osteochondritis affecting anterior tibial tuberosity. Also called apophysitis.

Paget disease: disease of excess bone removal and replacement with deformity; seen in older persons. Also called osteitis deformans.

Panner disease: aseptic necrosis; osteochondritis dissecans of capitellum of humerus.

Perthes disease: aseptic necrosis of the hips in children.

Pott disease: osteomyelitis; tuberculosis of the spine.

Scheuermann disease: osteochondritis affecting anterior vertebral body of apophysis; aseptic necrosis of vertebral bodies.

shepherd's crook deformity: characteristic deformity of proximal femur seen in fibrous dysplasia. The deformity has the appearance of a shepherd's crook.

Sinding-Larsen-Johansson disease: secondary center of ossification of inferior pole of patella.

Stewart-Morel syndrome: hyperostosis of frontal bone. Also called Morel syndrome.

Thiemann disease: avascular necrosis of proximal phalanges. Also called aseptic necrosis.

Tietze syndrome: chronic inflammation of the costochondral junction of a rib or ribs, causing pain.

Volkmann deformity: congenital dislocation of the ankle due to absent or defective fibula, not to be confused with Volkmann's ischemic contracture.

von Recklinghausen disease: congenital disease of fatty tumors, peripheral nerve tumors, areas of skin pigment changes, and other disorders. Also called neurofibromatosis.

Voorhoeve disease: osteopathia striata.

Waldenström disease: osteochondrosis of distal humerus at the radial side of elbow (capitellum).

Muscle diseases

Myo- (Gr. *mys*) is a combining form denoting relationship to muscle. The *myo-* root terms are listed first in this section, followed by miscellaneous muscle diseases, the muscular dystrophies (listed together for comparison), and other muscle disorders.

Myo- root terms

myasthenia gravis: syndrome of attacks of muscle weakness that are episodic and reversible. Also called Erb-Goldflam disease.

myatrophy: muscle wasting.

myoasthenia: lack of muscle strength. Also called amyosthenia.

myoblastoma: tumor of striated muscle consisting of groups of granular-appearing cells resembling primitive myoblasts.

myobradia: sluggish muscle reaction to electric stimuli.

myocele: herniation and protrusion of muscle through its ruptured muscle sheath.

myocelialgia: pain in abdominal muscles.

myocelitis: inflammation of abdominal muscles.

myocellulitis: myositis with cellulitis.

myocerosis: waxy-appearing degeneration of muscle.

myoclonus: any disorder in which rapid rigidity and relaxation alternate; myoclonia.

myocoele: the cavity within a myotome.

myocytoma: muscle tumor.

myodegeneration: muscle degeneration.

myodemia: fatty degeneration of muscle.

myodiastasis: separation of muscle.

myodynia: pain in the muscles; myalgia, myo-salgia.

myodystonia: disorder of muscle tone.

myoedema: edema, muscle swelling.

myofascitis: inflammation of muscle and its fascia, particularly of fascial insertion of muscle to bone.

myofibroma: a muscular and fibrous tumor; fibroma containing muscular elements.

myofibrosis: replacement of muscle tissue by fibrous tissue.

myogelosis: an area of hardening in a muscle.

myohypertrophia: muscular hypertrophy.

myoischemia: local deficiency of blood supply in muscle.

myokerosis: waxy degeneration of muscle tissue. Also called myocerosis.

myolipoma: fatty tumor of muscle.

myolysis: disintegration or degeneration of muscle tissue.

myoma: tumor made up of muscular elements.

myomalacia: pathogenic softening of muscle.

myomatosis: formation of multiple muscle tumors.

myomelanosis: black pigmentation of a portion of muscle.

myoneuralgia: muscular nerve pain.

myoneurasthenia: relaxed state of the muscular system in neurasthenia (lack of nerve strength).

myoneuroma: a nerve tumor containing muscle tissue.

myoneurosis: any abnormal nerve condition of the muscles.

myopachynsis: hypertrophy of muscle; thickening.

myopalmus: muscle twitching.

myoparalysis: paralysis of muscle. Also called myoparesis.

myopathy: any disease of the muscles.

myophagism: atrophy or wasting away of muscle tissue, with removal of tissue by inflammatory cells.

myopsychopathy: any muscular nerve affection associated with mental weakness or disorder.

myorrhexis: a muscle rupture.

myosarcoma: malignant muscle tumor.

myosclerosis: hardening, or sclerosis, of muscle.

myoseism: jerky, irregular muscle contractions.

myositis: inflammation of a voluntary muscle.

  myositis ossificans: ossification of muscle in response to trauma.

  myositis ossificans progressiva: a terminal process in which multiple muscles ossify; more specifically, fibrous dysplasia ossificans progressiva.

myospasia: clonic contraction of muscle.

myospasm: muscle spasm.

myospasmia: disease characterized by uncontrolled muscle spasms.

myosteoma: bony tumor in muscle.

myosynizesis: adhesions of muscle.

myostasis: stretching of muscle.

myotenositis: inflammation of muscle and its tendon insertion.

myotonia: increased muscular irritability and contractility with decreased power of relaxation; tension and tonic spasm of muscle.

Miscellaneous muscle diseases and conditions

amyoplasia congenita: disorder of fascia and muscle resulting in contracted joints during growth. Also called arthrogryposis.

amyotonia congenita: muscle disorder of the newborn, usually fatal; characterized by muscle degeneration with failure of replacement (congenital hypotonia, Oppenheim disease); several types include Werdnig-Hoffman disease (CNS origin), rod disease (microscopic rods forming within muscle cells), and central core disease, which is not fatal.

congenital myotonia: disorder, found at birth, in which initiation and cessation of voluntary movement are delayed. Also called Thomsen disease.

familial periodic paralysis: disorder of muscle metabolism in which periods of partial to nearly complete paralysis occur. Also called myotonia intermittens.

muscular dystrophy: a group of degenerative disorders of muscle resulting in atrophy and weakness. Also called Erb disease.

pseudohypertrophic: dystrophy of shoulder girdle and sometimes pelvic girdle muscles, beginning with hypertrophy in childhood, followed by atrophy. Also called Erb paralysis.

fascioscapulohumeral: marked atrophy of face, shoulder girdle, and arm muscles. Also called Landouzy-Déjèrine disease.

limb girdle: slow, progressive dystrophy, affecting mostly the back and pelvic muscles.

distal: dystrophy affecting mostly the distal muscles of the extremities and usually slowly progressive proximally.

ocular: dystrophy usually confined to the levator and other facial muscles. Also called progressive dystrophic ophthalmoplegia.

myotonic dystrophy: myotonia followed eventually by atrophy of face and neck muscles, ultimately extending to muscles of trunk and extremities.

muscle atrophy: a general loss of muscle from various causes; muscle wasting.

muscle cramps: uncontrolled contraction of muscle. Also called *charley horse.*

muscle guarding: involuntary contraction of muscle in effort to avoid pain that would be produced by moving the body part.

muscle spasm: sudden contraction of muscle, usually in reflexive response to stimulus from external source, for example, back spasm caused by a herniated disk.

muscle ischemia: decreased blood supply to a muscle; can be spontaneously reversible, if not,

ischemic contracture may develop.

muscle contracture: a condition of fixed high resistance to passive stretch of a muscle resulting from fibrosis of the tissues supporting the muscles or the joints, or from disorders of the muscle fibers.

ischemic c.: contracture and degeneration of muscle due to interference with circulation from pressure, as by a tight bandage or from injury or cold.

organic c.: contracture that is permanent and continuous.

postpoliomyelitic c: any distortion of a joint following an attack of poliomyelitis.

rhabdomyosarcoma: malignancy of muscle cells.

shin splints: a term that merely defines pain in the shin (anterolateral aspect of leg or along medial aspect of Achilles tendon); believed due either to an ischemia caused by lower extremity overexertion with compartment swelling or traumatic periostitis of the medial margin of the tibia.

Stewart-Morel syndrome: intermittent progressive muscular rigidity. Also called *stiff man syndrome.*

Cartilage diseases

Chondro- (Gr. *chondros,* gristle or cartilage) is a combining form denoting a relationship to cartilage. Cartilage serves a very important function in the growing process and joint motion. Healthy cartilage is essential for normal growth.

A growth plate called the epiphysis, a cartilage layer near or outside the joint, is essential to most of the longitudinal growth of bone during childhood. Disorders of this structure can lead to dwarfism or deformity. Cartilage is not apparent on x-ray film, and many cartilage diseases are not detected on x-ray film until sufficient degeneration to cause joint narrowing takes place. Often a disorder that affects cartilage affects bone as well, such as osteo/chondr/itis (inflammation of bone and cartilage) or osteo/chondr/oma (bone and cartilage tumor).

Since diseased cartilage cells affect the combined function of bones and joints, many cartilage disease terms are found in the sections on bone tumors and joint diseases. The cartilage-related diseases are categorized in this section as:

1. *Chondro-* root diseases
2. Abnormalities of the ends of bone
3. Mucopolysaccharidoses (metabolism effects)
4. Miscellaneous cartilage diseases

Chondro- root diseases

chondralgia: pain in cartilage; chondrodynia.

chondritis: inflammation of cartilage.

chondroblastoma: tumor cells that differentiate into cartilage cells. Also called chondroma.

chondrodysplasia: hereditary deforming abnormal cartilage formation. Also called dyschondroplasia.

chondrodystrophia: rare condition of nutritional abnormality of cartilage development. Also called dwarfism.

chondroepiphysitis: inflammation of epiphyseal cartilage.

chondrofibroma: fibroma with cartilaginous elements.

chondrolipoma: fatty tumor containing cartilaginous elements.

chondrolysis: degeneration of cartilage cells, ending in cell death.

chondroma: cartilage tumor; hyperplastic growth of cartilage tissue.

chondromalacia: softening of cartilage, as of the patella.

chondromatosis: multiple formation of chondromas. Also called synoviochondromatosis.

chondrometaplasia: condition in which cells that would normally form cartilage function abnormally.

chondromyoma: muscle tumor with cartilaginous elements.

chondromyxofibroma: mucous tumor with cartilaginous and fibrous elements.

chondromyxoma: mucous tumor with cartilaginous elements.

chondromyxosarcoma: sarcoma containing cartilaginous and mucous elements.

chondronecrosis: necrosis (death) of cartilage.

chondro-osteodystrophy: nutritional abnormality of bone and cartilage.

chondropathology: diseased state of cartilage.

chondropathy: disease of cartilage.

chondrophyte: excess cartilaginous growth at bone ends, at the margins of a joint.

chondroporosis: a normal growth process in childhood; in adults the formation of empty space in cartilage is a part of a disease process.

chondrosarcoma: malignant cartilage tumor in which cells are making cartilage.

chondrosarcomatosis: multiple chondrosarcomas; abnormal tumor cartilage.

chondrosteoma: tumor made up of bone and cartilaginous tissue.

Abnormalities of the ends of bone

dysplasia epiphysealis hemimelia: an osteochondroma arising from an epiphysis and projecting from the articular surface. This will usually interfere with joint function.

epiphyseal hyperplasia: condition in which the epiphyses form from multiple centers and become enlarged and misshapen.

multiple epiphyseal dysplasia: multiple irregular epiphyseal ossification centers causing enlargement and flaring. Also called dysplasia epiphyseal multiplex congenita.

spondyloepiphyseal dysplasia: inability to ossify normal epiphyseal centers, resulting in dwarfing and/or precocious osteoarthritis, primarily in spine and hips.

stippled epiphysis: radiologic sign of chondrodystrophia calcificans, a disease associated with multiple calcification of epiphyseal cartilage. A mild form of the condition may be called epiphyseal dysplasia.

Mucopolysaccharidoses

The mucopolysaccharidoses are a variety of heritable metabolic disorders of mucopolysaccharides presently called *proteoglycans*, manifested by excretion of these substances in the urine. A mucopolysaccharide is a specific ammoniated or sulfinated polysaccharide chain. *Muco-* signifies the gelatinous appearance of the pure aggregate of these molecules—it is a sticky material that is a part of joint fluid and intracellular spaces, cartilage, and some other tissues. Most disorders of mucopolysaccharide metabolism are autosomal recessive. For many types, eponymic designations are preferred because the metabolic nomenclature is complicated.

achondroplasia: inherited, familial, congenital dwarfism associated with deformed long bones and misshapen epiphyses; achondroplastic dwarfism, chondrodystrophia fetalis.

cartilage-hair hypoplasia: rare dwarfism, very similar to achondroplasia.

diastrophic dwarfism: autosomal recessive dwarfism with flattening subluxation of various epiphyses.

Hunter syndrome: similar to Hurler syndrome, but less severely deforming; sex-linked inheritance; type II mucopolysaccharidosis.

Hurler syndrome: severely deforming condition associated with blindness, mental retardation, and early death; type I mucopolysaccharidosis.

Maroteaux-Lamy syndrome: growth retardation, lumbar kyphosis, sternal protrusion; no mental retardation; type VI mucopolysaccharidosis.

Morquio syndrome: dwarfing disease affecting mostly the spine and hips; little or no mental retardation; type IV mucopolysaccharidosis, chondro-osteodystrophy.

Sanfilippo syndrome: mild skeletal deformity but more severe mental retardation than types I and II; type III mucopolysaccharidosis.

Scheie syndrome: no mental impairment but noted corneal clouding, aortic disease, and stiff joints; type V mucopolysaccharidosis.

Miscellaneous cartilage diseases

Maffucci syndrome: dyschondroplasia with hemangiomas, some of which have calcified walls as seen on x-ray examination.

Ollier disease: multiple enchondromatosis, usually unilateral benign cartilage tumors of bone.

synchondrosis: fusion of cartilage surfaces in a joint. This may be a disease state or a normal maturation process, depending on the location.

synoviochondromatosis: a process in which the joint lining forms small nodules of cartilage, which may break loose and be free in the joint.

Synonymous with synovial osteochondromatosis or osteochondromatosis

Diseases of other soft tissue

In addition to bone, muscle, and cartilage, other tissues surround a joint. The root terms for these tissues—*fibro-, lipo-, myxo-, muco-*—denote the relationships of the tissues to certain disease processes and disorders. Further clarification of these tissue types is given in the discussion of each category. For a discussion of soft tissue tumor staging, see the box on page 37.

Fibro- root diseases

Fibro- (L. *fibra,* fiber) is a combining form indicating the presence of or association with fibrous tissue such as tendons and ligaments. Such tissue contains collagen, which is the major supportive protein of bone, tendon, cartilage, and connective tissue. This elongated, threadlike structure may be subjected to the following abnormal processes.

fibroma: benign fibroblastic tumor.

fibromatosis: formation of multiple fibromas.

fibrosarcoma: malignant fibroblastic tumor.

fibrosis: proliferation of fibrous tissue.

fibrositis: inflammation of fibrous tissue.

fibrous dysplasia ossificans progressiva: a progressive and usually lethal process in which multiple muscles ossify. Also called myositis ossificans progressiva.

fibrous histiocytoma: a benign tumor of bone containing fibrous stroma, xanthomatous cells, and a round and spindle cell component. There is a malignant form called malignant fibrous histiocytoma.

malignant fibrous histiocytoma: a highly malignant soft tissue tumor of later adult life that is initially seen as a subcutaneous to deep muscle lesion. Also called malignant fibrous xanthoma, fibroxanthosarcoma, malignant giant cell tumor of soft tissue.

monostotic fibrous dysplasia: disease of bony remodeling, causing deformity of only one bone.

polyostotic fibrous dysplasia: disease marked by fibrous tissue replacement of bone with resulting

---

SOFT TISSUE TUMOR STAGING

In an effort to preserve functional limbs it has become important to have a standard staging system for tumors that arise from the soft tissues of the musculoskeletal system (sarcomas).

A intracompartmental
B extracompartmental

The Musculoskeletal Tumor Society staging for soft tissue sarcomas is graded by location and cellular appearance.

I low-grade malignancy
II high-grade malignancy

The staging of soft tissue sarcomas can also be based on a letter system, G, T, N, and M

G = grade of malignancy: G_1 well differentiated (low-grade malignancy), G_2 moderately differentiated, and G_3 poorly differentiated with high malignant potential.

T = size of the primary tumor: T_1 is less than 5 cm diameter, T_2 5 cm or more, and T_3 any size that involves bone or main vessel or nerve.

N = status of regional lymph nodes; N_0 no metastasis, N_1 metastasis.

M = distant metastasis: M_0 no metastasis, M_1 distant metastasis.

Staging is based on the cumulative information of the four parameters.

stage I	G_1		T_1 or T_2	N_0	M_0
stage II	G_2		T_1 or T_2	N_0	M_0
stage III	G_3		T_1 or T_2	N_0	M_0
	any G		any T	N_1	M_0
stage IV	any G	or	T_3	N_0	or	M_0 = IV
	any G		any T	N	or	M_1 = IV

Adapted from: Soft tissue sarcoma staging and management, Maryland Medical Journal 35(4):237, 1986.

---

deformities and clinical appearance of café-au-lait skin pigmentation and precocious puberty. Also known as Albright syndrome.

neurofibroma: abnormal proliferation of nerve sheath cells. Also called Schwann tumor.

periarticular fibrositis: inflammatory condition of fibrous tissue surrounding a joint.

periosteal fibroma: a fibrous tumor of bone covering tissue.

Lipo- root diseases

Lipo- (Gr. *lipos,* fat) is a combining form denoting relationship to fat and fatty tissue. There are several disease processes based on this root.

lipofibroma: a fibrous fatty tumor.

lipoma: a fatty tumor; tumor made up of fat cells.

liposarcoma: a malignant tumor arising from fatty tissue.

Myxo- root diseases

Myxo- (Gr. *myxa,* mucus) is a combining form denoting relationship to mucus. Myxomatous cells contain mucous material that is clear in appearance. These cells are naturally found in the intervertebral disks, but when seen elsewhere they usually represent an abnormality. Myxomatous cells contain the mucopolysaccharide (proteoglycan) material, which could rupture, causing mucous cysts to form. Terms containing *myxo-* indicate the presence of this type of cell.

chondromyxofibroma: tumor containing elements of cartilage, myxoid, and fibrous cells.

myxofibroma: tumor containing both fibrous and myxomatous tissue.

myxoma: tumor containing myxoid cells.

myxosarcoma: sarcoma containing myxomatous tissue.

Muco- related diseases

The Latin word *mucus,* for the purposes of orthopaedics, does not imply secretions but rather the association of tissues that contain certain chemicals called *mucopolysaccharides,* which, when sufficient collection of material occurs, are in the form of a clear jelly and seen in certain cysts. Elsewhere in medicine the terms *mucus* and *mucous* relate particularly to the gut and respiratory tract.

ganglion cyst: mucous cyst, a sac of mucopolysaccharides, usually near a joint, from 1 mm to over 5 cm in size.

mucopolysaccharidosis: any of a variety of heritable disease states resulting from abnormalities in mucopolysaccharide (sugars containing SO_4 and NH_2) metabolism. These affect mostly cartilage in terms of orthopaedic diseases and cause stunted growth.

mucous cyst: in orthopaedics, a benign cyst under the fingernail.

Ligament, tendon, bursa, and fascia diseases

Desmo- (Gr. *desmos,* ligament) is a combining form denoting relationship to a band, bond, or ligament. Ligaments are composed of fibrous tissue that binds the joints together. Desmogenous dysfunctions and diseases may be any of the following.

desmectasis: stretching of a ligament.

desmitis: inflammation of a ligament.

desmocytoma: now called fibrosarcoma.

desmodynia: pain in a ligament. Also called desmalgia.

desmoid: collection of fibrous tissue occurring at the insertion of a tendon (cortical desmoid) or arising from soft tissue of an extremity. The latter is a true tumor, recurrent but not malignant. Also called extra-abdominal desmoid.

desmoma: a fibroma; a benign fibrous tumor.

desmopathy: any pathologic disease of a ligament.

desmoplasia: formation and development of fibrous tissue.

desmoplastic: producing or forming adhesions.

desmorrhexis: rupture of a ligament.

desmosis: disease of connective tissue.

extraabdominal desmoid (fibromatosis): a desmoid tumor that recurs with extensions in fascial planes but with no metastasis.

Eponymic ligamentous diseases

de Quervain disease: tenosynovitis of the abductor pollicis longus and extensor pollicis brevis.

Duplay disease: capsulitis of the glenohumeral joint area. Also called *frozen shoulder.*

Marfan syndrome: defect in elastic tissue resulting in ligamentous laxity, spiderlike fingers, and dissecting aneurysms of aorta in adult years.

Pellegrini-Steida disease: ligamentous calcification of the medial collateral ligament of the knee.

Tendo-/teno- related diseases

Tendo- and *teno-* (L. *tendo;* Gr. *tenōn*) are combining forms denoting relationship to a tendon. A tendon is a fibrous cord of connective tissue in which the fibers of a muscle end and by which muscle is attached to bone.

tendinitis: inflammation of tendons and of tendon-muscle attachments. Also called tenontitis, tenonitis, tenositis.

tenodynia: pain in a tendon. Also called tenontodynia.

tenontagra: a gouty affection of tendons.

tenontophyma: tumorous growth in tendon.

tenontothecitis: inflammation of a tendon sheath.

tenoperiostitis: inflammation of muscle-tendon attachment to bone, for example, tennis elbow and golfer's elbow.

tenophyte: growth or concretion in tendon.

tenositis: inflammation of a tendon.

tenostosis: ossification of a tendon.

tenosynovitis: inflammation of a tendon sheath and synovial sac. Also called tendosynovitis.

Other tendo- related diseases

Albert achillodynia: discomfort felt around terminal segment of heel cord. Also called achillodynia and achillobursitis.

snapping tendons: affliction of the tendons of the thumb or fingers resulting in snapping on adduction.

tennis elbow: inflammation of the origin of the extensor carpi radialis brevis muscle, which is at the outer elbow. Also called epicondylitis.

Bursa- related diseases

Bursae (pl.) are closed sacs of fibrous tissue, lined with synovial membrane, filled with viscid fluid, and situated in places in tissue where friction would otherwise inhibit function, such as near joints. Most disorders of bursae are part of another disease process.

bursitis: inflammation of a bursa at site of bony prominences between muscles or tendons.

bursolith: a calculus or concretion in a bursa.

bursopathy: any pathologic condition of bursae.

Fascia- related diseases

Fasciae (L. *fascia,* band) are bands of fibrous tissue that lie deep within the skin and form an investment for muscles and various organs of the body. *Retinacula* are also thickened bands that bind into position muscles and tendons of distal portion of limbs. (Retinaculum, sing.) There are several processes that are problematic and disease related.

Dupuytren contracture: a thickening and contracture of the palmar fascia of the hand resulting in flexion deformities of the fingers.

fasciitis: inflammation of fascia. Usually an anatomic structure is named when describing the location of the fasciitis, for example, plantar fasciitis, inflammation of the fascia of the sole of the foot.

nodular fasciitis: a fasciitis resulting in the formation of nodules.

Joint diseases (arthro-, synovio-, capsulo-, ankylo-)

The terms discussed in this section relate to loss of joint function or a change in appearance of the joint. Joint function depends on its surrounding tissue. The joint *(arthro-)* has a smooth inner lining (synovium) and a stronger fibrous outer connective tissue *(capsulo-).* Affections of the joint cartilage, synovium, and capsule may result in transient or permanent functional changes. When motion is severely or completely lost, *ankylosis* is the result.

Disease or dysfunctions affecting the joint spaces are categorized in this section as:

1. *arthro-:* joint
2. *synovio-:* synovium or fluid sac
3. *capsulo-:* the capsule enclosure around joint area
4. *ankylo-:* abnormal fusion of the joint

Arthro- related diseases

Arthro- (Gr. *arthron,* joint) is a combining form denoting some relationship to a joint, the junction where two bones meet and articulate with one another. Articulatio (Latin) is a general term for joint. The *arthro-* related diseases are:

arthralgia: pain in a joint. Also called arthrodynia.

arthrempyesis: infection in a joint. Also called arthroempyesis.

arthritis: inflammation of a joint; pathologic and may be crippling; can be degenerative joint disease. Various types are osteoarthritis, gouty a., rheumatoid a., septic a., traumatic a., infectious a., allergenic a., and hemophilic a.

arthrocace: infected cavity of a joint; caries.

arthrocele: swollen joint.

arthrochalasis: abnormal relaxation or flaccidity of a joint.

arthrochondritis: inflammation of the cartilages of a joint.

arthrodysplasia: deformity of various joints; hereditary condition.

arthrogryposis: persistent flexure or contracture of a joint; usually related to a congenital neuromuscular disorder.

arthrokatadysis: limitation of motion of the hip resulting from protrusio acetabuli (deep-shelled acetabulum).

arthrokleisis: ankylosis of a joint.

arthrolith: deposit of calculus in a joint.

arthromeningitis: synovitis; inflammation of the membranous lining of joint.

arthroncus: swelling of a joint.

arthroneuralgia: nerve pain in a joint.

arthronosos: disease of joints.

arthropathy: any joint disease.

arthrophyma: swelling of a joint.

arthrophyte: abnormal growth in a joint cavity.

arthropyosis: suppuration, or formation of pus, in a joint cavity.

arthrorheumatism: articular rheumatism.

arthrosclerosis: hardening or stiffening of a joint.

arthrosis: disease or abnormal condition of a joint.

arthrosteitis: inflammation of the bony structure of a joint.

arthrosynovitis: inflammation of the synovial membrane of a joint.

arthroxerosis: chronic osteoarthritis.

Other joint diseases

diffuse idiopathic sclerosing hyperostosis (DISH): excess bone formation at the margins of large joints, particularly the lumbar spine and hips.

exarticulation: amputation of a portion of a limb at the joint.

flail joint: complete loss of ligamentous stability.

frozen shoulder: severe loss of motion in the shoulder joint resulting from inflammation of the capsule.

gouty arthritis: inflammatory joint changes associated with gout; may be associated with tophi.

gouty node: collection of uric acid crystals near joints.

hemarthrosis: extravasation of blood into a joint or synovial cavity.

hydrarthrosis: accumulation of watery fluid in the joint cavity.

hypertrophic arthritis: increased bone formation around the joint, as seen on x-ray examination; osteoarthritis.

internal derangement of joint: commonly named "internal knee injuries," particularly when the precise nature of the injury is unknown.

joint mice: loose pieces of cartilage or other organic material in the joint.

luxation: dislocation of bone or bones at joint site.

pauciarticular: involving a few joints as opposed to involving many joints.

polyarthritis: inflammation of many joints.

psuedarthrosis: false joints that result from nonunion of a fracture or from a pathologic bone condition.

pustulotic osteoarthropathy: pain, swelling, and x-ray findings of hypertrophy and sclerotic changes involving the sternum, ribs, and clavicle associated with a skin condition pustulosis palmaris et plantaris. The sacrum, spine, and peripheral joints may also show x-ray changes. The cause is unknown.

rice bodies: small, glistening, soft, loose bodies either in joints or bursae, loose fibrocartilage tissue.

suppurative arthritis: bacteria infection causing pain, swelling, tenderness, redness, and effusion; pyarthrosis.

synarthrosis: ankylosis and contracture; usually caused by arthritic joint disease.

villous lipomatous proliferation: rare disorder of synovial joint lining where there is fatty proliferation with the formation of numerous villous formations. The term *lipoma arborescens* was applied to this condition. Because it is not a neoplasm, the villous lipomatous proliferation term is preferred.

Eponymic joint diseases

Baker cyst: cystic lesion appearing in the popliteal fossa of the knee. In the adult this is usually a synovial fluid cystic extension due to intraarticular disease. This results in a new synovial-lined sac appearing in the popliteal fossa. In the child, the cyst is usually a ganglion arising from one of the tendons in the popliteal area.

Bechet syndrome: disease of undetermined etiology that may produce joint complaints predominantly in young people in the third decade of life. Marked by oral and genital ulcerations, and eye and skin lesions. Often arthritis, thrombophlebitis, gastrointestinal lesions, and central nervous system lesions may occur in some individuals.

Charcot joint disease: mechanical destruction of joints caused by lack of sensation (not to be confused with Charcot-Marie-Tooth disease).

Ehlers-Danlos syndrome: generalized joint capsular laxity occurring as a hereditary disease.

Kawasaki disease: a mucocutaneous lymph node

syndrome in children characterized by fever, exanthomatous skin disease, and sometimes arthritis (30% to 40%).

Lyme disease: inflammatory arthritis involving usually a few joints, particularly the knees, caused by an organism that is transmitted by a tick.

Reiter syndrome: arthritis of various joints, usually associated with one or more of the triad of urethral drip, conjunctivitis, and oral mucosal lesions.

Synovio- related diseases

Synovial fluid, or synovia, is an alkaline viscid transparent fluid resembling egg white that is found in joint cavities, tendon sheaths, and bursae and is responsible for lubrication and nourishment of these joint structures. Synovial membrane is the inner lining of a joint, which is a two-layer membrane on a bed of fat composed of certain cells that produce synovial fluid; other cells act as phagocytes. Related disease processes are the following.

synovial cyst: accumulation of fluid in the bursa or sac, causing a tumorlike cyst.

synovial osteochondromatosis: formation by the synovium of cartilage bodies, which develop into bone.

synoviochondromatosis: synovial formation of cartilage bodies.

synovioma: a benign or malignant tumor of the synovial membrane.

synovitis: inflammation of synovial membrane, which may be associated with swelling.

Miscellaneous synovial diseases

pigmented villonodular synovitis: inflammation of synovium with production of pigment, giant cells, and other characteristic cell types.

villous synovitis: inflammation of joint lining, resulting in long fronds of synovium.

Capsulo-related diseases

The capsule (L. *capsula,* small box) is the thick fibrous tissue surrounding the joint outside the synovium and defines the limits of the joint. There are two related dysfunctions.

adhesive capsulitis: inflammation of a capsule that results in limited joint motion. Also called *frozen shoulder.*

capsulitis: inflammation of the capsule.

Ankylo- related diseases

The combining form *ankylo-* means bent or deformed. It was originally used to describe untreated deforming loss of joint function. Now such terms apply to joints fused congenitally or those that are aligned normally because of surgical process. Therefore the implication of *ankylo-* is not necessarily bent or deformed but rather complete fusion of a joint or at least restricted motion.

ankylodactylia: adhesions of fingers or toes to one another.

ankylosis: consolidation and abnormal immobility of a joint.

  bony a.: abnormal union of bones at joint site; true ankylosis.

  extracapsular a.: caused by rigidity of structure exterior to joint capsule, usually a surgically implanted piece of bone.

  false a.: resulting from other causes not related to the abnormal union of bones comprising the joint.

  fibrous a.: caused by formation of fibrous bands within the joint.

  intracapsular a.: caused by undue rigidity of structure within the joint capsule.

  ligamentous a.: resulting from rigidity of ligaments.

  spurious a.: false ankylosis.

Blood vessel diseases and conditions

All tissues of the body are supplied with nutrients and oxygen by blood vessels. These vessels are subject to an assortment of disease processes. The larger named arteries are usually impaired by arteriosclerosis or trauma, the larger named veins are usually impaired by trauma or thrombosis, and the smaller unnamed vessels (on either side of the circulation) can be injured by arteriosclerosis, trauma or systemic degenerative disorders, for example, collagen vascular diseases. In addition to these, the heart itself can be afflicted with diseases of the arteries feeding the heart or with deterioration of the muscle (cardiomyopathy).

Trauma and arteriosclerosis (hardening of the arteries) are the two most frequent arterial conditions that are seen by the orthopaedic surgeon. However, the orthopaedist will often see a host of other vascular disorders or symptoms that influence the treatment of a musculoskeletal problem. The venous and arterial disorders, collagen vascular disorders, and blood vessel tumors are considered here.

Venous disorders

deep venous thrombosis (DVT): blood clots in the deep venous circulation usually of the lower extremity, in the calf, thigh, or pelvis. Portions of these clots may break off and lodge in the lungs, causing pulmonary embolus. These clots in the veins eventually destroy the valves of the veins and can cause chronic problems related to venous insufficiency.

embolus: (Gr. *embolos* plug) an undissolved clot that has broken free of a vessel wall and traveled to some distant point; a pulmonary embolus is a clot lodged in the lung. (See Arterial disorders.)

phlebitis: inflammation of a vein; may be a result of infection, inflammation, or trauma and is usually associated with thrombus in that vein (thrombophlebitis).

phlebothrombosis: a clot in a vein; phlebitis with secondary thrombosis.

postphlebitic syndrome: chronic venous insufficiency of lower limbs resulting from deep venous thrombosis. Develops with loss of function of valves in veins, allowing blood to pool and cause swelling, pain, leg ulceration, and varicose veins.

pulmonary embolism (PE): acute obstruction to circulation in lungs as a result of a clot that has migrated from the pelvic or leg veins and lodged in the lung. A life-threatening problem requiring anticoagulants and sometimes surgery.

thrombophlebitis: inflammation of a vein associated with thrombosis (blood clots) usually in the lower limbs. The clot can also become infected, becoming septic thrombophlebitis.

thrombus: a blood clot incompletely or completely occluding a blood vessel.

varices (*sing.* **-ix**): enlarged and tortuous (twisted) veins or lymphatic vessels, usually of the lower limbs; many types.

venous insufficiency (reflux): malfunction of venous valves that allow blood to flow in a retrograde (backward) direction. Also called postphlebitic syndrome.

Arterial disorders

aneurysm: a thin-walled dilated segment of a vessel wall that may be caused by degeneration from arteriosclerosis congenital abnormality or trauma. Complications of aneurysms include rupture, thrombosis, or breakoff of a blood clot that has collected in the aneurysm.

arterial insufficiency: inadequate blood flow to an organ or extremity frequently caused by arteriosclerotic narrowing or occlusion of the blood vessel.

arterial occlusive disease: hardening of the arteries. Also called arteriosclerosis.

anterior compartment syndrome: traumatized or overexerted anterior leg muscles, resulting in swelling and decreased blood supply with severe intracompartmental ischemia and edema. Known also as shin splints, a term applied to other disorders.

arteriosclerosis: name for degenerative process that affects most blood vessels in most people (in varying degrees) and begins in early teens. Its progression is related in part to genetics, diet, smoking, and high blood pressure. It can be exacerbated by injuries such as trauma or surgery; it causes narrowing and irregular surfaces in blood vessels or may cause aneurysmal disease. It is the most frequent problem in arteries. Also called atherosclerosis.

arteriovenous fistula (AVF): an abnormal communication between an artery and a vein. Also called AV fistula. See AV malformation.

atheroma: a localized collection of arteriosclerosis (thickened arterial intima) that has degenerated.

blue toe syndrome: a bluish or black tender and painful discoloration of a toe. It is the result of a localized acute ischemia of the toe caused by distal embolization of platelet aggregates or arteriosclerotic plaque, which then occludes the small end vessels. This represents a proximal embologenic source, for example, aneurysm or significant arteriosclerotic plaque.

Buerger disease: thromboangiitis obliterans: an inflammation of the arteries (and veins) in extremity causing severe ischemia; occurs usually in young smokers and is a pathologic variance of arteriosclerosis.

cerebrovascular accident (CVA): ischemia of a portion of the brain as a result of an occluded blood vessel from an embolus arising from the heart or great vessels of the neck; frequently the result of hardening of the arteries, a rupture of the blood vessel in the brain, or a tumor. Also called stroke.

chilblains: breakdown of skin and swelling of the hands and feet from overexposure to cold moisture; thermal injuries.

claudication: inadequate blood flow to large muscle groups of lower limbs resulting from hardening of the arteries, causing pain, numbness, or heaviness in muscle groups brought on by exercise and relieved by rest.

compartment syndrome: any generalized diminished oxygenated blood supply to a confined muscle compartment due to excessive use or trauma-related swelling. The syndrome may self-correct or progress with eventual muscle necrosis, loss of arterial blood supply, and loss of limb. The most commonly affected compartments are the anterior leg *(anterior compartment syndrome),* volar forearm (leading to Volkmann ischemic contracture), and anterior thigh *(rectus femorus syndrome).*

embolus: a blood clot or piece of atheromatous debris that blocks an artery or vein. Can also be made up of an air bubble, fat, portion of tumor, or piece of prosthetic material. This embolus, when traveling to the heart, may cause a heart attack; to the brain, could cause a stroke; and to the lower limbs, may cause acute ischemia.

fibromuscular d.: a poorly understood uncommon degenerative disease of the arteries frequently affecting the renal arteries of young females. The problem causes narrowing of the vessel with weblike deformities that appear as a string of beads on arteriography. Can also cause aneurysm.

fistula: abnormal communication between any two structures that normally do not communicate; can be the result of trauma, arteriosclerosis, or surgical procedure. An arteriovenous fistula may be created and used for hemodialysis.

frostbite: damage to tissue resulting from exposure to cold; may result in lowering blood supply sufficiently to cause permanent sensory loss, chronic pain, or partial limb loss.

infarct: small area of ischemic necrosis resulting from acute interruption of blood supply. This term is frequently applied to areas of the brain or heart.

ischemia: acute or chronic decreased blood flow to organ or limb caused by obstruction of inflow of arterial blood or by vasoconstriction. Acutely, the symptoms include the six p's: pain, pallor, pulselessness, paresthesias, paralysis, and poikilothermia (coldness).

kinking: bending of an artery, causing pain; result of trauma or body position.

malformation, arteriovenous (AVM): congenital arteriovenous connection often resulting in disfigurement or malfunction. Frequently seen as a discolored area on the skin, but may represent a much larger diversion of blood such that it interferes with organ function. Its continuing presence may interfere with the heart because of the large alteration in flow that it creates.

popliteal cyst: degeneration of the wall of the popliteal artery resulting in a cysticlike structure within the wall of the artery that can partially or completely occlude the artery. Usually occurs in the popliteal artery. This term should be popliteal arterial cyst to avoid confusion with the more common synovial or ganglion type.

popliteal entrapment: partial or complete occlusion of popliteal artery as a result of abnormal location of adjacent medial head of the gastrocnemius muscle. May include any one or all of the artery, vein, and nerve.

rest pain: distal foot pain caused by acute or chronic arterial ischemia representing a significant decrease in blood flow; usually from hardening of the arteries. The pain is burning, sharp in nature, and frequently begins by keeping the patient awake at night. May be relieved by dependent position.

rubor (dependent): dark purplish red color to foot when foot is hung over the edge of bed. It represents maximally dilated capillary beds that are responding to decreased arterial inflow and then their subsequent fill by gravity.

stroke: see cerebrovascular accident (CVA).

Sudeck atrophy: a vascular reflex in a limb, caused by minor trauma, resulting in a red, stiff, and severely painful limb; referred to as "causalgia" when caused by trauma involving a large area or affecting a larger nerve.

thrombosis: formation of blood clots, whereas *thrombus* is a blood clot.

transient ischemic attack (TIA): transient neurologic deficit that clears within 24 hours. Usually the result of decreased blood flow to the portion of brain from a blood clot from either the heart or extracranial carotid vessels. Usually from hardening of the arteries—atheromatous plaque breaks off and lodges in the vessels of the brain or eye.

varices (*sing.* **-ix**)**:** enlarged and tortuous (twisted) veins, arteries, or lymphatic vessels, usually of the lower limbs; many types.

Volkmann contracture: The final state of an unrelieved forearm compartment syndrome; decreased blood supply to forearm muscles resulting in muscle death, contractures of tendons to wrist and hand, and a claw-hand deformity. This usually starts out as a compartment syndrome that develops after an elbow or forearm fracture.

Collagen vascular and other disorders

Collagen vascular diseases are a series of disorders relating to the basic building blocks of the body, that is, collagen. The walls of blood vessels are made up of collagen, a type of protein seen in all connective tissue such as bone, cartilage, and tendon. Certain diseases affect the collagen, particularly in scattered blood vessels.

Through a variety of mechanisms, the immunologic system of the body begins to attack, thereby causing degeneration in small blood vessels and/or parts of the bony anatomy (joint capsule, synovial fluid of joint and synovium). The systemic inflammatory condition that results can be mildly inconvenient or severely disabling, or can result in death. Certain diseases such as rheumatoid arthritis affect this collagen and, as a result, interfere with the function of bones, joints, and blood vessels. The term *inflammatory joint disease* is often used to describe arthritis, but this general term is also applied to gout, pseudogout, and some other systemic causes of arthritis.

Dyscollagenoses and *systemic connectivitis* are terms specifically related to the immune connective tissue disorders of rheumatoid arthritis, systemic lupus erythematosus, Sjörgren syndrome, progressive systemic sclerosis, polyarteritis nodosa, polymyositis, dermatomyositis, and eosinophilic fasciitis. This spectrum of disorders represents the effects on the different collagens of the joint lining and vascular walls.

The treatment of these disorders is often complicated and frustrating for both patient and physician, frequently involves corticosteroids (antiinflammatory drugs) and nonsteroidal antiinflammatory drugs (ibuprofen, aspirin), and so forth, and often involves drugs that directly interfere with the immune mechanism of the body (antimetabolites). Terms associated with these various conditions are discussed here along with a series of other miscellaneous disorders.

ankylosing spondylitis: inflammatory joint disease affecting mostly the spine, hips, and pelvis. Seen most commonly in young men, this can lead to fusion of the spine with deformity, depending on the position of the spine during the fusion process. Seen in the child, the disorder is called Marie-Strümpell disease or rheumatoid spondylitis.

arteritis: inflammation of small arteries.

calcinosis circumscripta: the quadrad of calcium deposits in the skin (calcinosis cutis), Raynaud's phenomenon, scleroderma, and telangiectasia is seen in this collagen disease that has been considered a variant of scleroderma.

causalgia: a specific disease entity with pain and disability, caused by partial nerve injury, that may result in extreme pain in limbs, hypersensitivity, and paresthesias. On physical exam, thin, warm, dry skin with mild swelling or atrophy, may be present, with bluish discoloration and skin breakdown (minor scaling to frank ulceration). Usual patterns of patchy osteoporosis may accompany syndrome in affected limb. Also called reflex sympathetic dystrophy and Sudeck atrophy. *Mimocausalgia* refers to the same symptom complex but without obvious inciting nerve injury.

CREST syndrome (limited scleroderma): a complex of *c*alcinosis of articular tissue associated with *R*aynaud phenomenon, *e*sophageal dysmotility, *s*clerodactyly, and *t*elangiectasia. This condition appears to be less aggressive than scleroderma.

ergotism: acute or chronic effects of ergot alkaloids on the blood flow to an organ such as the brain or limbs. Ergot alkaloids are in some plants and medicines that are taken for headaches.

Felty syndrome: a combination of chronic rheumatoid arthritis, enlarged spleen, and a reduced number of granulocytes in the white blood count.

focal scleroderma: disease of unknown etiology characterized by circumscribed areas of fibrosis of the skin, subcutaneous fat, fascia, and muscle into bone. It is usually restricted to a limb and usually occurs in children and young adults. Also called *Addison's keloid*.

lupus erythematosus: disease, affecting not only the joints but also heart, heart lining, and circulation in bone. It is life threatening, although a protracted mild course is possible. This disease may be called *systemic lupus erythematosus* to distinguish it from discoid lupus, a more benign process.

Marie-Strümpell disease: a disease beginning in childhood, similar to rheumatoid arthritis, usually resulting in ankylosis of the spine and involvement of the liver and spleen. Also called rheumatoid or ankylosing spondylitis.

Mönckeberg sclerosis: calcification of the middle coat of small and medium-sized muscular arteries. Also called medial arteriosclerosis.

polyarteritis nodosa: a disease causing nodules in small arteries with some microscopic clotting, resulting in muscle cramps and eventual loss of muscle tone; can be severe.

Raynaud disease or phenomenon: an abnormal persisting coolness, blanching, or blueness in the hand, usually as a result of exposure to cold.

rheumatoid arthritis: generalized inflammatory joint disease. In children, it is called juvenile rheumatoid arthritis and Still's disease. The disease may result in mild, lifelong discomfort, or it may become severely crippling; in some cases, there is associated skin nodularity. Certain laboratory studies confirm the diagnosis. (Positive rheumatoid factor.)

scleroderma: disease causing a waxy thickening of the skin and classically affecting swallowing; tends to be severely progressive.

Sjögren syndrome: a group of conditions including keratoconjunctivitis sicca (dry eyes), arthritis, dry mouth, and enlargement of the parotid glands.

vasoconstriction: narrowing of vessel lumen caused by contraction of muscular vessel walls.

vasodilation: enlargement of vessel lumen caused by relaxing of muscular vessel wall.

vasospastic: localized intermittent contraction of a blood vessel.

Blood vessel tumors

hemangioma: any benign small vessel tumor of dilated blood vessels; may be flush with the skin with a violescent, patchy discoloration or elevated like a violescent or red mole. Size may vary from 1 mm to large area of the body.

hemangioendothelioma: tumor composed mostly of endothelial cells of the inner walls of capillary vessels.

hemangiopericytoma: a spindle cell tumor with a

rich vascular network; arises from pericytes.

hemangiosarcoma: a malignant blood vessel tumor; angiosarcoma.

Associated vascular terms

acrocyanosis: modeling of the skin of the extremity not produced by major vascular occlusions. May be related to an emotional change or temperature.

atrophy: reduction in size of an anatomic structure, frequently related to disuse or decreased blood supply.

arrhythmias: abnormal rhythm of the heart.

bradycardia: abnormal slowing of heart rate usually under 60 beats/minute.

bruit: abnormal sound on mediate auscultation over a blood vessel or the heart and indicates turbulence.

congestive heart failure: condition in which heart is unable to pump out venous blood returning to it, resulting in pooling of venous blood and accumulation of fluid in various parts of the body (lungs, legs, etc.)

cyanosis: discoloration of the skin or nail beds, bluish-purple in color; represents decreased blood flow to that area.

hypercholesteremia: an elevated blood cholesterol level.

hypertension: elevated blood pressure either temporary or permanent; may be an elevation of the systolic or diastolic blood vessels or pressure.

hypotension: blood pressure below normal.

hypovolemia: loss of normal amount of circulating blood volume; could be the result of hemorrhage from trauma (or from ulcer).

hypoxia: decreased amount of oxygen in any given tissue.

myocardial infarction (MI): acute or chronic blockage of blood vessels to the heart, resulting in localized area of ischemia (heart attack).

necrosis: pathologic definition of death of tissues caused by lack of blood supply to that part.

normotensive: normal blood pressure.

occlusion: closed or shut, such as an occluded artery or vein.

palpitation: sensation either by patient or examiner of irregular heartbeat.

stasis: decrease or absence of flow in the venous circulation.

stenosis: narrowing of lumen of blood vessel; a stricture.

tachycardia: abnormal increase in heart rate, usually over 100 beats/minute.

Neurologic diseases

Neuro- (Gr. *neuron,* nerve) is a combining form denoting the relationship to a nerve or nerves, or to the nervous system in general. Of all the specialties in medicine, neurology interrelates more frequently with orthopaedics than does any other. There are two reasons for this. First, the presenting symptoms of certain neurologic disorders may be quite similar to those of some orthopaedic disorders or diseases in that they result in muscular loss, altered function, and possible deformities, particularly in growing individuals.

In orthopaedic diagnoses the nervous system is considered in two portions, the central and the peripheral. The central portion is composed of the brain, spinal cord, and their covering soft tissues. The peripheral portion is composed of all the nerves in the body. Because some diseases affect both the central and peripheral nervous systems simultaneously, discussion of both is presented in an alphabetic listing of nerve disorders, except for some eponymic terms that belong to a specific category. The same term may be defined several times in this chapter to avoid cross-referencing elsewhere.

General neurologic diseases

amyotrophic lateral sclerosis (ALS): disease principally of the spinal cord, seen in adult life; results in loss of motor control and eventual death. Also called Charcot d., Lou Gehrig d.

apoplexy: old term used to describe a stroke, a bleeding into or loss of blood supply to the brain.

apraxia: loss of ability to perform purposeful movements even though parts concerned are not paralyzed.

ataxia: motor incoordinaton.

atonia: lack of tone or tension; relaxation, flaccidity.

axonotmesis: disruption of nerve plasma without disruption of the axon sheath, resulting in a recovery of nerve function over a period of up to 3 years.

causalgia: burning pain, associated with glossy skin; most frequently follows some type of nerve injury.

cerebral palsy (CP): a very general term applied to central nervous system disorders found at birth or infancy and affecting muscle control; can range from being almost undetectable to totally incapacitating and extremely deforming. There is mild to severe loss of motor control, which is called *diplegic CP* if it seems to affect primarily the lower extremities.

    spastic CP: most common form; attempts by victim to use affected muscles result in uncontrolled contractions.

    ataxic CP: additional elements of incoordination.

    athetoid CP: uncontrolled writhing movements.

    flaccid CP: a very severe form in which muscle contractions cannot be initiated.

chorea: continuing uncontrolled jerking motions caused by brain disease; may occur as a result of rheumatic fever or other diseases; may be inherited, which is called Huntington chorea; St. Vitus dance.

dural ectasia: often seen with neurofibromatosis, thickening of the dural tissues may occur. This can lead to dissolution of the spinal elements and eventual spinal instability.

entrapment syndrome: symptoms caused by entrapment of a nerve in soft or hard tissue, for example, occipital nerve entrapment syndrome, a chronic muscle irritation of the neck, causing impingement on occipital nerve.

epilepsy: disorder of nervous system characterized by seizures in which there may be clonic and tonic muscular contractions and loss of consciousness.

    grand mal e.: epilepsy marked by major convulsions, usually first tonic then clonic, oscillating eyeballs, feeble pulse, stupor, and unconsciousness.

    petit mal e.: mild or minor attack (small seizures) of epilepsy without convulsions other than slight twitching of muscles of the face or extremities.

    jacksonian e.: recurrent episodes of localized convulsive seizures or spasms limited to a part of the body, without loss of consciousness.

ganglioneuroma: tumor made up of ganglion cells.

glioma: tumor arising from specialized connective tissue found in brain and spinal cord.

glomus tumor: a benign tumor consisting of nerve and small vessel components. These small lesions often produce severe pain and local vascular effects. They are often found near the tips of digits of the hands and feet.

hemiplegia: paralysis of one side of the body.

locomotor ataxia: see Tabes dorsalis.

lumbar theco-peritoneal shunt syndrome: a syndrome following theco-peritoneal shunting for idiopathic communicating hydrocephalus. Characterized by severe, rigid, and progressive lumbar lordosis; severe bilateral restriction of straight leg raising; and abnormalities of stance and gait.

meralgia: pain in the thigh, usually caused by irritation of lateral cutaneous nerve of the thigh.

motor neuron disease: any disease caused by destruction of the nerve cells involved in voluntary muscle function.

    upper motor neuron d.: any brain disorder that affects the normal pathways leading to voluntary muscle function.

    lower motor neuron d.: disorder of the cells in the spinal cord, resulting in loss of motor function.

multiple sclerosis: slowly progressive disease of nervous system in which scattered areas of degeneration of the myelin occur; common in the spinal cord; cause unknown.

myopathy hand: a characteristic hand dysfunction due to spinal cord injury. A loss of adduction power, extension of the ulnar two or three fingers, and an inability to grip and release rapidly with these fingers distinguishes this hand weakness from other hand dysfunctions due to peripheral nerve disorders.

neural tube defect: a group of malformations of the brain and spinal cord that originate at various times during fetal development. The most commonly seen kind is meningomyelocele.

neuralgia: pain along the course of a nerve or nerves.

neuritis: inflammation of any nerve; usually painful.

neurogenic: occurring because of a nervous system disorder.

neurologic disease: any disease of the nervous system.

neurolysis: dissolution of the nerve tissue in disease process.

neuroma: benign tumor of the nerve.

traumatic n.: neuroma caused by a complete cutting of the nerve or by sufficient injury to cause excess scarring in the nerve.

amputation n.: a traumatic neuroma occurring after an amputation.

neuropathy: any disease of the peripheral nerves (those outside the brain and spinal cord).

neuropraxia: contusion of a nerve resulting in transient disruption of nerve function; less severe than axonotmesis or neurotmesis.

neurotmesis: complete transection of a nerve, resulting in cell death.

paralysis: loss or impairment of voluntary muscle function; palsy.

paralysis agitans: chronic nervous disease in later life marked by muscular tremor or by a peculiar gait; Parkinson disease.

paraplegia: paralysis of lower part of body or lower extremities.

paresis: incomplete loss of voluntary muscle function.

paresthesia: abnormal sensations such as numbness, burning, tickling, and crawling due to central or peripheral nerve lesions such as multiple sclerosis or locomotor ataxia.

pellagra: vitamin B_6 deficiency disease manifested by disorders of skin, alimentary tract, and nervous system.

peripheral neuropathy: diseases at or distal to the nerve root.

poliomyelitis: inflammation of gray matter of spinal cord; may result in loss of voluntary muscle control.

polyneuritis: inflammation of multiple nerves.

psychomotor: referring to mental origin of muscle movement.

quadriplegia: loss of voluntary muscle function in both arms and legs.

radiculitis: inflammation of intradural portion of a spinal nerve root prior to its entrance into the intervertebral foramen, or of the portion between that foramen and the nerve plexus.

radiculoneuritis: inflammation of nerve root and nerve.

radiculopathy: disease at the origin of a nerve, the spinal nerve root.

syncope: fainting or swooning caused by lack of oxygen or blood flow to the brain.

syringomyelia: disorder of spinal cord, marked by abnormal cavities filled with liquid.

tabes dorsalis: severe progressive disease of the central nervous system, caused by syphilis and characterized by demyelination of the dorsal columns of the spinal cord. Also called locomotor ataxia. Duchenne disease.

taboparesis: condition in which symptoms of tabes dorsalis and general paresis are associated. Also called neurosyphilis.

thoracic outlet syndrome: a mechanical problem related to the exit of arteries and nerves at the base of the neck leading down the arm, and can also involve the vein bringing blood back from the arm. Compression of these structures as they pass through a narrow foramen between the scalenus anticus muscle and first rib. Problem may be exacerbated by congenitally present additional cervical rib. Early signs are pain in the hand or shoulder. Arteries may be damaged in the process and cause an aneurysm in the area with possible break off of clot from the aneurysm.

tic: involuntary and usually quick repetitious contractions of a muscle or muscle groups; repeated twitching.

tic douloureux: a painful affliction (neuralgia) involving the trigeminal nerve.

tremor: involuntary trembling or quivering; shaking.

vertigo: loss of equilibrium.

Eponymic neurologic diseases

Bell palsy: loss of function of the facial nerves.

Brown-Séquard syndrome: injury to only one side of the spinal cord, resulting in loss of motion on one side of the body and loss of sensation on the opposite side.

Charcot joint disease: joint destruction caused by loss of normal sensation.

Friedreich ataxia: inherited disease with sclerosis of the dorsal and lateral columns of the spinal cord, attended by loss of coordination; usually apparent in early childhood; can be fatal.

Guillain-Barré syndrome: viral disorder involving spinal cord, peripheral nerves,and nerve roots; recovery of lost voluntary muscle function usually occurs, but the disease can be fatal.

Marie-Charcot-Tooth disease: spontaneous degeneration of neuromuscular complex; most commonly peroneal nerve, but also ulnar nerve. Also called Charcot-Marie-Tooth disease.

Morton neuroma: excessive proliferation of perineural tissue, usually at the third and fourth metatarsal heads.

Naffziger syndrome: scalenus anticus syndrome; pain in brachial plexus distribution, caused by muscle impingement.

Parkinson disease: see Paralysis agitans.

Parsonage-Turner syndrome: a condition of the brachial plexus resulting in sudden onset of pain and muscle weakness in upper limbs that may lead to muscle wasting (atrophy). Pain may occur simultaneously or after several weeks, and last 1 to 4 weeks or persist for 18 months. Cause unknown. Also called *neuralgic amyotrophy.*

Raynaud disease: disease in which the small arterioles of upper limbs, particularly of the fingertips, becomes extremely sensitive to cold, and the vessels undergo segmental spasm, in-

terrupting blood flow to tissue; occasionally progresses to necrosis and dry gangrene in fingertips.

schwannoma: neoplasm of a nerve sheath.

Sudeck atrophy: see Eponymic bone diseases.

von Recklinghausen disease: multiple neurofibromatosis.

METABOLIC DISEASES

There are thousands of chemicals in the body. Most of them are being rapidly destroyed and replaced as part of the essential chain of events that supplies energy, growth, and normal tissue replacement. There are conditions in which some of these chemicals may accumulate or be produced in inadequate quantity for normal function. Not all metabolic diseases can be identified at birth.

Gout is a disease in which uric acid accumulates in the soft tissues; it usually does not occur until middle adult life. Sickle cell anemia is the result of production of the wrong kind of chemical, causing changes in the shape of red cells and a subsequent decreased oxygen supply; this disorder is usually detected in infancy.

Many such disorders of chemical production and destruction (metabolism) have been defined elsewhere in this text because of certain characteristic tissues or extremity appearances. Some terms will be redefined here, with greater emphasis placed on the metabolic aspects.

Osteopenia is a term that defines abnormally diminished bone. It may occur regionally after immobilization, or be due to a systemic effect involving the entire skeleton. The term does not define the quality of the bone, but simply states that there is less of it (osteo = bone + penia = deficiency).

Osteoporosis is a condition where the mineral and organic content is normal, but there is less bone. The most common generalized osteoporosis is associated with aging (senile osteoporosis). Some metabolic conditions such as the postmenopausal state and abnormal gastrointestinal absorption are associated with a generalized osteoporosis. If no specific cause is found the condition is often referred to as *idiopathic osteoporosis.* In children it is called *juvenile osteoporosis*.

Osteomalacia describes softening of bone, resulting from vitamin D deficiency or kidney disease. Milk allergy, liver disease, excision of the ovaries, kidney disorders, and chronic intestinal problems may interfere with vitamin D metabolism, absorption of calcium, or other processes, resulting in abnormal bone formation and mineralization.

Diseases associated with osteomalacia

Fanconi syndrome: a severe form of vitamin D–resistant rickets, often fatal, and characterized by the presence of glucose, amino acids, and other chemicals in the urine.

hyperparathyroidism: abnormal increase in the level of parathyroid hormone, resulting in loss of calcium from bones.

hypoparathyroidism: abnormal decrease in the level of parathyroid hormone, either congenital or acquired, resulting in decreased bone formation and lowered serum calcium.

hypophosphatasia: an autosomal recessive inherited disease characterized by severe skeletal defects resulting from a failure of calcification of bone.

milk-alkali syndrome: osteoporosis and/or osteomalacia, usually resulting from excessive intake of milk and alkali to treat ulcer disease; changes in therapy have reduced the prevalence of this disorder.

pseudohypoparathyroidism: a condition resembling hypoparathyroidism; normal parathyroid hormone levels are present, but the response to the hormone is abnormal.

renal osteodystrophy: descriptive of a specific bone resorptive pattern seen in children and adults who have chronic kidney disease.

rickets: refers to the specific appearance of stunted growth, prominent rib cartilage (rachitic rosary), skull deformity (hot cross bun skull), and bowlegs; these appear during childhood and are characteristic of a variety of disorders that lead to a failure of normal calcification of bone. In the United States the cause is rarely nutritional, but the disease is still seen because many children are born with kidney problems that produce a bone salt loss.

vitamin D–dependent rickets (VDDR): rickets due to an autosomal recessively inherited deficiency, the vitamin D enzyme 1 alpha hydroxylase, or due to a general tissue resistance to the vitamin D metabolite.

vitamin D–resistant rickets (VDRR): rickets marked by normal-appearing kidneys that excrete excessive phosphorus into the urine; resistant to usual vitamin D therapy but responds to very high doses of vitamin D.

Diseases associated with osteoporosis

Cushing disease: disease caused by increase in corticosteroids from the adrenal glands or medication; may result in a characteristic vertebral body appearance and generalized osteoporosis.

hyperthyroidism: increased thyroid hormone production and increased general metabolism; may result in osteoporosis.

hypothyroidism: decreased thyroid hormone; may result in less bone production and osteoporosis.

Other metabolic diseases

diabetes: disorder of insulin and sugar metabolism, resulting in high blood glucose levels. Does not necessarily cause bone disorders, but in later life causes vascular compromise to the legs, possibly leading to amputation.

Down syndrome: mongolism; the condition is produced by chromosomal abnormality. Also called trisomy 21.

Ehlers-Danlos syndrome: inherited abnormality of elastic tissue, resulting in hypermobile joints.

gout: a disease process where crystals are deposited into the joint lining or inflammatory cells within the joint. The most common form is urate (monosodium urate monohydrate). Other forms include pyrophosphate (calcium pyrophosphate dihydrate), apatite (various calcium crystals), cholesterol, and oxalate (calcium oxalate monohydrate and dihydrate).

hemophilia: inherited disorder of coagulation; sex-linked; repeated hemorrhages may result in bone and joint deformity.

Klinefelter syndrome: failure of full sexual development in males, with development of some female characteristics; results from the fertilized egg receiving both female X chromosomes and the male Y chromosome.

lipid storage disease: inherited disorder resulting in multiple problems; bony disorders are secondary to displacement of the marrow by abnormal cells, resulting in avascular necrosis of the hip or irregular patterns on x-ray film. Also called lipid reticuloendotheliosis.

Marfan syndrome: inherited collagen defect in elastic tissue resulting in ligamentous laxity, spiderlike fingers, with joint and vessel disorders.

Milroy's disease: swelling of distal parts caused by a congenital disorder in which there is a retention of lymph fluid. Also called familial lymphedema.

mucopolysaccharidosis: hereditary condition affecting growth and resulting in abnormal urinary output of mucopolysaccharrides. There are at least six specific types of this disorder (listed previously in this chapter).

sickle cell anemia: autosomal recessive inherited disease that affects the shape of red cells (oatshaped erythrocytes); the result that most concerns orthopaedists is *salmonella bone infection* in infancy and bone infarcts in adults, particularly of the hip.

Stickler syndrome: a genetically dominant disorder often associated with small lower jaw, nearsightedness, thin limbs, mild scoliosis, and early degenerative arthritis.

thalassemia: autosomal recessive inherited disease of red cell structure; may result in skeletal deformity.

Turner syndrome: failure of development of some female characteristics in girls; results from failure of the fertilized egg to receive both female X chromosomes.

DISEASE PROCESSES BY ANATOMIC AREAS
Back and neck diseases

The spine is a complex organ that is a series of joints with attending bone, nerve tissues, muscles, and ligaments. In addition, there are two elements not common to other joints, namely, intervertebral disks and the spinal cord and nerves in the bony spinal canal. The nerves may be affected by either bone or disk disease; therefore this section is divided into discussions of diseases affecting bone, nerves, spinal cord, vertebral disks, and congenital disorders.

Diseases of the spine may be treated by other medical specialties, particularly neurosurgery in the case of spinal cord and nerve lesions and injuries. However, the orthopaedist treats many diseases and conditions of the spine such as scoliosis, spina bifida, and degenerative disk disease. Treatment may last for years in the correction of some deformities.

General bony diseases of the spine

The Latin word *vertebra* and the combining form *spondylo-* both denote the bony spinal segments. In some word combinations the root word is assigned only to a specific part of the vertebra, such as spondylolysis in which the defect is always at the pars interarticularis. However, spondylo- in general means vertebra.

Spondylo- root diseases

spondylalgia: pain in vertebra(e).

spondylarthritis: arthritis of the spine.

spondylarthrocace: tuberculosis of the spine. Also called spondylocace.

spondylexarthrosis: dislocation of a vertebra.

spondylitis: inflammation of vertebrae, including types such as ankylosing, rheumatoid, traumatic, and spondylitis deformans, and Kümmell and Marie-Strümpell disease.

spondylizema: depression or downward displacement of a vertebra, with destruction or softening of one below it.

spondylodynia: pain in vertebra(e).

spondyloepiphyseal dysplasia: disorder of growth affecting both the spine and the ends of long bones.

spondylolisthesis: displacement of a vertebral body on the one below. A general term with multiple distinctions:

anterior displacement: the forward movement of the superior segment on the inferior one.

sacral inclination: relationship of the sagittal plane of the sacrum to the vertical plane.

sagittal rotation: angular relationship between the body of the fifth lumbar vertebra and the sacrum. (Sagittal roll, lumbosacral kyphosis, slip angle.)

rounding of the cranial border: the relationship of the height to the width of the rounded portion of the superior sacrum.

wedging of olisthetic vertebra: the measure obtained by dividing the height of the anterior border of the fifth vertebra by the height of its posterior border, multiplied by 100.

sacrohorizontal angle: angle between the top of the sacrum and the horizontal line.

lumbosacral joint angle: angle between the inferior surface of the fifth lumbar vertebra and the top of the sacrum.

lumbar lordosis: angle made by lines drawn from the superior surface of the first and fifth lumbar vertebra.

spondylolysis: (Fig. 2-1) disruption of the pars interarticularis (a portion of bone between each of the joints of the back), allowing one vertebral body to slide forward on the next. May be referred to as pars interarticularis defect.

spondylomalacia: softening of vertebrae. Also called Kümmell disease.

spondylopathy: any vertebral disorder.

spondylopyosis: infection in vertebra(e).

spondyloschisis: congenital fissure (splitting) of vertebral arch.

spondylosis: bony replacement of ligaments around the disk spaces of the spine, associated with decreased mobility and eventual fusion. Also called *marginal osteophyte formation.*

Rachio- root diseases

Rachio-, as relating to spine, is less frequently used than more specific combining forms.

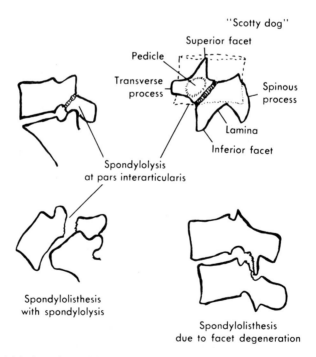

Fig. 2-1. Spondylolysis and spondylolisthesis seen in lateral view and oblique (Scotty dog) view.

rachialgia: pain in the vertebral column.

rachiocampsis: curvature of the spine.

rachiochysis: effusion of fluid within the vertebral canal.

rachiodynia: pain in the spinal column.

rachiokyphosis: humpbacked curvature of spine; kyphosis.

rachiomyelitis: inflammation of the spinal cord.

rachioparalysis: paralysis of the spinal muscles.

rachiopathy: any disease of the spine.

rachioplegia: spinal paralysis.

rachioscoliosis: lateral curvature of the spine.

rachisagra: pain or gout in the spine.

rachischisis: congenital fissure of the spinal cord.

Miscellaneous spinal bone disorders

alar dysgenesis: abnormality in development of the sacroiliac joint.

ankylosing spinal hyperostosis: an arthritic disorder in which bridging osteophytyes located anteriorly and posteriorly on the vertebral body bind two or more vertebrae together. Also called Forestier disease.

anterior spurring: ligament turning to bone on anterior side of vertebral body.

camptocormia: severe forward flexion of upper torso, usually an excessive psychologic reaction to back pain.

cervical rib: riblike structure in the seventh cervical vertebra that may cause nerve root irritation.

coccyalgia: pain in the coccyx region. Also called coccygodynia, coccyodynia, coccydynia.

cordoma: a malignancy usually occurring at the base of the skull or sacrum.

dysraphism: any failure of closure of the primary neural tube. This general category would include the disorder myelomeningocele.

facet tropism: asymmetrical orientation of the facets comparing right to left side.

flattening of normal lumbar curve: condition in which the hollow of the back becomes shallow or even straight.

functional scoliosis: any scoliosis that is caused by leg length or other functional disorder and not caused by a primary curvature of the spine.

interspinous pseudarthrosis: the formation of a false joint between two spinous processes.

kyphosis: round shoulder deformity; humpback; dorsal kyphotic curvature; may refer to any forward-bending area or deformity in the spine.

limbus annulare: a mass of bone situated at the anterosuperior margin of a vertebra. Arises from failure of fusion of the primary and secondary ossification centers.

lumbago: an archaic term meaning back pain.

lumbar kyphosis: reverse of the normal curve of the low back.

lumbarization: a partial or complete formation of a free-moving first sacral segment so that it looks like a lumbar vertebra.

marginal osteophytes: excess bone formation at the margin of the vertebral body. Also called spondylosis.

olisthy (Gr. *olisthanein*, to slip): a slipping of bone(s) from normal anatomic site, for example, a slipped disk.

paravertebral muscle spasm: spasm in the muscles on either side of the spinous processes (midline of the back); the term may be used to describe a physical finding or improperly used to define a disease process.

pseudoclaudication: increased pain and decreased strength in lower limbs associated with physical activity. Complaints are similar to those caused by an insufficient blood supply to the limb but are caused by diminished blood supply to the nerves in a narrowed spinal canal.

recurvatum: abnormal backward bending of a joint.

retrolisthesis: posterior displacement of the vertebra on the one below.

reversal of cervical lordosis: change in the normal curvature of the cervical spine as seen on lateral x-ray examination. This is usually a straightening of the normal lordotic curve or an actual reversal and is most commonly caused by muscle spasm, indicating cervical disk pathology.

rudimentary ribs: nubbins of ribs seen below the level where the last rib normally occurs.

sacralgia: pain in the sacrum.

sacralization: fusion of L-5 to the first segment of

the sacrum, so that the sacrum consists of six segments. Also called Bertolotti syndrome.

sacralized transverse process: one or both of the lumbar spinous transverse processes abnormally joining with the sacrum. Also called sacralization.

sacroiliitis: inflammation of the sacroiliac joint.

sciatica: pain radiating down the sciatic nerve into the posterior thigh and leg; can be caused by irritation of a nerve anywhere from the back to the thigh.

scoliorachitis: disease of the spine caused by rickets; abnormal bone mineralization.

scoliosis: a general term that applies to any side-to-side curve in the back, that is, a lateral and rotational deviation of the spine from the midline. Such a curve may be termed *fixed*, which means that any attempt to eliminate the curve by motion is not successful. Curves may be C-shaped or S-shaped (Fig. 2-2). A *compensated curve* has a flexible segment above or below the fixed curve; this compensation will place the spine (above or below) into a vertical position with the head at the midline. The rotation of the spinous process is away from the apex of the curve. *Levorotatory scoliosis* means that this rotation of the most dorsal element of the spine is to the left if one is looking at the patient from behind. *Dextrorotoscoliosis* is the opposite condition. The apex of a curve is called the *convex side*, for example, a right lumbar scoliosis is a lateral deviation of the spine in the lumbar region, with the apex of that curve to the right; the *concave side* of the curve is the opposite side.

Scoliosis may be associated with vertebral anomalies (missing parts of the vertebrae) and with forward bending (round back); the latter is called *kyphoscoliosis*. Scoliosis may occur at birth (*congenital*), occur from known causes or diseases (*acquired*), or occur from unknown causes (*idiopathic*). An example will best illustrate the terminology. In a right thoracic, left lumbar, *uncompensated rotatory scoliosis*,

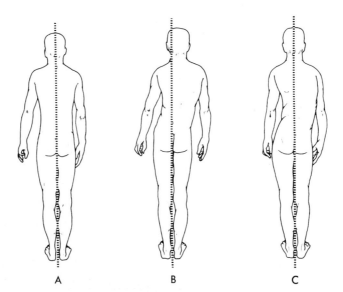

Fig. 2-2. Scoliosis. **A,** Normal. **B,** Right convex curve, uncentered. **C,** Right convex curve, centered. (From the American Orthopaedic Association: Manual of orthopaedic surgery, ed. 5, Chicago, 1979, The Association.)

viewed from behind, the upper back curves to the right and the lower back to the left; there is rotation of the spine, which may or may not be in both curves (unless so stated), and the center of the head is not in the midline when the patient is standing.

spina bifida: congenital absence of a large portion of the posterior spine, usually in the lumbosacral region. The severest form is myelomeningocele; see under Congenital diseases of the spine.

spina bifida occulta (SBO): congenital defect consisting of the absence of a vertebral arch of the spinal column; normally, there are no symptoms.

spinal stenosis: general term denoting narrowing of the spinal canal in the lumbar area leading to nerve root compromise; term often used for developmental abnormality that leaves a narrow, bony canal.

temporomandibular joint syndrome: complex of symptoms often seen in cervical sprain conditions. Symptoms include clicking in the jaw on opening and closing the mouth, soreness in the jaw, headaches, buzzing sounds, changes in hearing, stiffness in the neck and shoulders, dizziness, and swallowing disorders. It is believed that much of the reason for this symptom complex relates the change of the mandibular posture and the resultant change in cervical posture, or vice versa. Also called TMJ, craniomandibular cervical syndrome.

thoracic outlet syndrome: insufficiency of the outlet at the top of the rib cage, resulting in decrease in neurologic or vascular function to the arm on the affected side(s).

traction spur: a bony excrescence appearing on the anterolateral surface of the vertebral body near but not at the bony margin; arises as a result of disk degeneration.

transitional vertebra: a vertebra whose structure features some of the characteristics of the two adjacent vertebra. A common example is the fifth lumbar vertebra that has partial sacral components.

wedging: deformity of vertebral body, caused by trauma or gradual collapse, resulting in wedge-shaped vertebra; can also occur congenitally.

Eponymic spinal disorders

Marie-Strümpell disease: inflammation of the spine, occurring as a rheumatoid-type disease in children.

Pott disease: tuberculosis of the spine, usually in the lower thoracic segments.

Scheuermann disease: inflammation of the anterior cartilage of the bodies of the lower thoracic and upper lumbar segments, causing pain in some older growing children.

Schmorl nodes: developmental change resulting in inferior or superior extension of the intervertebral disk into the vertebral bodies.

Nerve root diseases of the spine

The nerve roots in the spinal canal lie in close contact with the vertebrae and emerge through openings called foramina. In the neck, nerve root irritation may be localized at the place where it exits through the foramen, whereas in the lumbar spine nerve root irritation usually occurs one level above that point.

Vertebrae and nerve roots of the spine are the same in number, except for the cervical spine—there are seven cervical vertebrae and eight cervical nerve roots (Fig. 2-3). This occurs because the first cervical nerve exits between the skull and the first cervical vertebra. Therefore between C7 and T1 the eighth cervical nerve makes its exit. After this level, all nerves exit in conformance with the vertebra above the point of exit. When the examiner speaks of the *nerve roots* of the spine, it is recorded singularly as C1 or C2, whereas if the examiner is speaking of the *intervertebral disk* between the vertebrae, it is recorded in combination as C1-2 or C2-3. The vertebrae are recorded individually as C1 or L4.

This section is concerned with the local spinal processes and the wide range of neurologic diseases seen by an orthopaedist and especially by a neurosurgeon.

cauda equina syndrome: sufficient pressure on the

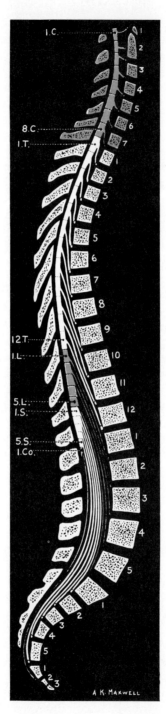

Fig. 2-3. Diagram showing the relation of the segments of the spinal cord and nerves to the segments of the vertebral column. (From Hamilton, WJ, editor: Textbook of human anatomy, ed. 2, London, England, 1976, The Macmillan Press, Ltd.)

nerves in the low back to produce multiple nerve root irritation and commonly loss of bowel and bladder control.

compression of nerve root: a mechanical process resulting from a tumor, fracture, or herniated disk; the resultant irritation is called *radiculitis* if there is actual inflammation around the nerve. Pain from this type of disorder is called *radicular pain*. A common lay term for pressure on the nerve is *pinched nerve*, as sometimes used by examiners. Following surgery and a normal healing process the patient may still have some irritation of the nerve, which is often referred to as *residual nerve root irritability. Sciatica* and *neuritis* may be used in describing these disorders, but the terms are not discrete in that the irritation of the nerve is not necessarily from within the spinal canal.

dermatomal: refers to the distribution of the loss of sensation or the presence of increased pain, tingling, or other sensory perceptions in the distribution of a specific nerve root. *Sclerotomal pain* is more diffuse and ill-defined pain arising from muscles in spasm. *Referred pain* is sclerotomal; the point of discomfort is caused by a disorder remote from that point; for example, patients who have bursitis in the shoulder commonly have elbow pain.

neurofibroma: fibrous tumor of a nerve, which may affect a nerve root and thus give the appearance of a herniated disk disease.

radiculopathy: any disease of the nerve root.

sacral cyst: abnormality in the spinal fluid sac in the sacrum.

Disk diseases

A disk is described as having a soft or fluidlike center (nucleus pulposus) and is surrounded by radial, circular, and longitudinal fibers that are firm, like gristle in meat. These intervertebral disks (IV disks) are situated between the vertebrae and act as shock absorbers. Any portion of the disk may herniate or extrude into the spinal canal, causing irritation and pressure on a nerve (Fig. 2-4).

cartilage space narrowing: narrowing of any cartilage space; also called disk space narrowing.

degenerative disk disease: gradual or rapid deterioration of the chemical composition and physical properties of the disk space. This may involve a simple increase in the rigidity of the nuclear material to be more involved with cellular removal of abnormal tissue and an inflammatory response. If the ligaments around the disk space ossify, they are often referred to as bony "spurs." Because the disk changes in its physical properties, some clinicians will describe the condition as a disorganized disk; that is, the normal property of a soft center surrounded by more rigid, fibrous tissue is disrupted. The inflammation and muscle spasm that may result over a prolonged period is often referred to as a chronic cervical sprain, reflecting the abnormal stresses on the ligaments.

diskitis: inflammation or infection of the disk space.

disk space infection: infection in the space normally occupied by an intervertebral disk.

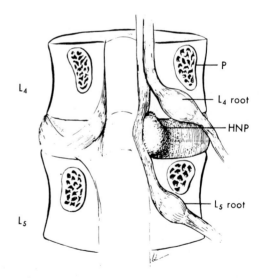

Fig. 2-4. Diagram of herniated nucleus pulposus *(HNP)* as seen from back with spinous processes and laminae removed from pedicles *(P).* Note that disk protrusion between fourth and fifth lumbar vertebrae impinges on fifth lumbar nerve root. (From Brashear RH and Raney BR: Shand's handbook of orthorpaedic surgery, ed 9, St Louis, 1978, The CV Mosby Co.)

herniated intervertebral disk (HID): outpouching of a disk. Also called HNP.

herniated nucleus pulposus (HNP): fibrous extrusion of semifluid nucleus pulposus through a ruptured intervertebral disk; damage results from pressure on the spinal cord or nerve roots, causing pain and disability. Also called HID, ruptured disk, slipped disk. There are four recognized degrees of disk diplacement:

intraspongy nuclear herniation: a bulge of the disk within the annulus fibrosus.

protrusion: the displaced nuclear material causes a discrete bulge in the annulus, but no material escapes through the annular fibers.

extrusion: the displaced material reaches the spinal canal through disrupted fibers of the annulus, but remains connected to the central disk material.

sequestration: the displaced material escapes as free fragment(s) which may migrate elsewhere.

intervertebral disk narrowing: narrowing of the space between any two vertebral bodies.

sciatica: sciatic nerve irritation with pain along course of posterior limb; may be caused by disk disease with a (usually) intervertebral disk pressing on the nerve.

Naffziger syndrome: intervertebral disk disease, cervical rib, or some other disorder causes the scalene muscles to go into spasm, resulting in pressure on the major nerve plexus of the arm, causing pain in the neck, shoulder, arm, and hand. Also called scalenus anticus syndrome.

Diseases of the spinal cord

Because *myelo-* is the Greek root for marrow, and because it was originally thought that the spinal cord was a part of the bone marrow, many words seem to denote bony diseases but actually refer to an affliction of the spinal cord. For that reason the term *myelitis* is not used alone in this discussion; for example, it may be used to denote a disease of the bone marrow (osteomyelitis) or a disease of the spinal cord (poliomyelitis). This section contains a mixture of terms, some of which may not necessarily relate to the spine. Disorders that are most commonly congenital problems are discussed in a following section.

Myelo- root diseases, acquired

myelalgia: pain in the spinal cord.

myelanalosis: wasting of spinal marrow. Also called tabes dorsalis.

myelapoplexy: hemorrhage within the spinal cord.

myelasthenia: loss of nerve strength caused by some disorder of the spinal cord.

myelatrophy: atrophy (wasting away) of spinal cord because of lack of nutrition, causing it to diminish in size.

myelauxe: abnormal increase in size of spinal cord.

myelencephalitis: inflammation of the brain and spinal cord.

myeleterosis: abnormal alteration of the spinal cord.

myeloencephalitis: inflammation of spinal cord and brain.

myelomalacia: softening of the spinal cord.

myelomeningitis: inflammation of spinal cord and meninges (spinal membranes).

myeloneuritis: inflammation of spinal cord and peripheral nerves.

myeloparalysis: spinal paralysis.

myelopathy: functional disturbance and pathologic changes in the spinal cord.

myelophthisis: wasting of the spinal cord; reduction of cell-forming function of bone marrow.

myeloplegia: spinal paralysis.

myeloradiculitis: inflammation of spinal cord and nerve roots.

myeloradiculopathy: disease of spinal cord and spinal nerve roots.

myelorrhagia: spinal hemorrhage.

myelosclerosis: hardening of the spinal cord.

myelosyphilis: syphilis of the spinal cord.

Other spinal disease or conditions

central cord syndrome: most common of the incomplete traumatic spinal cord syndromes characterized by motor impairment that is proportionately greater in the upper limbs than in the lower, with bladder dysfunction and a variable degree of sensory loss below the level of the cord lesion.

ependymoma: tumor of the spinal cord.

hematomyelia: effusion of blood (hemorrhage) into the substance of the spinal cord.

hematorachis: spinal apoplexy; hemorrhage into vertebral canal.

leptomeningitis: inflammation of the pia mater and arachnoid of the brain and spinal cord.

leptomeningopathy: disease of the arachnoid or pia mater of the brain and spinal cord.

meningioma: tumor arising from meninges, usually benign, does not recur if totally removed.

meningismus: apparent irritation of brain or spinal cord in which symptoms simulate meningitis but in which no actual inflammation of the membranes is present. Also called meningism.

meningitis: inflammation of the meninges of the brain or spinal cord, caused by infectious agents such as bacteria, fungi, or viruses.

meningocele: local cystic protrusion of meninges through a cranial fissure; may be congenital or acquired.

meningoencephalomyelitis: inflammation of brain and spinal cord and their membranes.

meningomyelitis: inflammation of spinal cord, its enveloping arachnoid and pia mater, and sometimes the dura mater.

pyriformis syndrome: a clinical diagnosis based on complaints of pain and abnormal sensations in the buttocks region with extension into the hips and posterior thigh as would be seen in sciatica. This is due to tightness of the pyriformis muscle with pressure on the sciatic nerve.

syringomyelia: cavities filled with fluid in spinal cord, usually involving upper segments initially and involving the shoulder muscles.

Congenital disease of the spine
Myelo- root diseases

myelatelia: imperfect development of the spinal cord.

myelocele: herniation and protrusion of substance of spinal cord through defect in the bony spinal canal.

myelocystocele: cystic protrusion of substance of the spinal cord through a defect in the bony spinal canal.

myelocystomeningocele: cystic protrusion of substance of the spinal cord, with meninges, through a defect in the spinal canal.

myelodiastasis: separation of the spinal cord.

myelodysplasia: defective development of any part of spinal cord.

myelomeningocele: herniation of cord and meninges through a defect in the vertebral column.

Other cogential back disease

diastematomyelia: congenital defect associated with spina bifida in which the spinal cord is split in half by bony spicules or fibrous bands, each half being surrounded by a dural sac.

Congenital anomalies of the vertebrae

failure of segmentation: failure of a portion or all of two or more adjoining vertebrae to separate into normal units.

hemivertebra: missing lateral portion of vertebral body, resulting in a wedge shape. If two hemivertebrae are near each other, they may be *balanced*, that is, the two wedges point in opposite directions, and a lesser curve or no curve results. *Unbalanced* means that there is no opposing wedge for one or more hemivertebrae, and the net result is an abnormal curve.

symmetric fusion: an equal fusion throughout the vertebral body.

unsegmented bar: a fusion on one side or the other of the vertebrae, which may involve the posterior elements or vertebral bodies; may occur at multiple levels and skip vertebral segments and may result in severe curves.

Eponymic congenital back disease

Arnold-Chiari syndrome: congenital combination of brain herniation and exposed spinal cord in the lower back.

Hip (coxa) diseases

The Latin term *coxa* refers to the part of the skeleton lateral to and including the hip joint. (Do not confuse coxa [hip] with coccyx [tailbone].) The most common adult problems of the hip are osteoarthritis, other arthropathies, and avascular necrosis. These are defined in the sections dealing with bone, cartilage, and joint disease.

congenital dislocated hip: hip dislocated at birth; the condition varies in severity.

congenital dysplasia of the hip: a failure of normal bony modeling of the hip socket (acetabulum) and/or ball (femoral head).

coxa breva: short hip with a small femoral head caused by premature closure of the epiphysis.

coxa magna: enlarged femoral head.

coxa plana: flat femoral head (osteochondrosis) of the capitular epiphysis of the femur. Also called Legg-Perthes disease.

coxa saltans (snapping hip): snapping of the hip due to tightness of the iliotibial tract over the greater trochanter.

coxa senilis: degenerative hip disease concomitant with old age; malum coxae senilis.

coxa valga: hip deformity in which the angle of axis of the head and neck of the femur and the axis of its shaft (neck shaft angle) is increased.

coxa vara: reduced neck shaft angle, usually caused by failure of normal bone growth; coxa adducta.

coxa vara luxans: fissure of neck of femur, with dislocation of the head developing from coxa vara.

coxalgia: hip pain, coxadynia.

coxarthrocace: fungus disease of the hip joint.

coxarthropathy: any hip joint disease.

coxarthrosis: degenerative joint disease or osteoarthritis of the hip joint.

coxitis: inflammation of the hip joint. Also called *coxarthria, coxarthritis.*

coxotuberculosis: tuberculosis of the hip joint.

Namaqualand hip dysplasia: autosomal dominant condition seen in African children from 3 to 20 years of age. There is a failure of growth in the femoral epiphysis, resulting in pain associated with an early degenerative arthritis of the hip.

observation hip: a group of symptoms referred to the hip that includes a limp, pain, and limited motion of the hip joint with normal x-rays. The condition is a diagnostic dilemma in that it may be due to toxic synovitis, infection, or an early avascular necrosis.

proximal focal femoral deficiency (PFFD): failure of normal formation of the thigh side of the hip; varies in severity.

Knee (genu) diseases

Genu is a Latin term for knee (pl. *genua*). It is also a general term denoting any anatomic structure that is bent like a knee. Specifically, it is the site of articulation between the femur and tibia. Knee-related problems are divided into three section:
1. The old genu descriptive terms
2. Joint injury
3. Other terms specifically related to the knee but not to a specific injury.

Genu terms

genu recurvatum (back-knee): ability of the knee to bend backward; caused by trauma or general joint laxity.

genu valgum: deformity in which knees are close together, with ankle space increased. Also called knock-knee.

genu varum: deformity in which knees are bowed out and ankles are close in; may be associated with internal tibial torsion (ITT).

Interrelationship and outcome of joint injury

The knee is an unusual joint because it contains *ligaments* within the joint. There are also medial and lateral *menisci* (crescent-shaped cartilages) that can be damaged (Fig. 2-5). Finally, the normal motions of the knee are very complex, including two planes of rotation; therefore it is very common to see multiple injuries.

A sprained knee is often a benign injury involving only mild damage to the ligament. However, a tear of the meniscus can occur in association with a sprain. *Meniscus tears* are described by their appearance, such as "parrot-beak" and "bucket-handle." The location of tears may be used to define a specific meniscus injury, for example, *posterior horn* or *anterior horn*. Meniscus injury commonly

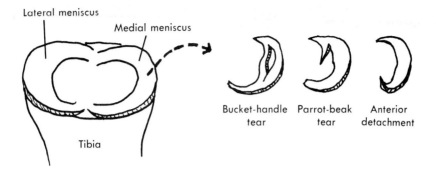

Fig. 2-5. Location of menisci and three typical derangements.

occurs as a result of a rotational injury. *Rotational instability* (rotatory or angular) is produced by rupture of specific anatomic structures. The normal up-and-down gliding mechanism of a patella may be disrupted, and the patella has a tendency to move out of its groove laterally *(subluxing patella)*. A subluxing patella need not be caused by injury but does commonly occur with rotational injury. All these disorders can result in a chronic reaction in the knee, similar to the eyes' response to a foreign body. The lining of the knee becomes inflamed and may allow fluid *(effusion)* to collect. If the effusion is persistent, a *pouch*, called a *Baker cyst*, may form behind the knee.

Another outcome of knee injury is the formation of loose fragments *(loose bodies)* of meniscal cartilage or other tissue, causing inflammation *(synovitis* or *meniscitis)*. The cartilage of the kneecap may become frayed *(chondromalacia patellae)*. However, not all cases of chondromalacia result from injury. If the inflammation persists long enough, the patient will eventually develop *degenerative arthritis*. Often the examiner is not sure of the exact problem of the knee but suspects that something is functionally incorrect. The general term then used is *internal derangement of the knee* (IDK).

A surgically excised meniscus sometimes grows back in part *(regenerated medial meniscus)*, or a portion may be left behind *(retained posterior horn)*.

Other terms related to the knee

Baker cyst: sac of usually clear fluid behind the knee, may occur spontaneously in childhood or later on in life resulting from injury.

bipartite patella: a patella that has bony maturation occurring from two centers rather than one center; usually congenital, causing no symptoms, but may be mistaken for a fracture.

congenital dislocation: a progressive anterior dislocation of the tibia caused by abnormal tissue remodeling; seen in infancy.

flexion contracture: formation of fibrous bands that prevent complete extension of the knee.

hamstrung knee: tight hamstrings during growth resulting in a slight knee flexion gait with subsequent synovitis and chondromalacia.

high-riding patella: see Patella alta.

housemaid's knee: prepatellar bursitis: inflammation of the bursa in front of the patella.

jumper's knee: tenderness in the area of the inferior pole of the patella; usually seen in volleyball and basketball players.

Osgood-Schlatter disease: a painful portion of bone just below the anterior knee, caused by inflammation of the anterior tibial apophysis; occurs during childhood.

patella alta: a high-riding patella, usually associated with knee complaints.

patella baja: a low-riding patella with a relatively shortened patellar tendon, usually associated with knee pain.

popliteal cyst: any cyst behind the knee. In adults this is usually an outpouching of the posterior knee joint area and is a sign of chronic inflammation in the knee. In the child and young adults, this may be a ganglion cyst arising from one of the tendons around the knee.

popliteal pterygium syndrome: severe flexion of the knee and equinus deformity of the foot associated with popliteal web extending from the ischium to the heel. Other concurrent deformities include toenail dysplasia, and cral cavity abnormalities such as cleft palate or lip pits.

thigh atrophy: loss of muscle tone of the quadriceps, causing dynamic instability.

Congenital limb absences

In the past, various nonuniform ways of describing congenital limb absences were used. Now there is a standard classification accepted by the orthopaedic community.* A congenital deficiency may be at the end of a limb (terminal) or somewhere in the middle (intercalary). In addition, it may be transverse or longitudinal; the transverse deficiency is a complete across-the-limb loss, and a longitudinal deficiency leaves a longitudinal portion of the limb intact.

Terminal transverse

acheira: absence of the hand (carpals, metacarpals, phalanges).

adactylia: absence of all five rays (metacarpals and phalanges).

amelia: complete absence of a limb.

apodia: absence of the foot.

complete aphalangia: absence of one or more phalanges from all five digits.

hemimelia: absence of the forearm and hand or leg and foot portion of a limb.

partial hemimelia absence of part of the forearm or leg.

---

*Frantz, C.H., and O'Rahilly, R.: Congenital limb deficiencies, J. Bone Joint Surg. **43**(8):1202-1224, 1961.

Terminal longitudinal

complete paraxial hemimelia: lengthwise loss of one side or the other of the forearm and hand or leg and foot.

incomplete paraxial hemimelia: similar to hemimelia, but a portion of affected bone remains, for example, complete absence of the ulna with a portion of the diameter of the radius intact.

partial adactylia: absence of one to four rays (phalanges and metacarpals).

partial aphalangia: absence of one or more of the three phalanges from one to four digits.

Intercalary transverse

complete phocomelia: presence of only a hand or foot.

distal phocomelia: hand directly attached to upper arm; or foot directly attached to thigh.

proximal phocomelia; presence of hand and forearm or leg and foot.

Intercalary longitudinal

complete paraxial hemimelia: absence of radius or ulna with intact hand or absence of tibia or fibula with intact foot.

incomplete paraxial hemimelia: similar to complete hemimelia, except a portion of affected bone remains intact.

partial adactylia: absence of all or part of the first through fifth rays.

partial aphalangia: absence of the proximal or middle phalanx from one or more digits, one through five. A common deformity is a complete loss of the radius with the rest of the arm and hand being intact—intercalary complete paraxial hemimelia. Proximal focal femoral deficiency (PFFD) is an absence of a portion of the hip and/or proximal femur.

Symbols

The following symbols are used for congenital limb absences:

-: transverse

/: longitudinal

I: intercalary

T: terminal

1, 2, 3, 4, 5: denotes ray involved

_: when line is used above a letter, indicates the lower extremity

‾: when line is used below a letter, indicates the upper extremity

TI: tibia, complete

ti: tibia, incomplete

FI: fibula, complete

fi: fibula, incomplete

R: radius, complete

r: radius, incomplete

U: ulna, complete

u: ulna, incomplete

Associated disease processes and related words

Descriptions of diseases of the musculoskeletal system are often accompanied by terms denoting symptoms or some qualitative nature of disease; these terms are frequently used in defining diseases.

Symptoms in themselves are often interpreted as the disease state. For example, arthritis means inflammation of the joints, but it can be argued that arthritis is not a specific disease. There are many associated terms used in describing diseases, but the list given here is concerned with those often related to orthopaedic terms.

abrasion: any superficial scraping of skin tissue or mucous membrane, mechanically or through injury.

abscess: a localized collection of pus in a cavity, which may form in any tissue.

acute: disease of recent onset or recurrence.

adenopathy: glandular swelling of the lymph nodes with morbid pathologic condition.

adhesions: tissue structures normally separated that adhere together because of inflammation or injury.

afebrile: without fever.

-agra (suffix): violent pain or seizure of acute pain.

-algia (suffix): painful.

allergy: hypersensitive state manifested by specific tissue changes after repeated exposure to particular allergens; an antibody-antigen reaction.

amniotic band syndrome: congenital presence of constricting bands that may affect trunk, limbs, and cranium; partial amputations may result.

analgesia: loss of sensitivity to pain.

analgia: absence of pain.

anastomosis: connection of two distinct parts of cavities forming a passageway; traumatic or surgical. An example is the reattachment of a ruptured blood vessel after the injured portion has been removed.

anesthesia: loss of feeling or sensation of pain with or without loss of consciousness.

anomaly: malformation; a deviation from normal, usually referring to a congenital or hereditary defect.

anteflexion: abnormal forward curvature.

anteversion: forward rotation, as commonly seen in the femoral neck.

aphasia: an either partial or complete transient or permanent inability to understand or speak the spoken word as a result of a central neurologic occurrence such as stroke or injury.

apraxia: impairment of goal-directed movements despite the absence of paralysis, for example, the inability to speak but ability to put thoughts on paper.

aseptic: free of bacterial or fungal contamination.

asphyxia: lack of oxygen.

aspiration: removal of fluids from some cavity, such as a bloody effusion in the knee; also, the accidental breathing of fluids or solids into the lungs.

astasia: motor incoordination with inability to stand or sit.

asthenia: lack of strength and energy.

asymmetry: dissimilarity between two corresponding parts of the body.

asymptomatic: absence of symptoms.

asynergia: disturbance of coordination.

ataxia: lack of coordination and muscle movement.

athetosis: involuntary writhing motions of the body (usually upper extremities).

atonia: lack of muscle tone (atonic, adj.).

atrophy: wasting away, as may be seen with lack of nutrition, nerve supply, or normal use of all or part of the body.

atypical: irregular; appearing abnormal.

avascular: absence of adequate blood supply.

avulsion: tearing away of a part or structure from its attachment.

benign: not causing destruction of life or limb; when used in reference to tumors, denotes the absence of metastasis.

bifurcation: the site at which any given structure divides in two.

bipartite: having two parts where only one is expected, for example, a bipartite patella.

bossing: a rounded prominence of bone that is abnormally visible under the skin.

bruit (pronounced bru-ee): abnormal sound heard on auscultation of a blood vessel or the heart.

cachexia: general ill health and malnutrition.

café-au-lait: brown-colored spots on surface of skin, often symptomatic of a systemic disease.

calcification: the deposition of calcium salts either in normal osteoid or abnormally in soft tissue.

callosity: hardening of the epidermis because of persistent pressure.

callus: formation of new bone around a fracture site.

caries: decay and death of bone from bacterial action.

causalgia: burning pain in the distribution of the peripheral nerve caused by some local injury.

cellulitis: swelling and inflammation of soft tissues; may be caused by bacteria or chemical irritation.

chronic: persisting over a long period of time.

cicatrix: scar, may be formed by healing of any wound or tissue injury.

claudication: muscle cramps associated with activity in lower limbs; usually caused by an insufficiency of blood supply to the involved limb or inadequate venous drainage.

clonus: uncontrolled spasmodic muscle jerking (as seen in epilepsy), with alternation of contractions and relaxation.

-coele (suffix): indicates a sac or cavity; -cele.

comatose: a semiconscious state; in a coma.

congenital: present at birth.

contracture: permanent shortening of muscle tissue due to paralysis, spasm, or fibrosis of tissue around a joint.

contrecoup: a blow to one side of the body that causes damage on the other, as often seen in head injuries.

contusion: bruise of any tissue but without disruption.

convalescence: any given period of recovery.

conversion disorder: a response to psychological conflict or need manifested by unintentionally produced signs of a physical disorder where there is no known identifiable cause.

convulsion: violent involuntary contractions of voluntary muscles; paroxysm, seizure.

crepitus: any crackling or creaking sound or sensation found on the examination of movements of joints, muscles, or tendons.

cyanosis: bluish discoloration of skin resulting from abnormally low levels of oxygen in blood; the actual cause is an excessive concentration of reduced hemoglobin (cyanotic, adj.)

cyst: any sac, normal or abnormal, containing liquid or semisolid material.

debridement: removal of foreign material or devitalized tissue from a wound.

decalcification: loss of calcium salts from bone or soft tissue.

decubitus ulcer: an area of breakdown of skin and/or subcutaneous tissue as a result of unrelieved pressure on a bony prominence or portion of the body resting on a firm surface for a long time. The lesions are staged as follows:

Stage I   only the dermis is involved
Stage II   dermis and subcutaneous fat is involved
Stage III   ulcer involves some deep fascia or muscle, bone not uncovered
Stage IV   bone is exposed

defervescence: a period of abatement of fever

degenerative: deterioration of quality of tissue; rarely refers to dead tissue; usually describes a state of abnormal remodeling or replacement of tissue, sometimes making it less functional.

dehiscence: splitting or separation of a part or all of a closed wound.

demarcation (demarcation line): zone between normal and abnormal tissue, most commonly used to denote area or line of normal appearing tissue next to gangrenous tissue in a devitalized limb. This term is also used in describing radiographic changes where the x-ray evidence of disease shows a clear line or zone of activity.

deossification: loss or removal of mineral matter from bone or osseous tissue.

derangement: displacement of position of any given anatomic part; commonly used in reference to joints.

diagnosis: describes a precise disorder or may be less precisely used in describing a symptom.

diffuse: widely distributed; used in association with symptoms or disease terms.

diverticulum: in orthopaedics, usually refers to outpouching of a joint or tendon sheath.

dowager's hump: round upper back deformity.

dynia (suffix): denotes pain.

dys- (prefix): denotes defective, difficult, or painful.

dysesthesia: pinprick sensations; painful touch perception.

dysfunction: impairment of function.

dysplasia: abnormal development or replacement of tissue.

dystrophy: failure of normal replacement of tissue; see Osteo-, chondro-, and muscular dystrophies.

eburnation (osteosclerosis): in degenerative joint disease, changes in subchondral bone render its substance dense, smooth, and ivorylike. The bone surface becomes exposed due to complete loss of cartilage surface.

ecchymosis: extravasation of blood under the skin, as seen in a bruise.

edema: excessive accumulations of fluid in soft tissues causing swelling; may be the result of heart failure, venous insufficiency, kidney failure, or malnutrition. (edematous, adj.).

effusion: collection of fluid in a cavity such as the joint space.

elastofibroma: a benign tumorlike growth usually seen in the back. It is a painless, slow-growing, firm, subcutaneous mass not attached to skin and microscopically appears as an nonencapsulated proliferation of collagen and elastin fibers with few fibroblasts. The most common location is subscapular.

emaciation: wasted condition of the body; malnutrition.

enucleation: removal, either surgically or traumatically, of a tissue, organ, or foreign body.

erosion: uneven wearing away of a surface, as seen on x-ray films of diseased bones.

erythema: redness of skin, as seen in sunburn; caused by an increased blood supply (capillary congestion).

eschar: scab.

esthesia: perception, feeling, sensation.

etiology: study of cause of a disease, based on what is presently known about that disease process.

exacerbation: aggravation of symptoms or increased severity of disease.

exudate: escape of fluid, cells, or debris from blood vessels into soft tissue, cavities, or wounds.

factitious injury: the unconscious production of symptoms or actual physical injury for purposes of secondary gain, that is, attention or preferential treatment.

Fanconi anemia: radial club-hand deformity associated with dwarfism, brownish pigmentation of the skin, anomalies of the thumb, and then at 5 to 10 years of age a diminished number of all blood cells develops. Also called congenital pancytopenia, idiopathic refractory anemia.

febrile: with fever.

fibrillation: involuntary contraction of small groups of muscle fibers as occurs with nerve root irritation.

fissures: groove or natural division in tissue; also, ulcerlike sore.

flaccid: lacking muscle tone, whether voluntary or involuntary muscle.

flail: absence of motor control, as seen in a flail

joint, may connote an abnormal mobility associated with loss of normal control such as flail chest, which is a chest crush injury.

foreign body: anything within a tissue that may lead to infection, inflammation, or scarring, requiring removal.

friable: tissue that is easily crumbled or separated.

fusiform: spindle shaped, tapered at ends.

gangrene: death of tissue caused by loss of blood supply (ischemia), bacterial infection or both.

granulation: reddish, moist, new tissue along edges of a healing wound.

hemorrhage: abnormal bleeding into soft tissues or a cavity; should this process form a discrete pocket of blood, it is called a hematoma; if the blood is evenly distributed in the tissue, it may appear as petechiae (very small), purpura (up to 1 cm size), or ecchymosis (larger than 1 cm).

Holt-Oram syndrome: atrial septal defect or other cardiac abnormality associated with a radial club-hand deformity.

hypalgesia: diminished sensitivity to pain; hypoesthesia.

hyperalgesia: increased sensitivity to pain; hyperesthesia.

hyperextension: excessive extension of joint.

hyperglycemia: abnormally high blood glucose level increasing risk of infection.

hypertension: high blood pressure.

hypertonia: excessive tension of muscles or arteries.

hypertrophy: increase in size of structure.

hypoglycemia: abnormally low blood glucose level.

hypoplasia: a defective or incomplete development of tissue or an organ.

hypotension: low blood pressure.

idiopathic: disease process with an unknown cause.

impingement: pressure transmitted from one tissue to the next, such as nerve impingement.

induration: firmness of soft tissue caused by extravasation of fluids and/or cells from blood vessels.

infarct: local area tissue death resulting from reduced or completely obliterated blood supply.

infection: an invasion into tissue of any microorganisms (for example, bacteria) with a reaction to the viable irritant. The terms *infection* and *inflammation* are not interchangeable. The distinction is important in that inflammation is a vascular response that may not specifically or necessarily be due to infection.

inflammation: localized increase in blood supply, resulting in small vessel dilatation and/or migration of white blood cells into the tissue; common examples are bloodshot eyes, bursitis, arthritis, and tennis elbow.

insidious: undetectable development of symptoms or disease, usually gradual in onset.

ischemia: insufficient blood supply to a tissue or organ.

laceration: a cut, any wound made by a sharp or blunt object.

lesion: circumscribed area of tissue altered by structural or functional disease; many types.

line of demarcation: a zone of inflammatory reaction separating a gangrenous area from healthy tissue.

lipping: development of excess bone at the margins of a joint, as seen in arthritis.

lytic: denoting dissolution of tissue; used to refer to radiographic appearance of bone that has been displaced by some pathologic process.

maceration: softening or loss of surface tissue caused by constant exposure to moisture.

malaise: subjective feeling of being ill.

malignant: disease resistant to treatment resulting in eventual destruction of tissue; in tumors, implies that the tumor spreads by seeding itself in distant regions of the body or by local uncontrolled invasion.

malingering: pretending to be ill on knowingly being observed.

metastasis: the spread of malignant cells to other organs or tissues—a malignant tumor is said to metastasize.

morbid: the disease state; however, the term may denote ready visibility, such as "morbid anatomy."

morbidity: conditions inducing disease with untoward results; could be congenital, acquired, iatrogenic.

mucopurulent: denotes an exudate containing mucus and pus.

mucosanguineous: denotes an exudate containing mucus and blood.

necrosis: death of tissue.

neoplasm: abnormal new growth of tissue, either benign or malignant.

nevus: mole or birthmark.

nidus: place or source of infection or reaction.

node: confined tissue swelling or mass that can be readily seen or palpated, for example, lymph node.

nodule: small node, usually hard.

obesity: abnormal accumulation of body fat.

occlusion: obstruction.

occult: hidden, not observable unless closely examined.

-odynia (suffix): pain.

onco-: combining form denoting relationship to swelling, mass, or tumor.

-orrhagia (suffix): hemorrhage.

-orrhea (suffix): discharge.

-orrhexis (suffix): rupture.

-osis (suffix): abnormal condition.

pectus caranatum: pigeon chest.

pectus excavatum: central depression of breast bone.

petechiae: tiny hemorrhages into the tissue; when seen in the skin, they appear as little violet-colored dots.

-phyma (suffix): swelling produced by exudate to subcutaneous tissue.

polyps: protruding growths from mucous membranes.

prognosis: prediction of the outcome of disease or surgery.

prophylaxis: prevention of disease

proprioception: sensibility to position, whether conscious or unconscious.

purulent: pus-forming.

pyogenic: having the ability to produce pus.

pyrexia: fever.

quiescence: the discontinuation of symptoms or a disease, the connotation being an expectation of the return of symptoms or disease.

rarefaction: decrease in density, usually used to refer to appearance of bone on radiograph.

recrudescence: relapse or recurrence of symptoms.

regressive remodeling: removal and replacement of bone such that the replacement occurs progressively away from the original maximal border of bone, for example codfish vertebrae.

rhizomelic: short proximal end of a limb, such as seen in achondroplastic dwarfism.

rigidus: stiffness.

rubor: redness of the skin.

rudimentary: the insufficient development of a part or the development of an extra part such that no function is served by its presence; a rudimentary limb is so deficient that it serves no function, and a thirteenth rib similarly serves no function and is rudimentary.

rupture: discontinuity of tissue, usually referring to muscles and tendons.

sanguinous: bloody, as in a wound. This is in contrast to serosanguinous fluid, which is serous fluid containing some red cells.

saponification: the calcification that occurs with the breakdown of fatty acids in the avascular area of aseptic necrosis.

sebaceous: secreting a greasy substance, as in oily skin or sebaceous cyst.

sepsis: denotes the presence of infection caused by bacteria.

septicemia: bacteria in the blood. It should be noted that blood poisoning often refers to the red streaks seen in a limb that has an infection; however, this condition is more accurately a lymphangitis.

sequelae: consequences of disease, denoting that one pathologic condition leads to another discrete pathologic condition; for example, muscle spasticity is a sequela of cerebral palsy.

seropurulent: denotes an exudate containing both pus and serous material.

serosanguineous: denotes an exudate containing both blood and serous material.

serous: denotes an exudate that is usually yellow,

fairly fluid, and possibly blood-tinged.

slough: spontaneous separation of devitalized tissue from living tissue.

somatization disorder: in some patients with chronic pain, there are recurrent somatic complaints without apparent significant physical disorder. Physical symptoms are related to anxiety, and the patient may seek medical attention over a period of years.

spasm: sudden or violent involuntary contractions of muscle.

spastic: characterized by spasm.

spurs: abnormal projection of bone at the margin or joints or strong ligamentous or tendinous attachments.

stenosis: stricture or narrowing of a canal or opening.

stigma: physical mark that aids in the identification of an abnormal process.

subliminal: below the threshold of sensation; weak; no muscle contractions.

supernumerary: an excess number of anatomic parts, for example, six fingers on one hand.

suppurative: producing pus.

syncope: fainting.

TAR syndrome: *t*hrombocytopenia *a*genesis *ra*dius; the coincidental findings of bilateral failure of formation of the radius associated with petechiae, black stools, and other signs of thrombocytopenia resulting from a failure of normal formation of platelets. This autosomal recessive disorder improves with proper support, leaving the skeletal deformity as the primary problem.

tonus: the involuntary continued contraction of a muscle after the patient has attempted voluntary relaxation.

toxic: poisonous.

trauma: any injury to tissue or psyche; can result from chemical, physical, or temporal events.

tumefaction: swelling, puffiness, edema.

tumor: a swelling, in the most generalized sense. However, the term connotes a neoplasm, that is, a new uncontrolled growth of tissue.

turgid: swollen or congested, describing a physcial finding on palpation.

ulcer: a penetrating disruption of mucous membrane of skin.

VATER association: the term is an acronym for a nonrandom group of occurrences that include *v*ertebral segmentation and fusion, *a*nal atresia, *t*racheoesophageal fistula, *e*sophageal atresia, and *r*adial ray defects. Other defects may occur.

vestigial: remnants of a structure that functioned in a previous stage of species or individual development.

wryneck: torticollis; stiff condition of the neck caused by spastic muscle contractions.

3

X-ray films and scanning techniques

Roentgenograms (x-ray films) are an indispensable diagnostic tool in the orthopaedic examination of a patient in detecting a fracture, dislocation, or pathologic changes; however, occult (hidden) fractures, early infection, and certain other conditions in which the bone has not reacted sufficiently may not be visible on film examination. The advent of diagnostic imaging is rapidly changing radiologic procedures. Film techniques that look at a structure being examined are now being aided by nuclear medicine techniques that not only identify the anatomic site but also obtain images of the physiology within and surrounding this site.

A roentgenogram is an image made by means of roentgen rays (an x-ray), with the roentgen being a unit of x-radiation. It is the proper name for taking films, but usually shortened to x-ray film or just film in general conversation. A radiograph is a record or photograph made by radioactivity and refers only to scans. A radiogram is a message sent only by radio waves. It is important to distinguish these differences as the word *x-ray* is not synonymous for roentgenogram, radiography for roentgenography, nor radiograph for roentgenogram. Only roentgenology and radiology are synonymous.

The radiologist (roentgenologist), a board-certified specialist in radiology, is often consulted by the orthopaedist and other physicians to give interpretations of the more complicated pathology on x-ray film. They are assisted by qualified technicians who have learned the fundamentals of positioning the patients, working with the x-ray equipment, and developing film.

Most orthopaedic offices have x-ray equipment

available so an x-ray film examination can be made on the first visit. Follow-up views determine changes in bone, such as those seen in fracture healing or those as in soft tissue lesions and osteoarthritis, indicating a progression or isolation of the disease process as a result of bony reaction.

This chapter deals with the specialized terminology of invasive and noninvasive radiologic techniques, and nuclear medicine studies used in the orthopaedic examination. It has been expanded on to include a section on x-ray film signs, a grading system for avascular necrosis of the femoral head, a more detailed definition of magnetic resonance imaging (NMR), and a section on radiotherapy. The descriptive terminology used in radiographic interpretations are as follows.

The *angulation* of the fracture is designated by the direction of the apex of the fracture points. *Fragments* themselves are designated as proximal and distal.

When broken ends of the principal fragments are touching, they are said to be in *apposition*. Accuracy or degree of apposition is defined in percentages, such as 50%, indicating at least one x-ray film view.

The *site* may be diaphyseal, metaphyseal, or epiphyseal portions of a specific bone, or may be intraarticular. *Extent* may be described as complete, incomplete, cracked, hairline, buckled, or greenstick. The *configuration* may be transverse, oblique, or spiral and is referred to as comminuted when more than two fragments are present. The *fracture fragments* may be undisplaced or displaced.

Thus a fracture is described by referring to its site by bone name, extent, configuration, relationship of fragments to each other, relationship to the external environment, and finally the presence or absence of complications.

There are many types of film techniques, but the following list pertains more specifically to those used in orthopaedics, including x-ray lines, angles, and methods.

ORTHOPAEDIC X-RAY TECHNIQUES

AP: anteroposterior view of a part (x-ray beam passes from front to back).

apical lordotic view: usually a chest x-ray view for the apices of the lungs, but taken if a patient's symptoms suggest an orthopaedic problem, such as of the clavicle.

apical view: apex, tip, or point of subject x-rayed.

arthrography: x-ray procedure showing interior outline of a joint after radiopaque medium and/or air has been injected intra-articularly; tendon, ligament, or meniscal tears can be detected in this manner; arthrogram.

baseline films: refers to x-ray films taken at time of first examination and compared with those taken later.

bone density: a procedure where the relative density of bone can be determined by several different radiologic techniques. Plain x-ray films can have a density gradient plate placed on the film at the same time the x-ray study of the part is being made. From this plate, a comparative density of the bone may be made. This is most commonly done with the spine. Photons from a single emitting source can be used to directly measure the density of bone, most commonly the distal radius and lumbar spine. These studies can then be compared to age-matched normal values. This procedure is called *photon densitometry.*

bone marrow pressure (BMP): measurement taken to detect bone necrosis. The pressure is taken while a venography and core decompression are performed to aid in diagnosis of ischemic necrosis of the femoral head (INFH), forming an early basis for treatment.

Breuerton view: special view of hand to search for early joint changes in rheumatoid arthritis.

Carter-Rowe view: x-ray view of the hip taken at a 45-degree oblique angle to determine size of bony fragment in a posterior acetabular hip fracture or other abnormality of the pelvis.

clenched fist view: to demonstrate scapholunate instability, an AP x-ray is taken with the fist clenched.

choppy sea sign: an apparent but not real tear of a meniscus seen on arthrogram.

coned-down view: close-up of a particular area, with radiation shielded from the rest of the patient's body.

contrast medium: opaque material given intravenously, intramuscularly, orally, or rectally to examine internal structures during x-ray procedure; many kinds are presently used in x-ray examinations to differentiate the organs or areas being examined.

diskography: visualization of the cervical and lumbar intervertebral disk after direct injection of a radiopaque dye into the disk; diskogram.

epidurography: x-ray examination following introduction of radiopaque contrast material into epidural space to demonstrate compromise.

femoral arteriography: x-ray examination of the femoral artery of the leg and its branches following injection of a radiopaque medium; determines the presence of defects in the arterial system or can be useful in outlining extent of a tumor. Also called arteriogram.

fluoroscopy: direct visual x-ray procedure by use of x-ray tube, fluoroscopic screen, and television monitor for intensification; used in myelograms and arthrograms so that the patient may be positioned properly for regular x-ray films.

Hobb view: for sternoclavicular joint, while standing the patient bends over end of x-ray table and cassette with hands on head, neck parallel to table, and chest about 45 degrees to table. The x-ray beam is vertical to the cassette.

Hughston view: x-ray view of the knee with knee flexed to 60 degrees and taken at a 55-degree angle to show a cartilage-osseous fracture of the femoral condyle or subluxing patella.

intraosseous venography: a test done on bone to denote increased bone marrow pressure (BMP) as related to necrosis of bone.

inversion ankle stress: an AP radiograph of the ankle, which is stressed in inversion to test the integrity of the lateral collateral ankle ligaments.

KUB (kidneys, ureters, bladder)**:** generally not an orthopaedic x-ray procedure but taken occasionally to study the abdominal wall and/or suspected masses.

lateral view: x-ray view taken side to side, left or right.

lumbosacral series: a group of x-ray views of the lumbar and sacral spines (AP, two oblique, lateral, and lateral spot of L-5 to S-1).

lymphangiography: x-ray examination following introduction of radiopaque material into peripheral lymphatic vessels to determine presence of blockage or tumor in proximal lymphatic vessels.

metrizamide myelography: an iodine-based water-soluble contrast medium for myelogram. The material does not have to be withdrawn after completion of the study, giving some advantages over the oil based material which is withdrawn.

mortise view: x-ray view of the ankle rotated internally until medial and lateral malleoli are parallel to film; demonstrates the talus, tibia, and fibula without superimposition; used for comparison with normal AP view and to detect joint abnormalities.

myelogram: x-ray examination taken with air or contrast medium injected into the spinal column under fluoroscopy to examine the spinal cord and canal for possible disk protrusions or lesions. Also called myelography.

Neer trans-scapular (Neer lateral): a posterior oblique scapular projection to help obtain a lateral view of the shoulder in trauma.

opaque: nontransparent.

PA: posterioanterior view (from back to front).

Pantopaque: trade name for an iodinated oil used in producing contrast x-ray films, as in myelography.

phlebogram: x-ray examination following introduction of radiopaque contrast material into a peripheral vein to detect presence of venous blockage such as thrombophlebitis; venogram.

plantar axial of foot: a view that offers visualization of the plantar aspect of the metatarsal heads.

pneumoarthrogram: injection of air into a joint before x-ray examination to determine internal outline, as in meniscal tear or other injuries and abnormalities.

push-pull ankle stress: a lateral view of the ankle which is stressed in an attempt to evaluate the anterior talofibular ligament.

radiolucent: permitting free passage of radiant energy (x-ray) through an area, with dark appearance on film.

radiopaque: preventing passage of radiant energy (x-ray), thus allowing the representative area to appear light or white on exposed film.

scanography: x-ray examination of the hips, knees, and ankles with a ruler on one film to determine leg lengths; used for leg length discrepancy. Also called scanogram.

scout film: a general term for an x-ray examination of an anatomic area that will subsequently undergo contrast study. Purpose is to check x-ray techniques and look for bony or soft tissue abnormalities.

serendipity view: for sternoclavicular dislocation, an AP view taken with patient supine, and tube angled upward 40 degrees from the vertical position.

sinogram: an x-ray examination for sinus tract infection in bone, taken after injection of water-soluble contrast after saline cleanser, to determine the course of a deep draining wound.

sunset view: x-ray view of patella with knee bent to permit a profile view; used for examination of patellar and adjacent femoral surfaces. Also called sunrise view, tangential view.

tangential view: sunset view.

tomography: used to show detailed images of structures lying in a predetermined plane of tissue, while blurring or eliminating details of images of structures in other planes as in polytomogram, planogram, or zonogram; tomogram.

translucent: allowing some light to pass through but not clearly transparent, for example, soft tissue appears as a light shadow on an x-ray film when compared with bone.

true lateral: perfectly positioned lateral projection without rotation.

tunnel view: x-ray view of tibia, fibula, and femur only with patella out of the way; a knee notch or intercondylar view; the x-ray examination is done with the tibia and fibula straight and the femur at a 45-degree angle.

von Rosen view: x-ray view of the hips in abduction and internal rotation for determining dislocation of the hip(s).

wet reading: as implied. Today, films are dried automatically and are read dry. In the past, if an immediate interpretation of the film was required, it was read while still wet. Thus a request for an immediate interpretation is still called *wet reading*.

windshield wiper sign: x-ray view outlining the shadow of a prosthesis with the appearance of a windshield wiper; with a loose internal prosthesis, there is bone absorption and formation secondary to a to-and-fro motion of the stem of the prosthesis in the shaft of the bone.

ROUTINE X-RAY VIEWS

Following is a list of routine x-ray views required for an area of chief complaint. The number of views varies and is often determined by the history and physical examination. For instance, an AP view may be unremarkable, but on lateral view may reveal a fracture or dislocation, depending on the angle of view taken. A complaint of hip pain could well be originating in the knee, exacerbating symptoms in the hip, and so forth. Asymmetry of two identical bones (femur-femur) can also relate an underlying abnormality. Therefore, more than one film is usually required to diagnose the chief complaint.

Thoracic region

chest: PA, lateral.
clavicle: AP, apical lordotic, tangential.
ribs:
    anterior: PA, obliques, lateral.
    posterior: AP, obliques, lateral.
scapula: AP, oblique, lateral.

shoulder: AP, internal rotation; AP, external rotation; axillary lateral; transthoracic lateral.
sternum: PA, right anterior oblique, lateral.

Upper limbs

elbow: AP, lateral.
hands/fingers: AP, lateral, oblique.
humerus: AP, lateral, transthoracic lateral.
radius/ulna: AP, lateral.
wrist: AP, lateral, oblique, AP with ulnar and radial deviation (for scaphoid fracture), carpal tunnel.

Spinal region

C-spine: AP, lateral, both obliques, open-mouth odontoid.
coccyx: AP, lateral.
L-spine: AP, lateral, both obliques, coned down L-5 to S-1 lateral.
pelvis: AP.
SI joints: AP, both obliques.
sacrum: AP lateral.
T-spine: AP, lateral.

Lower limbs

ankle: AP lateral, and mortise oblique.
femur: AP, lateral.
foot/toes: AP, lateral, oblique.
hip: AP, frogleg, and/or crosstable lateral.
knee: AP, lateral, tunnel, Hughston.
patella: tunnel, sunset, lateral, PA.
tibia/fibula: AP, lateral.
calcaneus: lateral plantodorsal.

Additional views requested may be views in flexion and extension, special views of the skull, "push-pull" films of hips for piston sign, and cine (movies) of x-ray images.

X-RAY ANGLES, LINES, SIGNS, AND METHODS
Angles

The anatomic description is taken directly from anatomic points using the intersection of two straight lines to form the angle.

acromial angle: angle between clavicle and head of humerus.
Baumann angle: angle of capitellum in reference

to distal humeral epiphysis seen in AP view, usually 75 degrees from the vertical.

Böhler angle: the two superior surfaces of the calcaneus.

carrying angle: the AP angle of the extended elbow, that is, the angle of the forearm when arm is extended.

CE (center edge) angle: angle created by two lines drawn from the center of the femoral capital epiphysis, one line being vertical and the other extending to the acetabular edge.

Codman angle: discrete angle at edge of the bone cortex produced by periosteal elevation and reactive bone in the area of a tumor. Also called Codman triangle.

Hilgenreiner angle: angle of the acetabular slope to the Y-line (horizontal line drawn through both acetabular centers).

Kager's triangle: a triangular space anterior to the Achilles tendon normally visible on x-ray film as a radiolucent area.

Konstram angle: for gibbus deformity, the obtuse angle created by the intersection of the two lines drawn parallel to the surface of the superior vertebral body above and inferior surface of vertebral body below the deformed segment(s).

Laurin angle (lateral patello-femoral angle): acute angle created by intersection of line drawn from medial to lateral condylar points and a line parallel to the lateral undersurface of the patella.

Merchant angle: created by intersection of two lines drawn from intracondylar apex of patella to center and a line perpendicular to plane of condyles. Also called sulcus a.

Mikulicz angle: angle of declination formed by the neck of the femoral epiphysis and diaphysis center lines.

neck shaft angle: angle created by intersection of a line drawn through the femoral shaft and a line through the femoral head and neck.

Pauwels angle: angle of a femoral neck fracture in reference to the horizontal line of a standing patient.

pelvic femoral angle: angle of inclination formed by the pelvis with line of femoral shaft.

Q angle: made by intersection of lines drawn from anterosuperior iliac spine (ASIS) to midpatella and from midpatella to anterior tibial tuberosity.

sacrovertebral angle: angle obtained by junction of lines through lateral projection of sacrum and lumbar spine.

Lines and ratios

Line is defined here as a line seen or drawn directly on the x-ray film to help in the interpretation of the film, and anatomic lines of reference.

Blackburne ratio: for a patella alta, with the knee flexed at 30 degrees the ratio is measured A:B. A is the distance from the point parallel to the tibial condylar surface to the inferior weight-bearing surface of the patella. B is the height of the weight-bearing portion of the patella. The noncartilagenous inferior pole portion of the patella is eliminated from the measurement.

Blumensaat line: line parallel to superior part of intercondylar notch as seen on lateral x-ray examination used to judge the relative height of the patella.

fracture line: any line thought to be the result of a fracture.

Frankel line: line around outer margins of bony epiphysis, seen in scurvy.

Harris line: a straight, thin radiodense line across the metaphysis of bone resulting from a previous change in growth rate of that bone; most commonly seen after a fracture. Also called growth arrest line.

Heuter line: a line drawn horizontal to the medial epicondyle of the humerus, passing tip of olecranon when elbow is extended.

Insall ratio: for patella alta, with the knee flexed at 30 degrees the ratio is the length of the patella tendon to the height of the patella. A number greater than 1.0 indicates patella alta.

Kohler line: a slanted line drawn from the acetabular "tear drop" to the most lateral tangent of the pelvic ring.

lead line: a radiodense thin line in metaphysis of bones affected by lead poisoning.

Nélaton line: line drawn from the anterosuperior iliac spine to the ischial tuberosity; normally goes through the greater trochanter.

Ogston line: line drawn from adduction tubercle to intercondylar notch; used as a guide for transection of condyle in osteotomy for knock-knee deformity.

Shenton line: a curved line seen in x-ray examinations of a normal hip joint, formed by top of obturator foramen and medial femoral neck to lesser trochanter.

Ullmann line: the line of displacement in spondylolisthesis.

Wegner line: radiographically relatively dense thin line at the junction of the epiphysis and diaphysis of a long bone; characteristically seen in vitamin C deficiency.

Winberger line: infraction (appearing as a radiolucent line) in the metaphysis, as seen in syphilis.

Y-line: line drawn through both triradiate cartilages at the acetabular center.

X-ray film signs

anterior hiatal sign: for posterior ligament ankle instability, a lateral x-ray shows a wedge-shaped opening at the anterior dome of the talus when the foot is flexed and pushed backward.

Ashhurst sign: for ankle diastasis, a widening of the normal overlap of the distal anterior tubercle and fibula at the ankle joint.

codfish vertebrae: the x-ray appearance of vertebrae severely involved with osteoporosis, where the central portion has a marked concave impression, similar to a codfish.

crescent sign: x-ray finding in avascular necrosis where there is a space between the subchondral plate and impacted bone of the femoral head, leaving a crescent-shaped area that is less dense on x-ray.

Hawkins sign: for avascular necrosis of the talus, zone of radiographic translucency beneath the subchondral plate of the dome of the talus.

posterior hiatal sign: for anterior ligament ankle instability; a lateral x-ray with the foot pulled forward shows a wedge-shaped opening at the posterior dome of the talus.

Risser sign: for skeletal maturity, the degree of capping of the iliac apophysis from beginning (Grade 1) to completion (Grade 4).

rugger jersey spine: the appearance of alternate light and dense zones seen in spine x-rays of patients with osteomalacia.

Methods

Bone age: In pediatric orthopaedics, refers to x-ray studies of skeletal changes of bone and the development of ossification centers from infancy to adulthood. These studies observe the size of bone, proportionate sizes between different bones in the wrist, texture changes, contour of bony margins, and bone markings. These are then contrasted to photographic plates that show bone and joint maturation of the wrist in 3-month age increments. Standard sets of plates are found in Gruelich and Pyle (1959) and Todd (1937).

Catterall hip score: for pediatric avascular necrosis of the femoral head, or Legg-Perthe disease.

I	no finding on AP, compression on frog leg lateral
II	central compression on both AP and frog leg lateral
III	lateral femoral head compression seen on AP x-ray, not covered by acetabulum, and medial femoral head is intact
IV	entire femoral head involved

Cobb method: for measuring angle or degree of curvature in scoliosis, using horizontal lines to vertebral bodies.

Fairbanks changes: a grading scale for the changes seen on the AP x-rays of osteoarthritic knees, originally used in postmeniscectomy patients seen in long-term followup.

Fergusson method: for measuring angle of degree of curvature in scoliosis, using vertical lines through spinous processes.

Ficat and Marcus: for avascular necrosis of the femoral head, two similar grading scale systems are currently used.

Arlet Ficat	Marcus	
I	I	mottled densities, may be obscure, anterosuperior weight-bearing area of femoral head
II	II	well-demarcated infarction, rim of increased density of bone at base of area of infarction
III	III	subtle flattening of femoral head or subchondral radiolucent crescent

IV   pronounced collapse of avascular segment

IV   V   degenerative arthritis with loss of cartilage space

VI   marked degenerative changes.

Mose concentric rings: for avascular necrosis of femoral head in children, a system using concentric rings with 2-millimeter separations.

Singh index: an index of osteoporosis accomplished by a grading system using the three major trabecular patterns in the femoral intertrochanteric and head region. Grades I through VI with lowest grade being the most osteoporotic.

Stulberg method: a system for measuring concentricity of femoral heads in Perthes' disease.

Ward triangle: a relatively radiolucent area of bone in the intertrochanteric area of the femur.

MAGNETIC RESONANCE IMAGING (MRI)

Formerly called a nuclear magnetic resonance study (NMR) the name was changed because people misunderstood the term and thought that harmful ionizing radiation was used. Instead, it is a safe and painless procedure. This technique allows observation of anatomic detail in soft tissue and bone that is not apparent on x-ray. It will also demonstrate the quality of the tissue such as in degeneration or infarction. In orthopaedics, the spinal disks, meniscal tissues, and tumors draw the most attention.

The patient is exposed to harmless strong magnetic fields. After a short time in a longitudinal magnetic field, a second pulsating magnetic field that is transverse to the other field is introduced. The movements of protons, which are usually random, are at first aligned and then that alignment is changed by the pulsating magnetic field, a radio wave. When the radio wave is turned off, the protons become realigned and emit a weak radio signal. With the use of "search coils" and a computer, cross-section images can be made for specified regions of the body. Hydrogen is the most common radio wave-emitting element used. This technique has a terminology unique to the system.

magnetic resonance spectroscopy: technique using magnetic resonance to determine the relative amounts of specific chemicals in an anatomic part. One such study is the evaluation of chemical reactions involving phosphate in the muscle. This type of evaluation helps to determine the metabolic adequacy of the muscle.

T_1 **weighted image:** an image in which the contrast is strongly affected by the longitudinal magnetic relaxation time, T_1. Such images are usually produced with a spin-echo pulse sequence having relaxation time (TR) about 500 milliseconds and an echo time (TE) less than or equal to 30 milliseconds.

T_2 **weighted image:** an image in which the contrast is strongly affected by the transverse magnetic relaxation time, T_2. Such images are usually produced with a spin-echo pulse sequence having the relaxation time (TR) greater than or equal to 2000 milliseconds and the echo time (TE) greater than or equal to 80 milliseconds.

INVASIVE AND NONINVASIVE TECHNIQUES

Bone scans, a special procedure and the most commonly employed nuclear medicine study in orthopaedics, consist basically of an x-ray film taken from "inside out." A radioactive material (radioisotope) is attached chemically to a substance that, when injected into the body, goes to bone collagen. The minute radioactivity coming from the bone can be detected by special instruments that will make a picture of the area of interest or of the entire skeleton. Although the detail is far from being as clear as that of an x-ray film, the bone scan has the advantage of showing places where bone is actively being made. An x-ray examination simply shows where bone is present.

CAT scan (computerized axial tomography): a computer that composes a three-dimensional picture. A series of x-ray beams rotated a degree at a time around an area of anatomic interest with each "slice" making a picture depicting the difference in tissue density. This allows visualization of pathologic lesions that have contrasting densities, such as tumors, blood clots, or hemorrhage. The advantage of this technique is that it is noninvasive and provides a sharp, detailed picture. This method is best for patients who cannot handle rigorous x-ray studies.

cineroentgenogram: recorded x-ray motion studies for relative motion of bones in a joint, for example, to detect carpal instability.

dual photon densitometry: used in estimating bone density, the part being measured is exposed to two beams of photons of different intensity. A two-dimensional picture of bone density is obtained with calculated subtraction of soft tissue density. The results are expressed in grams of bone mineral per square centimeter.

gallium scan (^{67}Ga): Radioactive gallium 67 is introduced intravenously and localizes in areas of concentrated granulocytes; used to detect hidden infections, such as osteomyelitis.

gamma camera: instrument used for radionuclear scans that comprises many Geiger counters so that radiation from the patient can be directed by different metal apertures to produce a picture.

indium scan (indium leukocyte scan): radioactive indium 111 is incubated with white cells taken from the patient. It is then reinjected into the circulation and localizes in areas of acute osteomyelitis. The test is insensitive for chronic osteomyelitis.

sonogram: use of high-frequency sound to outline soft tissue planes (not an x-ray examination). Normally used in orthopaedics to outline intrapelvic or intraabdominal masses, such as tumors or hemorrhage. Ultrasonograms and echograms are also sonograms used by other specialties.

SPECT (single photon emission computerized tomography): use of a single beam emission source to make two-dimensional images revealing relative areas of bone density. May be used in disorders such as avascular necrosis.

technetium scan (^{99m}Tc): used as a bone tracer when attached to polyphosphate or diphosphonate; a radioactive material study to determine pathologic conditions such as tumors, infection, and stress fractures.

Lung scans are most commonly used to detect pulmonary embolus, a blood clot to the lung. The same tracer that is used for a bone scan can be used in this study. However, the tracer is on a different chemical "tag" than the one used for bone.

ultrasound: mechanical radiant energy having a frequency beyond the upper limits of perception by the human ear (20,000 cycles/second). Can be used to detect abnormalities of human anatomy (rotator cuff tear) or function (cardiac ejection fraction).

VASCULAR DIAGNOSTIC STUDIES

Following routine history and physical examination that may include specific maneuvers performed by the physician (Chapter 4), other tests may be required regarding peripheral circulation affecting the limbs. These specific tests, while performed by vascular surgeons, are often made in conjunction with an orthopaedic problem and are added for information. These studies fall into two categories: invasive tests and noninvasive tests.

invasive tests: tests in which entrance into the body may be by medicine (injection of radioactive material) or by instrument (venipuncture). Examples would be:

arteriogram: invasive diagnostic procedure that employs injection of radiopaque material into the arteries in an effort to examine the blood supply to an area or understand the anatomic arrangement. Also called angiography.

phlebogram: invasive radiographic procedure where radiopaque material is injected into a vein to visualize possible blockage or other abnormalities. Also called venogram.

noninvasive tests: tests in which external techniques are applied and the body is not entered (ultrasound). This method frequently provides dynamic information. The various types are:

ankle-arm index: a ratio of arm and ankle blood pressures calculated by dividing the arm blood pressure by the ankle Doppler pressure. Values less than 1.0 indicate a variable amount of decreased blood flow.

Doppler: a diagnostic instrument that emits sound waves into the body. These sound waves are reflected back at a different velocity; it is this change in velocity that changes electrically to sound waves (strip recorder) and the conversion of these changes in velocity are read out as information regarding blood flow. A test for arterial pressure. A *bidirectional Doppler* is an instrument capable of determining a change in direction of blood flow.

electrocardiogram: graphic recording of electrical activity of the heart.

plethysmography: a noninvasive instrument that measures limb blood flow in an artery or vein on the basis of changes in volume of part or all of the extremity. Various types employ air, water, light, or mild electric current to measure these changes.

  impedance plethysmograph: an instrument to measure changes in electrical impedance in a limb, which indicates changes in blood content and limb volume.

  oculoplethysmography (OPG): a noninvasive diagnostic procedure measuring carotid artery pressure indirectly by measuring blood pressure in the eyes. The medium of measurement may either be air (oculopneumoplethysmography) or water (oculohydroplethysmography).

  photoplethysmography (PPG): noninvasive instrument that uses light to measure blood flow to skin and thereby measure blood in larger vessels that may be occluded by arteriosclerosis.

phleboreography (PRG): noninvasive instrument that records movement of blood in veins. Useful in helping diagnose deep venous thrombophlebitis. Also called venous phleboreography, venography.

pulse volume recorder (PVR): segmental air plethysmograph to determine changes in limb blood flow by change in cuff pressure.

TW$_2$ bone age: method of assessing skeletal maturity and relative bone age by use of a chart of comparative x-rays for different ages.

Radiotherapy

Ionizing radiation causes molecules to split when the radiation particle or wave hits the molecule. This event can cause injury to cells, particularly those that are dividing such as in tumors, the blood, and normal gastrointestinal lining.

As a result, ionizing radiation for diagnostic purposes is kept at a minimum, and treatment is made focal by a variety of techniques. The terminology listed here is restricted to techniques commonly applied to orthopaedic conditions and to some dosemetry terms.

dysprosium 165: a rare earth element with a half-life of 2.3 hours that when attached to ferric hydroxide microaggregates can be injected into rheumatoid joints to produce a synovectomy response.

RAD (roentgen absorbed dose): the actual energy absorbed by the local tissue, measured in ergs/gm. This is not a whole body count of absorbed dose but is a number that looks at each tissue system or organ.

REM (roentgen equivalent man): biologic effectiveness of radiation in a human subject. For diagnostic purposes, RAD is equal to REM.

Roentgen: the charge resulting from the exposure of air to radiation.

4

Orthopaedic tests, signs, and maneuvers

Tests, signs, and maneuvers provide some of the most frequently used terms in orthopaedics. Unfortunately, the terms involved possess the greatest possibility for confusion and typographic error because of similar names or meanings. Thus the newcomer to orthopaedics meets a challenge at the very onset of his or her career.

Eponyms for certain examinations vary from locale to locale or among institutions within the same area. Such variations are a reflection of the training center's influence, where the names of prominent local physicians are frequently used for these examinations. Occasionally, the same test is given two or more names, or the name can apply to more than one test or sign. In a problem-oriented situation, eponyms are routinely used in the physical evaluation process. Familiarity with the terms and techniques used in determining regional problems enables physicians and their assistants to record and clarify an orthopaedic examination.

The physical examination can be performed by using all the physical senses. The most common is a direct visual observation, although there may be some auditory findings on auscultation of the arterial pulses. Palpation, the use of hands in determining firmness, shape, and motion of a part, is also very productive. The way a patient walks (gait) or how he uses his upper and lower limbs can also be informative. The combination of these findings is described in this chapter.

A *test* may be part of the physical examination in which direct contact with the patient is made, or it may be a chemical test, x-ray examination, or other study. All tests described in this chapter will relate to the physical examination only.

A *sign* may be elucidated by a test, maneuver, or simply a visual observation, for example, a "list." It is an indication of the existence of a problem as perceived by the examiner.

A *maneuver* is a complex motion or series of movements used either as a test or treatment. It is also referred to as a method or technique.

A *phenomenon* is any sign or objective symptom, any observable occurrence or fact.

This chapter describes the physical examination by specific anatomic areas to include the neck, back, shoulder, upper limbs, hands, hips, lower limbs, knees, feet and ankles, neurologic, metabolic, and general. In addition to many new terms, a table has been included on Knee Instability Tests, an area that receives much attention. Scales and ratings, as pertains to pre- and postoperative assessment of joints and degree of functional impairment, have been expanded on to include a neurologic assessment grading system for spinal cord injury. The alphabetized list of tests, signs and maneuvers is provided to assist the reader in easily identifying the proper name by specific anatomic area (in parentheses).

TESTS, SIGNS, AND MANEUVERS

Abbott method (back)
Achilles bulge sign (feet, ankles)
Achilles squeeze test (lower limb)
Addis test (lower limbs)
Adson maneuver (neck)
Allen maneuver (neck)
Allen test (hands)

Allis maneuver (hips)
Allis sign (hips)
Amoss sign (back)
Anghelescu sign (back)
antecedent sign (general)
anterior tibial sign (lower limb)
anvil test (neck, hips)
Apley test and sign (knees)
Apprehension test (shoulder)
artifact (general)
Babinski sign and reflex (back, neurologic)
bayonet sign (knees)
Beevor sign (neurologic)
Bekhterev test (back)
bench test (back)
bowstring sign (lower limb)
bracelet test (hands)
Bragard sign (back)
British test (knees)
Brudzinski sign (neck, neurologic)
Bryant sign (shoulders)
café-au-lait spots (general)
Callaway test (shoulders)
camelback sign (knees)
Chaddock sign (neurologic)
Chiene test (hips)
Chvostek sign (metabolic)
circumduction maneuver (hands)
Cleeman sign (lower limb)
Codman sign (shoulders)
cogwheel phenomenon, sign (general)
commemorative sign (general)
Comolli sign (shoulders)
contralateral sign (neurologic)
contralateral straight leg raising test (back)
Coopernail sign (back)
Dawbarn sign (shoulders)
Déjèrine sign (back)
Demianoff sign (back)
Desault sign (hips)
dimple sign (feet, ankle)
doll's eyes sign; Cantelli sign (neurologic)
double camelback sign (knees)
drawer sign (knees)
drop arm test (shoulder)
Dugas test (shoulders)

Dupuytren sign (general)
Ely test; femoral nerve stretch test (hips, neurologic)
Erichsen sign (back)
external rotation recurvatum test (knees)
fabere sign; Patrick test (back)
fadire test (back)
fan sign (neurologic)
femoral nerve traction test (back)
finger to nose test (neurologic)
Finkelstein sign (hands)
flexion rotation drawer test (Noyes) (knees)
Fournier test (neurologic)
Fowler maneuver (hands)
Fränkel sign (neurologic)
Froment paper sign (hands)
Gaenslen sign (back)
Galeazzi sign (hips)
Goldthwait sign (back)
Gower sign (general)
grimace test (knees)
Guilland sign (neurologic)
Hamilton test (shoulders)
Helbing sign (feet, ankles)
hemodynamics (general)
Hirschberg sign (neurologic)
Hoffmann sign (neurologic)
Homans sign (lower limbs)
Hoover test (back)
Hueter sign and line (general)
Hughston jerk test (knee)
Huntington sign (neurologic)
Jansen test (hips)
Jendrassik maneuver (neurologic)
Kanavel sign (hands)
Keen sign (feet, ankles)
Kernig sign (neurologic)
Kerr sign (neurologic)
knee instability tests (knees)
Kocher maneuver (shoulders)
Lachman test (knees)
Langer line (general)
Langoria sign (hips)
Lasègue sign (back)
Laugier sign (upper limbs)
lead line; Burton sign (metabolic)

Leadbetter maneuver (hips)
Leichtenstern sign (neurologic)
Leri sign (neurologic)
Lhermitte sign (neurologic)
Linder sign (back)
list (back)
long tract sign (neurologic)
Lorenz sign (back)
Ludloff sign (hips)
McMurray sign; circumduction maneuver (knees)
Maisonneuve sign (hands)
Marie-Foix sign (feet, ankles)
Mendel-Bekhterev sign (neurologic)
Mennell sign (back)
Meyn and Quigley maneuver (upper limbs)
Milgram test (back)
Mills test (upper limbs)
Minor sign (back)
Moro reflex sign (neurologic)
Morquio sign (neurologic)
Morton test (feet, ankles)
Murphy sign (feet, ankles)
Naffziger sign (back)
Nélaton line (hips)
nuchocephalic reflex (neurologic)
Ober test (hips)
objective sign (general)
Oppenheim sign (neurologic)
Ortolani sign (hips)
paratonia (neurologic)
Parvin maneuver (upper limbs)
patellar retraction test (knees)
Patrick test (back)
Payr sign (lower limbs)
pelvic rock test (back)
Phalen test and maneuver (hands)
piano key sign (hands)
Piotrowski sign (neurologic)
piston sign; Dupuytren sign (hips)
pivot-shift test (MacIntosh) (knees)
posterior drawer test (knees)
postural fixation (back)
pronation sign (neurologic)
pseudo-Babinski sign (neurologic)
quadriceps test (general)
quadriceps active test (knees)
Queckenstedt sign (neurologic)

radialis sign; Strümpell sign (neurologic)
Raimiste sign (neurologic)
Raynaud phenomenon (general)
reverse Bigelow maneuver (hips)
reverse pivot shift (Jacob) knees
Romberg test and sign (neurologic)
Rust sign (neck)
Sagittal stress test (feet, ankles)
Sarbo sign (neurologic)
Schlesinger sign (lower limbs)
Schreiber maneuver (neurologic)
Sharp-Purser Test (neck)
Slocum test (knees)
somatic sign (general)
Soto-Hall sign (back)
spine sign (back)
sponge test (back)
Spurling test (neck)
stairs sign (neurologic)
station test (neurologic)
Stimson maneuver (hips)
straight leg raising test (back)
Strunsky sign (feet, ankles)
tendon reflexes (neurologic)
Tensilon test (metabolic)
Thomas sign (hips, neurologic)
Thompson (Simmonds) test (lower limbs)
thumbnail test (knees)
tibialis sign (neurologic)
Tinel sign; distal tingling on percussion sign (neurologic)
toe spread sign; Nelson sign (feet, ankles)
tourniquet test (lower limbs)
Trendelenburg test (hips)
Turyn sign (back)
Valsalva maneuver (back)
Vanzetti sign (back)
Wartenberg sign (hands)
Watson test (hands)
Wilson test (knees)
Yergason test (shoulders)

NECK

Adson maneuver: for scalenus anticus syndrome, noted on obliteration of radial pulse; upper limb to be tested is held in dependent position while head is rotated to the ipsilateral shoulder.

Allen maneuver: for same diagnosis as Adson m., except the forearm is flexed at right angle with the arm extended horizontally and rotated externally at the shoulder, with the head rotated to the contralateral shoulder.

anvil test: for vertebral disorders; a closed fist striking blow on top of the head elicits pain in the vertebra(e).

Rust sign: for caries or malignant disease of the cervical vertebrae; the patient supports his head with his hands while moving his body.

Sharp-Purser test: for chronic subluxation of the first on second cervical vertebra; with the patient sitting, the head is tilted forward and then backward with the examining finger on the first cervical spinous process.

Spurling test: for cervical spine and foraminal nerve encroachment; compression on the head with extension of the neck causes radicular pain into the upper extremities.

BACK

Abbott method: for scoliosis of the spine; traction is applied to produce overcorrection, followed by casting.

Amoss sign: for painful flexure of the spine; pain is produced when the patient places his hands far behind him in bed and tries rising from supine position to sitting position.

Anghelescu sign: for testing tuberculosis of the vertebrae or other destructive processes of the spine; in the supine position the patient places weight on his head and heels while lifting his body upward; inability to bend the spine indicates an ongoing disease process.

Bekhterev test: for nerve root irritability in sciatica; while sitting up in bed, the patient is asked to stretch out both legs; with sciatica he cannot sit up in bed this way; he can only stretch out each leg in turn.

bench test: for nonorganic back pain. In normal hip motion, the patient should be able to bend over and touch the floor kneeling on a 12-inch high bench; not being able to implies a nonorganic (or psychologic) back pain. Also called Burns test.

bowstring sign: with leg raised with knee bent in same position, pain is felt in the back of limb pressing on the popliteal fossa. Increased pain is sign of nerve irritability.

Bragard sign: for nerve or muscular involvement; with the knee stiff, the lower extremity is flexed at the hip until the patient experiences pain; the foot is then dorsiflexed. Increase in pain points to nerve involvement; no increase in pain indicates muscular involvement.

contralateral straight leg raising test: for sciatica; when the leg is flexed, the hip can also be flexed, but not when the leg is held straight. Flexing the sound thigh with the leg held straight causes pain on the affected side. Also called Fajersztajn crossed sciatic sign.

Coopernail sign: for fracture of pelvis; ecchymosis of the perineum, scrotum, or labia indicates a pelvic fracture.

Déjèrine sign: for symptoms of a herniated nucleus pulposus (HNP); a Valsalva maneuver produces aggravation of symptoms of radiculitis by coughing, sneezing, and straining at stool.

Demianoff sign: for differentiation of pain originating in the lumbosacral muscle from lumbar pain of any other origin; the pain is caused by stretching of the lumbosacral muscle.

Erichsen sign: for sacroiliac disease; when the iliac bones are sharply pressed toward each other, pain is felt in the sacroiliac area.

fabere sign: for testing lower back or sacroiliac joint disorder by using a forced position of the hip; the letters stand for *f*lexion *ab*duction *ex*ternal *r*otation in *ex*tension. Also called Patrick test, faber test, figure of 4 test.

fadire test: forced position of the hip causing pain; the letters stand for *f*lexion *ad*duction *i*nternal *r*otation in *ex*tension. Also called Patrick test, fadir sign.

femoral nerve traction test: for radiculopathy of the second through fourth lumbar nerves; with patient prone, the knee is flexed, causing back or thigh pain.

Gaenslen sign: for sacroiliac disease; pressure on hyperextended thigh with the opposite hip held in flexion elicits pain, indicating a sacroiliac problem.

Goldthwaite sign: for distinguishing lumbosacral from sacroiliac pain: with the patient supine, his leg is raised with one hand, while the examiner's other hand is placed under the patient's lower back; leverage is then applied to the side of the pelvis. If pain is felt by the patient before the lumbar spine is moved, the lesion is a sprain of the SI joint; if pain is not felt until after the lumbar spine is moved, the lesion is in the SI or lumbosacral articulation.

Hoover test: for a supposed malingering back disorder. While lying supine, the patient is asked to raise one leg with the knee straight and with the examiner holding the opposite heel. Any active effort to do this will result in pressure of the opposite heel against the examiner's hand. The lack of such effort implies malingering. Excessive pressure of the heel against the examiner's hand implies abdominal muscle weakness.

Lasègue sign: for sciatica; flexion of thigh upon hips is painless, and when the knee is bent, such flexion is easily made. If painless, there is no hip joint disease. If test produces pain when the leg is held straight, nerve root irritation or lower back disorder may be present. See straight leg raising test.

Linder sign: for sciatica; with the patient sitting or recumbent with outstretched legs, passive flexion of the head will cause pain in the leg or lumbar region.

list: said of a patient who leans to one side or another when standing or walking; most commonly seen in lumbar disk disease.

Lorenz sign: for ankylosing spondylitis (Marie-Strümpell disease); ankylotic rigidity of the spinal column, especially thoracic and lumbar segments.

Mennell sign: for spinal problems; examiner's thumb is taken over the posterosuperior spine of sacrum outward and inward for noting tenderness, which may be caused by sensitive deposits in gluteal aspect of posterosuperior spine; ligamentous strain and sensitivity.

Milgram test: for a lesion within the dural sac; while lying supine, the patient flexes both hips so that the knees are straight and both feet are lifted by only several inches. If the patient is able to hold this position without pain for 30 seconds, there is no problem within the dural sac. However, a positive test may occur for both intrathecal and extrathecal disorders.

Minor sign: for sciatica; patient rises from sitting position; supporting himself on healthy side, placing hand on back, and bending affected leg, revealing pain.

Naffziger sign: for sciatica or herniated nucleus pulposus; nerve root irritation is produced by external jugular venous compression by examiner.

Patrick test: for pain in lumbosacral area or hip. See Fabere sign and Fadire test.

pelvic rock test: for sacroiliac joint disorder, forcible compression of the iliac crest toward the midline will produce pain.

postural fixation: a sign noted on range of motion of the back; any postural deformity (stiffness) noted does not reverse with range of motion.

Soto-Hall sign: for lesions in back abnormalities; with the patient supine, flexion of the spine beginning at the neck and going downward will elicit pain in the area of the lesion.

spine sign: for poliomyelitis; the patient is unable to flex the spine anteriorly because of pain.

sponge test: for detecting lesions of the spine; the examiner passes a hot sponge up and down the spine, and the patient feels pain over the lesion.

straight leg raising (SLR) test: for determining nerve root irritation; the supine patient elevates his leg straight until there is back or ipsilateral extremity pain or until the pain is increased with dorsiflexion of the foot. Also called Lasègue sign.

Turyn sign: for sciatica; when examiner bends the patient's great toe dorsally, pain is felt in the gluteal region.

Valsalva maneuver: for determining nerve root irritability within the spinal canal. This maneuver is also used for many other unrelated reasons. The patient takes a deep breath and then on bearing down, such as one does when lifting a heavy object, notes pain.

Vanzetti sign: for sciatica; the pelvis is horizontal

in the presence of scoliosis. In other scoliotic conditions the pelvis is inclined.

SHOULDER

apprehension test: for anterior subluxing or dislocating shoulder, the arm is held abducted and extended while in external rotation. The patient is apprehensive in a positive exam.

Bryant sign: for dislocation of the shoulder with lowering of the axillary folds, as noted on visual examination.

Callaway test: for dislocation of the humerus; the circumference of the affected shoulder measured over the acromion and through the axilla is greater than that on the opposite, unaffected side.

Codman sign: for rupture of the supraspinatus tendon; the arm can be passively abducted without pain, but when support of the arm is removed and the deltoid muscle contracts suddenly, pain occurs again.

Comolli sign: for scapular fracture; shortly after injury, there is triangular swelling, reproducing the shape of the body of the scapula.

Dawbarn sign: for acute subacromial bursitis; with arm hanging by side, palpation over the bursa causes pain; when the arm is abducted, pain disappears.

drop arm test: for rotator cuff tear, the patient is unable to actively control bringing the arm down from a full abducted position past 90 degrees. The arm drops at 90 degrees.

Dugas test: for dislocation of the shoulder; placing hand of affected side on opposite shoulder and bringing elbow to side of chest, a dislocation may be present if the patient's elbow will not touch side of his chest; Dugas s.

Hamilton test: for luxated shoulder; a rod applied to the humerus can be made to touch the lateral condyle and acromion at the same time to determine a dislocation.

Kocher maneuver: for reducing anterior dislocations of the shoulder; done by abducting the arm, externally rotating, adduction, and then internally rotating.

Yergason test: for subluxation of the long head of the biceps tendon. While pulling distally on the elbow, the patient holds it flexed at 90 degrees with supination and forced external rotation of the shoulder against resistance by the examiner. Painful subluxation of the tendon can be palpated.

UPPER LIMBS

Laugier sign: for a displaced distal radial fracture; condition in which the styloid process of radius and ulna are on same level.

Meyn and Quigley maneuver: for dislocation of the elbow, the patient lies prone with the arm resting on the examining table and the elbow flexed at 90 degrees. The forearm is pulled distally while the opposite hand guides the olecranon.

Mills test: for tennis elbow, with wrist and fingers fully flexed and the forearm pronated, complete extension of the elbow is painful.

Parvin maneuver: for dislocated elbow, the patient lies prone with the arms and forearm over the edge of the examining table. Traction is applied on the wrist in a distal direction while the opposite hand pushes on the anterior distal arm in a posterior direction.

HANDS

Allen test: for occlusion of radial or ulnar artery. A method of determining if radial and ulnar arteries communicate through the two palmar arches. Both arteries are occluded digitally. First one artery is released, then the other, to observe pattern of capillary refill in the hand. This can be performed with a Doppler placed on the digits during test. The test is valuable prior to an invasive procedure on the arteries at the wrist.

bracelet test: for early rheumatoid arthritis involving the distal radioulnar joint; compression of the lower ends of the ulna and radius elicits moderate lateral pain.

circumduction maneuver: a maneuver for the thumb; any general test or motion involving a rotation action of a group of joints; a range of motion examination.

Finkelstein sign: bending the thumb into the palm to determine synovitis of the abductor pollicis longus tendon to wrist.

Fowler maneuver: a maneuver for testing rheumatoid arthritis; tight intrinsic muscles in ulnar deviation of the digits and a heavy, taut, ulnar band are demonstrated when the digit is held in its normal axial relationship.

Froment paper sign: for ulnar nerve loss; flexion of the distal phalanx of the thumb—with a sheet of paper held between the thumb and index finger, the thumb flexes on the side of the index finger.

Kanavel sign: for infection of a tendon sheath; there is a point of maximum tenderness in the palm 1 inch proximal to the base of the little finger.

key pinch: the strength in the ability to grasp, as in holding a key; lateral pinch.

Maisonneuve sign: for Colles' fracture; there is marked hyperextensibility of the hand.

Phalen test and maneuver: for carpal tunnel syndrome; irritation of the median nerve is determined by holding the wrist flexed or extended for 30 to 60 seconds, reproducing symptoms.

piano key sign: for dorsal subluxation of the distal ulna in rheumatoid arthritis or trauma; if examiner pushes the ulnar styloid (piano key) down, the patient will express a small exclamation (note).

prehension: the ability to grasp with the fingers and thumb.

pulp pinch: the strength in the position one would use to pick up a piece of paper.

Wartenberg sign: for intrinsic muscle weakness of the hand, while the fingers are extended there is an inability to bring together the ring and little finger.

Watson test: for scapholunate instability. The examiner can elicit a painful wrist click by compressing the scaphoid while the patient moves the wrist.

HIPS

Allis maneuver: for reduction of anterior hip dislocation, the supine patient has the knee flexed, hip slightly flexed with longitudinal traction, and an assistant stabilizes the pelvis while applying a lateral traction force to the medial thigh. The surgeon then adducts and internally rotates the femur.

Allis sign: for femoral neck fracture; relaxation of the fascia between the crest of the ilium and the greater trochanter.

anvil test: for early hip joint disease or diseased vertebrae; a closed fist striking a blow to the sole of the foot with leg extended produces pain in the hip or vertebrae.

Chiene test: for determining fracture of the neck of the femur by use of a tape measure.

Desault sign: for intracapsular fracture of the hip; alternation of the arc described by rotation of the greater trochanter, which normally describes the segment of a circle but in this fracture rotates only as the apex of the femur rotates about its own axis.

Ely test: for determining tightness of the rectus femoris, contracture of the lateral fascia of the thigh, or femoral nerve irritation; with patient in prone position, flexion of the leg on the thigh causes buttocks to arch away and leg to abduct at the hip joint.

Galeazzi sign: for congenital dislocation of the hip; the dislocated side is shorter when both thighs are flexed to 90 degrees, as demonstrated in infants; in an older patient a curvature of the spine is produced by shortened leg.

Jansen test: for osteoarthritis deformans of the hip; the patient is asked to cross the legs with a point just above the ankle resting on the opposite knee. If significant disease exists, this test and motion are impossible.

Langoria sign: for symptoms of intracapsular fracture of the femur; relaxation of the extensor muscles of the thigh is present.

Leadbetter maneuver: for slipped capital femoral epiphysis, a maneuver to get the epiphysis in place.

Ludloff sign: for traumatic separation of the epiphysis of the lesser trochanter; swelling and ecchymosis are present at the base of Scarpa triangle, together with inability to raise the thigh when in sitting position.

Nélaton line (x-ray and physical examinations): for detecting dislocation of the hip; a line from the anterosuperior iliac spine to the ischial tuberosity, which normally passes through the greater trochanter.

Ober test: for tight tensor fascia lata, with patient lying on side with hip and knee flexed on the surface, the opposite hip is extended while the knee is flexed. Inability to place the knee being tested on the table surface indicates a tight fascia lata.

Ortolani sign: for congenital dislocated hip; an audible click is heard when the hip goes into the socket; noted in infancy; if the sign is elicited; the dislocation should be corrected at that time to avoid hip dysfunction later. Also called Ortolani click.

piston sign: for congenital dislocation of the head of the femur; if positive, there is up-and-down movement of the head of the femur. Also called Dupuytren sign.

reverse Bigelow maneuver: for anterior dislocation of the hip, two maneuvers are done, both starting in hip flexion and abduction: In the first maneuver, while lifting on the lower leg of the supine patient there is a quick jerk on the flexed thigh; the second maneuver involves traction in the line of deformity with the hip then being adducted, sharply internally rotated, and extended.

Stimson maneuver: for posterior hip dislocation, the patient is placed prone on a table with the involved hip flexed and the opposite hip extended. With the involved knee flexed downward, pressure is applied to the calf, resulting in reduction of the dislocation.

Thomas sign: for hip joint flexion contracture; when the patient is walking, the fixed flexion of the hip can be compensated by lumbar lordosis. With the patient supine and flexing the opposite hip, the affected thigh raises off the table. Also called Strümpell sign, Thomas test.

Trendelenburg test: for muscular weakness in poliomyelitis, ununited fracture of the femoral neck, rheumatoid arthritis, coxa vara, and congenital dislocations. With the patient standing, weight is removed from one extremity. If gluteal fold drops on that side, it signifies muscular weakness of the opposite weight-bearing hip. Also called Trendelenburg sign.

LOWER LIMBS

Achilles squeeze test: for Achilles tendon rupture; squeezing the calf muscle fails to produce plantar flexion of the ankle joint.

Addis test: for determination of leg length discrepancy; with patient in prone position, flexing the knees to 90 degrees reveals the potential discrepancies of both tibial and femoral lengths.

anterior tibial sign: for spastic paraplegia; involuntary extension of the tibialis anterior muscle when thigh is actively flexed on the abdomen.

Cleeman sign: for distal fracture of femur with overriding of the fragments; shows creasing of the skin just above the patella.

Homan's sign: pain in calf on dorsiflexion of foot (active or passive). Once considered a reliable test in diagnosing deep vein thrombophlebitis, but no longer considered valid. (See *phleboreogram*, Chapter 3.)

Payr sign: early sign of impending postoperative thrombosis, indicated by tenderness when pressure is placed over the inner side of the foot.

Schlesinger sign: for extensor spasm at the knee joint; with patient's leg held at the knee joint and flexed strongly at the hip joint, there will follow an extensor spasm at the knee joint with extreme supination of the foot.

Thompson test: compression of calf muscle with foot at rest results in ankle flexion if Achilles tendon is intact. Also called Simmons test, Achilles squeeze test.

tourniquet test: for phlebitis of the leg; tourniquet is applied to the thigh and pressure gradually increased until the patient complains of pain in the calf; result is compared with the effect on the opposite leg.

KNEES (Table 1)

Apley test: for differentiating ligamentous from meniscal injury; tibial rotation on femur with traction or compression with the patient prone and knee flexed; Apley s.

bayonet sign: lateral placement of infrapatellar

Table 1. Knee instability tests

Instability	Positive test	Deficient structure
Medial	valgus stress at 30 degrees	medial collateral ligament
Lateral	varus stress at 30 degrees	minor lateral complex tear
Anterior	anterior drawer at 90 degrees, neutral rotation	anterior cruciate and partial medial and lateral collateral ligaments
Posterior	posterior drawer at 90 degrees	posterior cruciate, arcuate complex, posterior oblique ligament
Anteromedial	Slocum at 30 degrees external rotation accented	medial capsular ligament tibial collateral ligament posterior oblique ligament anterior cruciate ligament
Anterolateral	Slocum at 15 degrees internal rotation accented jerk test lateral pivot shift	lateral capsular ligament arcuate complex anterior cruciate ligament
Posterolateral	reverse pivot shift	arcuate complex lateral capsular ligament popliteus tendon some posterior cruciate ligament
Posteromedial (controversial)	medial tibial plateau shifts posterior on stress	tibial collateral ligament medial capsular ligament posterior oblique ligament semimembranosus anterior cruciate ligament

tendon with a valgus knee produces a bayonet appearance in the quadriceps patellar tendon complex.

British test: for knee pain and/or injury; compression of patella during active quadriceps contraction as knee is extended elicits pain.

camelback sign: an unusually prominent infrapatellar fat pad of the knee and hypertrophy of the vastus lateralis.

double camelback sign: prominence of a high-riding patella and infrapatellar fat pad, producing the appearance of a camel back.

drawer sign: for ligamentous instability or ruptured cruciate ligaments; with the patient supine and knee flexed to 90 degrees, the sign is positive if knee is not displaced abnormally in a posterior direction with knee pulled forward. Also called an *anterior drawer sign*, meaning the anterior cruciate is lax or ruptured.

external rotation recurvatum test: with the patient supine, the knee is brought from 10 degrees of flexion to maximum extension while palpating for external rotation of the tibia.

flexion rotation drawer test (Noyes): with the knee extended and the thigh relaxed, there is anterolateral tibial subluxation. The knee is gradually flexed with reduction of the subluxation occurring at about 30 degrees of flexion.

grimace test: for knee pain or crepitus; if compression of the patella elicits pain or crepitus is noted, the patient will grimace.

Hughston jerk test: for anterolateral instability of the knee noted by starting at 90 degrees flexion with tibia internally rotated and applying valgus force while rotating fibula medially. There is a jerk at about 20 degrees from full extension.

Lachman test: with the patient supine and the knee flexed to 20 degrees, the tibia is pulled anteriorly. A "give" reaction or mushy end point indicates a torn anterior cruciate ligament.

McMurray circumduction maneuver: for noting joint menisci tears or tags; there is cartilage clicking medially or laterally on manipulation of the knee; McMurray s.

patellar retraction test: for synovitis; compression of patella causes pain when the patient attempts to set the quadriceps muscles with the knee in full extension.

pivot shift test (MacIntosh): with the knee extended, the examiner internally rotates the leg and with a valgus stress gradually flexes the knee. There is a shift at 30 degrees to 40 degrees.

posterior drawer test: with the hips at 45 degrees and the knees flexed at 90 degrees the examiner sits on the foot and pushes the tibia backward; also with the hips and knees flexed at 90 degrees the heels are held together and the two knees observed for comparison of relative posterior sag of the tibia.

quadriceps active test: with the patient supine the involved knee is flexed at 90 degrees and the foot rests on the table. With one hand, the examiner supports the thigh and palpates the relaxed quadriceps muscle; the other hand stabilizes the foot. When the patient is asked to slide the foot down the table, the proximal leg is pulled forward by the patellar tendon, indicating a posterior cruciate tear with resulting posterior sagging of the leg.

reverse pivot shift (Jacob): with the patient supine, the lateral tibial plateau shifts from posterior subluxation to reduction as the knee is brought from flexion to extension.

Slocum test: for rotary instability of the knee; the examiner pulls on the upper calf of a supine patient with the knees flexed 90 degrees. Then, while the examiner sits on the patient's foot, he or she pulls anteriorly comparing the amount of give with the foot turned in 15 degrees neutral and turned out 30 degrees.

thumbnail test: for patellar fracture; fracture is felt as a sharp crevice when the examiner's thumbnail is passed over the subcutaneous surface of the patella.

Wilson test: with knee extended from 30 degrees with valgus stress and internal rotation of the foot, a click is heard in cases of osteochondritis dissecans.

FEET, ANKLES

Achilles bulge sign: seen in ankle instability, a bulging Achilles tendon occurs when the foot is pulled forward while the leg is pushed backward with the knee flexed. Also known as heel-cord sign.

dimple sign: for ruptured lateral collateral ligament of ankle, an anterior force is directed on the heel while a posterior force is directed on the distal leg. In the case of a ruptured ligament, a dimple will appear.

Helbing sign: for flatfoot; medialward curving of the Achilles tendon as viewed from behind.

Keen sign: for Pott fracture of the fibula; if fracture exists, there is increased diameter around the malleoli area of the ankle.

Marie-Foix sign: for central nervous system disorder; withdrawal of the lower leg on transverse pressure of the tarsus or forced flexion of toes, even when the leg is incapable of voluntary movement.

Morton test: for metatarsalgia or neuroma; transverse pressure across heads of the metatarsals causes sharp pain in the forefoot.

Murphy sign: for Achilles tendon bursitis at the heel, dorsiflexion of the foot produces pain.

sagittal stress test: for ankle instability, with the knee flexed to at least 45 degrees the foot is pulled forward while the leg is pushed backward. If the usual concavity of the Achilles tendon is flattened or reversed, the sign is positive for an instability of the anterior fibular collateral ligament.

Strunsky sign: for detecting lesions of the anterior arch of the foot; sudden flexing of the toes is painless in a normal foot, but painful if inflammation exists in the anterior arch.

toe spread sign: for Morton neuroma; disproportional spreading of the toes, comparing one foot with the other. Also called Nelson sign.

GAITS

A patient's walking pattern (gait) is very important in the evaluation of disorders, particularly those affecting the lower limbs. A limp is more apparent in the stance phase of walking. Of the various gait patterns, some have very specific characteristics, such as

antalgic gait: due to pain in the stance phase (while walking through on the foot), the time spent on the affected side is shortened compared to the normal side.

gluteus maximus gait: due to weak or nonfunctioning hip extensor muscles, the patient thrusts his or her thorax posteriorly to maintain hip extension.

gluteus medius gait (abductor lurch): due to weak or nonfunctioning hip abductor muscles, the patient lurches toward the weak side to place the center of gravity over the hip.

slap foot (drop foot) gait: due to weak or nonfunctioning ankle dorsiflexor muscles, the foot slaps down after heel strike.

NEUROLOGIC

Babinski reflex: for loss of brain control over lower extremities; scraping the soles causes toes to pull up. Also called Babinski reflex, toe sign.

Babinski sign: for testing sciatic nerve pain; also for loss or lessening of the Achilles tendon reflex in sciatica, distinguishing it from hysteric sciatica.

Beevor sign: for segmental nerve disease involving T5 to T12 or L1 nerve roots, the patient does an active sit-up with the arms held behind the head. In a positive examination the umbilicus moves toward the segment that is weak.

Brudzinski sign: for meningitis; flexion of the neck forward results in flexion of the hip and knee; when passive flexion of the lower limb on one side is made, a similar movement will be seen in the opposite limb. Also called neck sign, contralateral sign.

Chaddock sign: for upper motor neuron loss (brain); the big toe extends when irritating the skin in the external malleolar region; indicates lesions of the corticospinal paths. Also called external malleolus sign, Chaddock reflex.

contralateral sign: see Brudzinski sign.

doll's eye sign: for testing normal or abnormal brain function, the normal coordinated eye motions seen when passively turning the head of an unconscious patient. Also called Cantelli sign.

Ely test: for L3 and L4 nerve root irritation; flexing thigh with patient prone causes back and/or thigh pain. Also called femoral nerve stretch test, Ely sign.

fan sign: for central nerve problems; stroking the sole of the foot with a needle causes toes to spread; part of Babinski reflex examination.

finger to nose test: for cerebellar disease; when the patient attempts to put a finger on his nose and then to the examiner's finger, back and forth rapidly, any incoordination indicates test to be positive. Also called coordination extremity test.

Fournier test: for determining ataxic gait; it is noted with the patient moving about abruptly in walking, starting, and stopping.

Fränkel sign: for tabes dorsalis; noted by diminished tonicity of muscles about the hip joint.

Guilland sign: for meningeal irritation; when the contralateral quadriceps muscle group is pinched, there is brisk flexion at the hip and knee joint.

Hirschberg sign: for pyramidal tract disease; internal rotation and adduction of foot on rubbing inner lateral side.

Hoffmann sign: for testing digital reflex; nipping of three fingernails (index, middle, ring) produces flexion of terminal phalanx of thumb and second and third phalanx of some other finger; digital reflex.

Huntington sign: for lesions of the pyramidal tract; patient is supine, with legs hanging over the examining table, and is asked to cough; if coughing produces flexion of the thigh and extension of the leg in the paralyzed limb, a lesion is indicated.

Jendrassik maneuver: to enhance a patellar reflex; the reflex is tested when the patient hooks hands together with flexed fingers and pulls apart as hard as possible.

Kernig sign: for meningitis; in dorsal decubitus, the patient can easily and completely extend the leg; in sitting or lying down with thigh flexed upon the abdomen the leg cannot be completely extended.

Kerr sign: for spinal cord lesions; alteration of the

texture of the skin below the somatic level in eliciting location of lesions.

Leichtenstern sign: for cerebrospinal meningitis; tapping lightly on any bone of the extremities causes patient to wince suddenly.

Leri sign: for hemiplegia; passive flexion of the hand and wrist of the affected side shows no normal flexion at the elbow.

Lhermitte sign: for cervical cord injuries or cord degeneration; transient dysesthesia and weakness are noted in all four limbs when the patient flexes the head forward.

long tract sign: any sign that one would see in affection of either sensory or motor tracts in the spinal cord. For example, Babinski reflex, Romberg test.

Mendel-Bekhterev reflex: for organic hemiplegia; using a percussion hammer, the examiner notes flexion of the small toes if the dorsal surface of the cuboid bone is truck.

Moro reflex: for testing normal early neurologic development or the failure to progress neurologically; the infant is placed on a table, then the table is forcibly struck from either side, causing the infant's arms to be thrown out as in an embrace; should disappear as infancy progresses.

Morquio sign: for epidemic poliomyelitis; the supine patient resists attempts to raise trunk to a sitting position until the legs are passively flexed.

nuchocephalic reflex: for diffuse cerebral dysfunction as in senility; when the shoulders are turned to the left or right there is a failure of the head to turn in that direction within .5 seconds.

Oppenheim sign: for pyramidal tract disease; dorsal extension of the big toe is present when the medial side of the tibia is stroked in a downward direction.

paratonia: for diffuse cerebral dysfunction as in senility; the patient is asked to relax with the elbow passively flexed and extended. Intermittent opposition is abnormal.

Piotrowski sign: for organic disease of the central nervous system; percussion of tibialis muscle produces dorsiflexion and supination; anticus sign or reflex.

pronation sign: for central nervous disorders; there is a strong tendency for the forearm to pronate. Also called Strümpell sign.

pseudo-Babinski sign: in poliomyelitis the Babinski reflex is modified so only the big toe is extended, because all foot muscles except dorsiflexors of the big toe are paralyzed.

Queckenstedt sign: for detecting a block in the vertebral canal; compression of veins in the neck on one or both sides produces rapid rise in pressure of cerebral spinal fluid of a healthy person and quickly disappears, but in a patient with blockage in vertebral canal, pressure of cerebrospinal fluid is little or not at all affected by this sign.

radialis sign: for nerve impairment; inability to close the fist without marked dorsal extension of the wrist. Also called Strümpell sign.

Raimiste sign: for paretic condition; patient's hand and arm are held upright by examiner; a sound hand remains upright on being released, but a paretic hand flexes abruptly at the wrist.

Romberg test: for differentiation between peripheral and cerebellar ataxia; increase in clumsiness in movements and in width and uncertainty of gait when patient's eyes are closed indicate peripheral ataxia; no change indicates cerebellar type. (NOTE: Romberg sign is similar in testing but used for noting tabes dorsalis.)

Sarbó sign: for locomotor ataxia; analgesia of peroneal nerve is noted.

Schreiber maneuver: for patellar reflex testing; rubbing the inner side of the upper part of thigh enhances the reflex.

stairs sign: in locomotor ataxia there is difficulty or failure of ability to descend stairs.

station test: for coordination disturbance; feet are planted firmly together; if the body sways, lack of coordination is indicated.

tendon reflexes: for testing continuity of normal muscle to spinal cord to muscle reflex arc. Any tendon may be so tested, but the most common are the deep tendon reflexes (DTRs):
Achilles r.: ankle jerk.
quadriceps r.: patellar tendon or knee jerk.
biceps r.: elbow jerk.

triceps r.: elbow jerk.

mental r.: jaw jerk or reflex.

Thomas sign: for cord lesions; pinching of the trapezius muscle causes goose bumps above the level of the cord lesion.

tibialis sign: for spastic paralysis of the lower limb; there is dorsiflexion of the foot when the thigh is drawn toward the body. Also called tibial phenomenon.

Tinel sign: for noting a partial lesion or beginning regeneration of a nerve; tingling sensation of the distal end of a limb when percussion is made over the site of divided nerve as in carpal tunnel impingement on the median nerve of the hand. Also called formication sign, distal tingling on percussion (DTP) sign.

METABOLIC

Chvostek sign: for determining low serum calcium leading to tetany; tapping the cheek near the facial nerves causes the muscles to twitch or go into spasm. Also called *Chvostek* test, *Chvostek-Weiss* sign, *Weiss sign, Schultze-Chvostek sign*.

lead line: a blue line seen in the gums of a patient with lead poisoning. Also called *Burton sign*.

Tensilon test: for myasthenia gravis; a chemical test for denoting muscle strength or weakness; injection of endrophonium chloride (Tensilon) will reverse the symptoms in patients whose muscle weakness is caused by myasthenia gravis.

GENERAL

antecedent sign: any precursory indication of a malady.

artifact: a feature of a *test* which stimulates pathology or interference with the correct results of the test.

café-au-lait spots: for neurofibromatosis; hyperpigmented areas of skin indicate this ongoing problem. Also called *von Recklinghausen disease*.

cogwheel phenomenon: jerky motions produced on testing a muscle's strength; the jerks are neither rhythmic nor equal and represent malingering or protection from pain. Also called *cogwheel* sign.

commemorative sign: any sign of a previous disease.

Dupuytren sign: for determining sarcomatous bone; a crackling sensation on compression of that area is noted.

Gower sign: for progressive muscular dystrophy and tabes dorsalis; abrupt intermittent oscillation of iris under light is the indication of ongoing process.

hemodynamic test: to determine interrelationship of blood flow in normal anatomic structures versus disease.

Hueter sign: for indication of fracture; absence of the transmission of osseous vibration in fractures as heard by a stethoscope, where the fibrous material is interposed between the fragments.

Langer line: the normal tension lines of skin commonly used to define direction of scar, as to how the scar runs with or across those lines.

objective sign: one that can be seen, heard, measured, or felt by the diagnostician to confirm or deny an ongoing symptom. Also called *physical sign*.

quadriceps test: for hyperthyroidism or debilitating condition; while standing, the patient is asked to hold leg up and straight out; a disease is present if patient cannot maintain this position for 1 minute.

Raynaud phenomenon: pallor or blueness of fingers, toes, or nose brought about by exposure to cold and less commonly by other stresses.

somatic sign: any sign presented by trunk or limbs rather than sensory apparatus.

SCALES AND RATINGS

To have a reproducible presentation of the preoperative and postoperative condition of certain joints, various scales and rating systems have been developed. The scales and ratings are usually based on pain and the degree of functional impairment.

American shoulder and elbow system (ASES): a system for rating function in terms of activities of daily living, work, and sports; graded 0 to 4 from unable to function to no disability.

Frankel neurological assessment: for spinal cord injury.

Complete (A): No motor power below the level of the lesion

Sensory (B): No motor power but some sensation below the level of the lesion

Motor useless (C): Some motor power below the level of the lesion, but of no functional use to the patient

Motor useful (D): Motor power of functional use below the level of the lesion; the patient is able to walk with or without aids.

Recovery (E): Full motor power, normal sensation and no sphincter disturbance, although reflexes may be abnormal.

Mazur ankle rating: grading system for the ankle using pain and function as a basis for the rating.

Harris hip scale: a 100-point scale with 40 points for function and 60 for pain in the hip.

Lynholm knee-scoring scale: knee scale incorporating pain, swelling, function, and stability.

Marshall knee-scoring scale: knee scale including symptoms, function, and examination references

OTHER PHYSICAL EXAMINATION NOTATIONS

The portions of a physical examination that are not described as a test, sign, or maneuver include tests for ranges of motion, muscle strength and sensation, and sensory examinations. These tests are found under Physical medicine and rehabilitation and occupational therapy (Chapter 11).

5

Laboratory evaluations

Prerequisites for the diagnosis of musculoskeletal complaints are a thorough history and a clinical examination of the patient and, when necessary, an x-ray examination. From this information further carefully selected tests can be obtained from the laboratory.

This chapter discusses the examination of the blood and its components, synovial fluid, and the urine. The first section deals with those tests commonly performed as part of the routine evaluation of outpatients or preoperative patients. The next section discusses the laboratory findings of specific diseases as related to orthopaedics, taking into account that some generalized diseases result in orthopaedic problems. The definitions are designed to be comprehensive. Normal ranges of laboratory values must be reported according to accreditation and regulation with each laboratory result. Since normal values are dependent on the patient population, test methodology, and laboratory standardization, such values are not considered useful when published in textbooks, because they are likely to be misleading. Therefore, normal values have been deleted with this edition, and the initial statement or sentence in either section should be an adequate overview for those not concerned with the complete nature of the study.

Care must be exercised when using laboratory terminology, decimal points, significant figures in laboratory data, and other specific information. Forms are provided for most tests requested. Laboratory results should never be given over the telephone except in emergency situations. Requests may be emergency (stat), urgent, or routine.

A blood test may examine the quantity and type of cells, the level of chemicals in the serum, and (rarely) the chemical composition of the blood cell. For each laboratory test, the definition states what portion of blood is tested. For example, if it is a test on both cells and fluid of the blood, the phrase "whole blood" will be used.

The third and final section gives a list of laboratory abbreviations, normal laboratory results, and annotation of units.

ROUTINE EVALUATIONS (BLOOD, URINE, AND HEART)
CBC (complete blood count)

The CBC is a series of whole blood tests to determine the quantity or quality of blood cells. Some physicians prefer only a hemoglobin, hematocrit, and white count. Most laboratories use automated machines to provide all of the parameters as a part of a standard report, and a limited study such as an "H&H" is not cost-effective. The comprehensive CBC may include the following tests.

Hgb (Hb, hemoglobin): the percentage of iron-carrying protein in the blood depending on age and sex.

Hct (Hc, hematocrit): the volume of the blood occupied by red cells (the percentage of the volume of the blood).

H&H (hematocrit and hemoglobin): determination of hematocrit and hemoglobin levels only.

RBC (red blood count): the number of red cells (erythrocytes).

MCV (mean corpuscular volume): average volume per red cell.

MCH (mean corpuscular hemoglobin): the average amount of hemoglobin in each cell.

MCHC (mean corpuscular hemoglobin concentration): the average concentration of hemoglobin in the red cells and not of clinical value.

WBC (white blood count): number of white cells per cubic millimeter.

diff. (differential) percentage of white cell types: neutrophils (segmented and/or bands), lymphocytes, monocytes, eosinophils, basophils, and occasionally others. With present laboratory technology, the differential count may be performed manually by a technician using a microscope and counting chamber, or by an automated machine.

platelets (Plt): a blood test measuring the number of platelets (thrombocytes) per cubic millimeter of blood. Platelet counts are routinely done by automation. The values are an indication of a significant proportion of the patient's clotting capability.

bone marrow biopsy: laboratory test performed on bone marrow from the medullary cavity, such as the superior iliac crest, to determine under microscopic examination how blood-producing cells are performing.

Basic chemistry profile (formerly SMA-6)

This is a six-part test of blood chemistries of the serum.

Na (sodium): a major blood ion.

Cl (chloride): a blood salt (NaCl).

K (potassium): a blood salt.

HCO_3 (bicarbonate): a blood buffer.

glucose: a blood sugar.

BUN (blood urea nitrogen): a test for determining level of metabolic waste product normally cleared by the kidney, usually 10 to 20 mg/dl.

Expanded or general chemistry profile (formerly SMA-12)

The expanded chemistry profile uses 12 or more tests to produce a chemical profile. The following blood chemistry analyses are usually included in such a profile. Normal values may vary among laboratories and with age and sex.

total blood protein: total percentage of protein.

albumin: total albumin, as opposed to fractions of albumin. The amount of albumin compared with globulin (usually the rest of the protein) is called the *A/G ratio*.

Ca, P: calcium and phosphorus, the latter as phosphate in general, constitute the two main bone salts. The blood levels of these two elements do not necessarily denote bone problems.

cholesterol: a steroid-based fat that has been associated with predisposition to coronary artery disease. The level of cholesterol is dependent upon both genetic and dietary factors.

BUN: see basic chemistry profile.

UA (uric acid): metabolic by-product generally seen in high amounts in cases of gout. Elevated levels of uric acid are not necessarily correlated with acute attacks of gout.

Cr (creatinine): a metabolic by-product used as an index of kidney function.

total bilirubin: metabolic by-product of liver metabolism of hemoglobin.

ALP (serum alkaline phosphatase): enzyme present in bone, liver, and other organs.

LDH (lactic dehydrogenase): enzyme present in many organs.

AST (aspartate transaminase): enzyme present in many organs, particularly the liver.

ALT (alanine aminotransaminase): a nonspecific enzyme present in several organs, but generally used to measure evidence of liver damage.

Gamma GT (gamma-glutamyltransferase, gamma-glutamyltranspeptidase, GGTP): serum enzyme that is increased only in liver disease.

Urinalysis (UA, R & M [routine and microscopic])

The routine urinalysis includes a notation of the color, turbidity (appearance), specific gravity, pH (acidity or alkalinity), and sometimes the presence or absence of glucose, protein, bilirubin, ketone bodies, urobilinogen, and occult blood. A microscopic examination may be done on some sediment, and the material seen may be described as white cells, red cells, epithelial cells, and a variety of crystals and casts (microscopic debris usually from diseased kidneys). The quantity of cells and crystals is expressed in the number of observed objects per high-powered field (HPF) of the microscope, for example, six white cells per HPF, whereas the quantity of casts is expressed in the number of observed objects per low-powered field (LPF).

RESULTS OF LABORATORY FINDINGS

The general orthopaedic and related laboratory examinations and results found in this section are grouped according to similar disease processes, such as arthritis, infection, metabolic disturbances, and hematologic disorders, and also for assessment of spinal fluid and liver function.

However, these categories are not used as unit headings because the tests are often used to study a variety of problems, depending on the clinical circumstance. The orthopaedic laboratory workup may include any or all of the following.

sedimentation rate (sed. rate, erythrocyte sedimentation rate, ESR):

modified Westergren method: Test performed on anticoagulated whole blood to determine the speed of settling of cells in 1 hour. Three stages of sedimentation occur: (1) initial aggregation and rouleaux formation, (2) quick setting, and (3) packing. The normal ESR rate for males is 0 to 15 mm/hour and for females, 0 to 20 mm/hour. The test is nonspecific, similar to determination of temperature or pulse. An increased sedimentation rate may indicate certain conditions, particularly inflammation. Therefore this test is often used in evaluating bone and joint infections and other inflammatory disease. This rate may be corrected from values obtained from tables to take into account changes resulting from the amount of red cells (hematocrit) present. The corrected sedimentation rate is represented as follows: 21/11, meaning the sedimentation rate is 21 mm/hour, but because of anemia, it is corrected to 11 mm/hour.

bentonite flocculation test (BFT): for rheumatoid arthritis; usually given in terms of tube dilution ratios.

HLA factor: precisely, the HLA-B27 factor present in patients with ankylosing spondylitis.

CRP (carbohydrate reactive protein, C-reactive protein): a general serologic test that indicates the presence of inflammatory disease.

rheumatoid factor (RA factor): a serologic test to determine the presence of certain antibodies. This may be done in test tubes or on a slide (RA slide test). Some centers refer to this as a *rheumatoid arthritis agglutinin (RAAGG) test*. All these are screening tests and are reported as positive or negative. Also called *latex fixation test.*

Rose-Waaler test: a dilution test of serum, reported in fractions; a dilution of 1/32 or greater is considered significant. This means that the serum can be diluted five times and still be positive.

ASO titer (antistreptolysin O): this test is done mostly on children with joint complaints who are suspected of having rheumatic fever. The most significant finding for this test is an increase in the values over a period of a week. The reports may be given as a tube dilution ratio, such as 1/256, or in Todd units, which is the inverse number. A value of 160 Todd units or less is considered normal.

antinuclear factor (ANF): an immunologic screening test that reveals the presence of serum antibodies against cellular nuclear material (DNA); usually reported as positive or negative. The disease most commonly associated with significant positive values is lupus erythematosus.

antidouble stranded (native) DNA: test for antibodies against the genetic chemical information in the cell; a refined test for diagnosing systemic lupus erythematosus.

LE prep (lupus erythematosus preparation): specific test for lupus erythematosus. A blood smear of white blood cells is inspected under the microscope for large intracellular collections of nuclear material; reported as either positive or negative.

synovial fluid evaluation: evaluation of synovial fluid for the type and quantity of cells in the fluid. The normal white count of synovial fluid is considered to be 200 cells/microliter as the upper limit of normal. The leukocyte count is performed in a standard hemocytometer. In septic arthritis, the leukocyte count is almost always greater than 50,000 cells/μl. However, an occasional patient with gout, pseudogout, or rheumatoid arthritis may have counts in this range. Noninflammatory synovial findings reveal a white count of up to 5,000 with less than 30% polymorphonuclear leukocytes. In inflammatory synovitis, a 2,000 to 200,000 white count can be anticipated with greater than 50% polys. In infectious or septic arthritis, greater than 90% polymorphonuclear leukocytes can be expected. In crystal-induced arthritis, the synovial cell count can be 500 to 200,000 with less than 90% polymorphonuclear leukocytes. In hemorrhagic arthritis 50 to 10,000 white cells may be present, but fewer than 50% are polymorphonuclear leukocytes.

Gram stains are routinely performed for the detection of infectious arthritis, and, under certain circumstances, fungal and mycobacterial cultures are done. Viscosity is useful, usually indicating a noninflammatory process, when associated with a normal-appearing synovial fluid. Inflammatory (nonseptic) synovitis usually results in a synovial fluid that clots while standing. Polarization microscopy is useful in distinguishing the two types of crystal-induced arthritis. These include gout and pseudogout allowing the distinction between uric acid crystals seen in gout and certain calcium salt crystals in pseudogout.

C&S (culture and sensitivity): bacteria from a wound, urine, blood, throat, or any other source are placed into a tube or on a plate. The results of bacterial cultures are usually listed by organism and its antimicrobial sensitivity.

typical bacterial species reports: the following bacterial species are encountered in laboratory studies; they are listed for spelling purposes, without definitions. The term *common flora* denotes the presence of normal, nonpathogenic bacteria in throat cultures.

Staphylococcus aureus (Staph. aureus)
Streptococcus organisms
Escherichia coli (E. coli)
Pseudomonas organisms
Klebsiella organisms
Salmonella organisms
Neisseria gonorrhoeae (gonorrhea)
Mycobacterium tuberculosis
Mycobacterium organisms (atypical)

Common fungal organisms are:
Actinomyces
Blastomyces
Histoplasma
Coccidiodes

colony count (CC): the placement of a known amount of urine on culture media; the report is usually given in number of bacteria per milliliter of urine.

anaerobic culture: bacterial culture grown in the absence of oxygen (obligate anaerobes), or minimal free oxygen (facultative anaerobes). Certain organisms require this environment for growth, in contrast to the standard aerobic cultures grown in the presence of normal oxygen.

special culture: various specific growth media are used for certain organisms (that is, bacteria causing gonorrhea and tuberculosis, and fungi). A bacteriology text should be consulted for more specific information.

Gram stain: a general stain used on microscopic slide specimens to aid in seeing various organisms and to estimate their numbers. Depending on their color after the processing, they will be described as gram-positive or gram-negative. This aids in the initial selection of antibiotics that are likely to be useful. Also, white blood cells should be noted in sputum and wound specimens to indicate whether one is dealing with colonization or actual infection.

acid-fast bacillus (AFB): refers to the bright red appearance of mycobacteria when stained with a specific chemical and observed under a microscope. A more efficient method involving fluorescence microscopy is now available.

FTA (fluorescent treponema antibody): serologic test for syphilis; usually interpreted as positive or negative, but may be reported in dilutions. Other tests commonly used are the VDRL (Venereal Disease Research Laboratories), STS (serologic test for syphilis), and *dark-field microscopic examination*, a direct visualization of the live syphilis organisms in penile and perineal chancre preparations.

tine test: a skin test for tuberculosis. Four small pinpricks are made in the skin; 48 to 72 hours later the reaction is observed; usually reported as postive or negative.

PPD (purified protein derivative): a subcutaneous injection of various strengths (most commonly intermediate) of inactive tubercular material; the reactions may be read as positive or negative 48 to 72 hours later. However, the size of the erythematous response or induration may be recorded in millimeters.

FBS (fasting blood sugar): test most commonly done to detect diabetes. Blood sample has to be obtained at least 6 to 12 hours after the last meal. In the past, a glucose tolerance test (GTT) was a 2-to 5-hour study of both the blood and urine obtained from a patient who had taken 75 grams of sugar after fasting. The most efficient GTT is a fasting and 2-hour postprandial (after eating) blood glucose. If these values are abnormal according to the expected values for that particular laboratory, diabetes mellitus can be diagnosed.

Three different sets of criteria are available for interpreting the plasma glucose levels in the GTT. These include the NDDG (National Diabetes Data Group), the WHO (World Health Organization) criteria, and age-related expected values for glucose criteria. Those values are available on request from your laboratory. There is no value in performing a 3-to 5-hour GTT.

T_3, T_4 (thyroxin), and TSH (thyroid stimulating hormone): measures of a level of thyroid active hormones and the pituitary hormone-controlling thyroid function. There are various methods for determining these levels to help recognize hyper- and hypothyroidism. A caution in interpreting such values should be made in chronically ill patients.

ALP (alkaline phosphatase, alk PO_4 tase): test to determine the level of this enzyme. The most common sources of high values are rapid growth or fracture healing. In any growth spurt the value may be as high as two and one-half times normal. Other bony disorders causing alkaline phosphatase include Paget's disease, primary bone tu-

mors, some metastatic diseases, and osteomalacia. Because elevations in alkaline phosphatase can result from liver disorders, two additional tests may be performed: (1) heating the enzyme will destroy it if it comes from the liver, and (2) abnormally high values of *serum gamma glutamyl transpeptidase (gamma GT)* indicate liver disease. Isoenzymes of alkaline phosphatase can be measured indicating the organ of origin.

serum calcium (Ca): measures serum calcium concentration. Serum calcium levels are increased in hyperparathyroidism, while there is a concurrent decrease in serum phosphorus (PO_4). The phosphorus determination in parathyroid disease is dependent on renal function. Determination of calcium and phosphorus levels is commonly done as a screening measure; many diseases will affect the blood levels of these two chemicals.

serum lead level: in cases of lead poisoning the serum can be measured for that element specifically. Because lead is a heavy metal, the heavy metal screening test is used to determine the presence of lead poisoning.

mucopolysaccharides: test done on the urine to determine the excretion of abnormal amounts of specific mucopolysaccharides that are seen in diseases causing dwarfism, mental retardation, and other congenital problems.

CPK (creatine-phosphokinase): a test of serum enzyme. In muscle disorders, particularly muscular dystrophy, it is elevated. In the cases of suspected acute myocardial infarction, isoenzyme determinations are helpful.

creatinine: by-product of metabolism that is cleared by the kidney. A 2-hour creatinine clearance (Ccr) can be performed.

salicylates: a test that can be done on the blood to determine the specific levels of salicylate or on the urine as a screening test for the presence of aspirin. This can be done to follow the treatment of arthritis or in the event of an accidental overdose.

APTT (activated partial thromboplastin time): a sensitive test for monitoring patients receiving heparin to retard blood clotting.

pro time (prothrombin time): a test for blood

clotting commonly done to monitor patients taking blood thinners such as warfarin sodium (Coumadin).

PTT (partial thromboplastin time): test of the clotting mechanism in the blood, usually used to monitor a patient in anticoagulant therapy.

hemoglobin electrophoresis: a test to determine types of protein and red cell hemoglobin. Abnormalities are present in sickle cell disease, thalassemia, and other red cell disorders. The results of this test are reported as normal or described by the specific abnormality.

ALT (alanine transaminase): a serum test of an enzyme normally found increased in patients with liver disease.

ACP (acid phosphatase): a serum assay test for acid phosphatase activity. Elevations are usually associated with disease of the prostate, particularly cancer. Prostate specific antigen is increased in prostatic disease, particularly in prostatic cancer.

SPE (serum protein electrophoresis): a serum test to determine the presence and amount of particular protein; used to detect multiple myeloma—a report of a high gamma M or monoclonal pattern may indicate myeloma. An *immunoelectrophoresis* is a similar test reporting mg/dl of IgG, IgA, and IgM. The various components of the serum protein electrophoresis pattern and immunoelectrophoresis pattern can now be determined accurately.

reticulocyte count: a blood cell test to determine the increase in number of young red blood cells often seen in patients with anemia. When observed under the microscope, only 1 out of 100 red cells will normally show a particular stain within the cell wall. If there is more than 1%, there is probably increased blood formation.

blood volume: test of whole blood, usually done with radioactive tracers and reported in liters. The normal findings vary with the size and age of the patient. A *cell volume* can be done in a similar fashion.

blood gases: a measurement of the vapor pressure of oxygen (O_2) and carbon dioxide (CO_2) in the blood. The oxygen is usually presented with a percent saturation value, which is normally above 90%. The pH of the blood is simultaneously determined.

CSF (cerebrospinal fluid): a study that includes the following:

protein: normally 45 mg/dl.

glucose: normally two thirds that of the blood; decreased in bacterial infections.

cells: normally 0/cu mm to 3/cu mm; when an increased number of cells are present, they are divided into polys and lymphs.

culture: some fluid is placed on a growth medium to see if any organisms are present; occasionally, a slide is made from a smear of the fluid and a stain done directly to determine the presence of bacteria.

latex agglutination test: for various bacterial pathogens in cerebrospinal fluid, this allows a very rapid diagnosis of the bacterial causes of meningitis.

flow cytometry: for evaluation of tumors, a suspension of cells is passed by the path of an optical device that is able to measure the relative amounts of DNA. This may help in the relative grading of the tumor cells.

Blood bank procedures and products*

T&C (type and crossmatch): red blood cell products are tested for the antigenic components and antibody components; the most common are the ABO group and the Rh group. There is subgrouping for the Rh factors and for many other antigenic components. For this reason each unit of blood to be given to a patient must be crossmatched with the recipient's serum to the donor blood. A report is normally not given unless the request for specific blood type is made.

T&S (type and screen): the potential blood recipient is tested for most of the various antigenic components and antibodies likely to lead to hemolytic transfusion reaction. If the need arises for actual transfusion, crossmatch is then performed, or under emergency circumstances, the blood can be released without crossmatch.

---

*Prepared in part by Patrick Monaghan, PhD. Associate Professor, Clinical Pathology, George Washington University Medical Center, Washington, D.C.

direct Coombs test (direct antihuman globulin test): performed on patient's red blood cells to detect the presence of antibodies or complement components attached to the cells. The red cells with attached antibodies or complement components usually have a shortened life.

indirect Coombs test (indirect antihuman globulin test): performed on patient's serum to detect the presence of abnormal circulating antibodies. Presence of these atypical antibodies may cause a transfusion reaction. If present in women of childbearing age, these antibodies may be the etiologic agent in hemolytic disease of the newborn (erythroblastosis fetalis).

isoantibodies: circulating, naturally occurring antibodies, which are usually of the IgM classification of immunoglobulins. Group O individuals usually have isoantibodies A and B in their plasma.

alloantibodies: circulating atypical antibodies that are the result of prior antigenic stimulation from previous transfusion of blood products or pregnancy. The presence of these antibodies may cause delay in locating compatible blood products.

autologous blood: the patient's own blood that has been collected for elective surgery. It can be stored in the liquid state at 39.2° F (4° C) for 21 to 35 days, or the red cell concentrate may be frozen at −112° F (−80° C) for 3 years.

MSBOS (maximal surgical blood order schedule): a number of hospitals are establishing limits on the quantity of blood that is crossmatched or typed and held for various elective surgical procedures. These limits are based on the actual quantities of blood transfused per procedure, for example, total hip replacement, recommended type and screen (T and S).

HB$_s$Ag(HADD): test performed on donor blood to detect the presence of the hepatitis B surface antigen. This is also necessary in preventing transmission of hepatitis to a blood recipient. Its presence is detectable in certain patients who currently have, or have previously had clinical or subclinical hepatitis B. This test is negative in patients with hepatits A, or non-A, non-B hepatitis.

anti-human immune virus (anti-HTLD III): test for antibodies to the virus causing *auto*immune *de*ficiency *s*yndrome (AIDS). It is performed mainly in potential blood donors to prevent the transmission of this disease to blood recipients. In patients, it is used to detect those who are suspected of having AIDS.

intraoperative autologous transfusion (IAT): the intraoperative recovery of red cells for reinfusion during the course of surgery. The efficiency of this system has been improved with a hemodilution technique.

factor VIII and factor IX: blood coagulant factors that may be absent or significantly reduced in hereditary hemophilia A&B. These factors and certain specially prepared blood products are available for replacement in acquired disorders of the labile coagulant system.

Blood bank products

red cells: the main blood component remaining after plasma and platelets have been removed from whole blood. It has the identical red cell mass as whole blood and therefore provides the same oxygen-carrying capacity in a smaller volume. The removal of plasma also reduces the risk of transfusion reaction caused by donor isoantibodies and alloantibodies. Red cell products may be stored at 39.2° F (4° C) in the blood bank as packed red blood cells. Recent technologic advances also make it feasible to store this product in a frozen state at −112° F (−80° C) for 3 years. Patients who have a history of febrile reaction to bank-stored packed red cells should receive washed and thawed frozen red cell concentrates.

fresh frozen plasma (FFP): approximately 220 to 250 ml of fresh human plasma, which contains all of the known coagulation proteins. All these coagulation proteins are maintained at 80% to 100% levels for 1 year when the plasma is frozen; used for the replacement of coagulation proteins.

platelet concentrate: contains approximately 5.5 x 10^{10} platelets in 30 to 50 ml of volume. One unit of platelet concentrate is that quantity fractionated from one unit (450 ml) of whole blood. The shelf life of a unit of platelet concentrate is

72 hours depending on the storage. Platelet concentrates are transfused into bleeding patients who exhibit thrombocytopenia (decrease in number of platelets), for example.

cryoprecipitate: a blood plasma product that contains clotting factor I (fibrinogen), factor VIII (antihemophiliac factor in 10 to 25 ml of volume), and factor XIII. It is stored in a frozen state at $-0.4°$ F ($-18°$ C) or lower for 1 year; used in the treatment of classic hemophilic, von Willebrand disease, and fibrinogen replacement. Each unit (bag) of cryoprecipitate contains approximately 80 to 110 units of clotting factor VIII. Cryoprecipitates may also be a rich source of opsonic proteins.

albumin: a commercial product prepared from fractionated human plasma; generally available in concentrations of 5% to 25%; used for blood volume expansion and replacement of protein.

immune serum globulins: various gamma (IgG) globulins produced from sensitized individuals whose serum contains these antibodies; used for disease prophylaxis or attenuation, for example, $Rh_O(D)$. Immune globulin is given to $Rh_O(D)$-negative women to prevent the sensitization to the Rh antigen and the resulting potential for Rh hemolytic disease of the newborn.

blood plasma substitutes: synthetic plasma substances used for blood volume expansion, for example, dextran, hydroxyethyl starch (HES), and Ringer's lactate.

LABORATORY ABBREVIATIONS
Whole blood or clotting

CBC: complete blood count
Hct, Hc: hematocrit
Hgb, Hb: hemoglobin
H&H: hematocrit and hemoglobin
WBC: white blood (cell) count
wbc: white blood cell
diff: differential
   polys: neutrophils, polymorphonucleocytes, granulocytes
     segs: segmented
     nonsegs: nonsegmented, bands, stabs, juveniles

   lymphs: lymphocytes
   monos: monocytes
   basos: basophils
   eos: eosinophils
RBC: red blood (cell) count
rbc: red blood cell
MCV: mean corpuscular volume
MCH: mean corpuscular hemoglobin
MCHC: mean corpuscular hemoglobin concentration
Plt: platelet (thrombocyte)
T&C: type and crossmatch
T&S: type and screen
Rh: rhesus monkey factor ($Rh_O[D]$)
ABO: groups A, B, AB, and O blood
FFP: fresh frozen plasma
IAT: intraoperative autologous transfusion
MSBOS: maximal surgical blood order schedule
ESR: erythrocyte sedimentation rate
CSR: corrected sedimentation rate
LE prep: lupus erythematosus preparation
APTT: activated partial thromboplastin time
PTT: partial thromboplastin time
PT (pro time): prothrombin time

Serum chemistries

Na: sodium
Cl: chloride
K: potassium
HCO_3: bicarbonate
BUN: blood urea nitrogen
FBS: fasting blood sugar
Ca: calcium
PO_4: phosphorus (inorganic)
Chol: cholesterol
UA: uric acid (or urinalysis)
CR: creatinine
Alb: albumin
Glob: globulin
A/G: albumin/globulin ratio
ACP: acid phosphatase
ALP: (alk Po_4tase) alkaline phosphatase
GGTP: gamma glutamyltranspeptidase, same as gamma glutamyltransferase
AST: aspartate transaminase
ALT: alanine transaminase
LDH: lactic dehydrogenase

Bil: bilirubin
GTT: glucose tolerance test
CPK: creatine phosphokinase
SPE: serum protein electrophoresis

Serology

RA slide: rheumatoid arthritis slide test
RF: rheumatoid factor
RAAGG: rheumatoid arthritis agglutination
ASO: antistreptolysin O
ANF: antinuclear factor
anti-DNA: anti-deoxyribonucleic acid
FTA: fluorescent treponemal antibody
VDRL: Veneral Disease Research Laboratory
STS: serologic test for syphilis
SPE: serum protein electrophoresis
HB-Ag: hepatitis B antigen
anti HLTD III: antibody screen in testing for AIDS
HIV: human immunodeficiency virus. (Cause of AIDS—*auto*immune *d*eficiency *s*yndrome)

Urine

UA: urinalysis
R&M: routine and microscopic (of urine)
Ccr: creatinine clearance
pH: concentration of hydrogen ions
GLU: glucose and other reducing agents
Ace: acetone
Prot: protein
sG or sp gr: specific gravity
HPF: high-power field
HDF: high dry field

Other

PPD: purified protein derivative (TB skin test)
C&S: culture and sensitivity
CC: colony count
T_3: L-triiodothyronine (thyroxin)
T_4: L-tetraiodothyronine (thyroxin)
TSH: thyroid stimulating hormone
EKG or ECG: electrocardiogram
AFB: acid-fast bacteria
spec: specimen
CSF: cerebrospinal fluid
MSBOS: maximum surgical order schedule
IAT: intraoperative autologous transfusion

ANNOTATION OF UNITS
Weights

ng: nanogram = 1/1,000,000,000 gram
μg, mcg: microgram = 1/1,000,000 gram
mg: milligram = 1/1,000 gram
gm: gram (454 gm = 1 pound)
kg: kilogram = 1,000 grams = 2.2 pounds

Volume (fluid or gas)

μl, mcl: microliter = 1/1,000,000 liter
ml: milliliter = 1/1,000 liter
L: liter = 0.943 quarts (1 quart = 1.06 L)
dl: deciliter = 1/10 liter

Volume (space)

$μm^3$: cubic micrometer
mm^3: cubic millimeter
cc: cubic centimeter, cm^3
M^3: cubic meter

Length

μm: micrometer = 1/1,000,000 meter
mm: millimeter = 1/1,000 meter
cm: centimeter (0.39 inches; 2.54 cm = inch)
M: meter (39.37 inches)

Other parameters

mg/dl: milligrams per deciliter or milligram percent; the number of milligrams per 100 ml of fluid.
gm/dl: gram per deciliter or gram percent; the number of grams per 100 ml of fluid.
mEq: milliequivalent, 1/1,000 equivalent.
Eq: equivalent, 6.23 x 10_23 ionic charges.

Units

U: units, not to be confused with μ, which denotes 1/1,000,000.
IU: International Units; a new system of annotation of metric units agreed upon internationally and being instituted in the United States. Basically, the notation grams per 0.1 liter (gm/dl) is replacing grams percent (gm%) or grams per 100 cubic centimeters (cu cm or cc) of fluid. Certain specific rules have been recommended for use of the system, called the SI System from

Le Système Internationale d'Unitès, or the International System of Units.

1. Omit periods in abbreviations (kg, mm, ml, mg).
2. Omit plurals (70 kg, not 70 kgs).
3. Avoid commas as a spacer in expressing large numbers. (In some countries, the comma is used as a decimal.)
4. Compound prefixes should not be used (10^{-9} x meter = nanometer, not millimicrometer [mμm]).
5. Omit degree sign for Kelvin scale (310 K, not 310° K).
6. Multiples and submultiples are used in steps of 10^3 or 10^{-3}.
7. Only one solidus (/) may be used when indicating "per" or a denominator: acceleration = velocity per second; m/s^2, not m/s/s.
8. When the compound unit is derived from the multiplication of two base units, a point (·) is used to so indicate. Torque is the newton-meter, therefore N·m, not Nm.
9. The preferred spelling is meter not metre, liter not litre, kilogram not kilogramme.

F: Fahrenheit.
C: Centigrade; Celsius.

Routine physiologic parameters

vital signs: the easily measurable sustaining functions, which include temperature, pulse, respiration (rate), and blood pressure. These vital signs have been and will continue to be the major index of a patient's general progress.

height and weight: taken into consideration in an orthopaedic workup, since many back problems are related to the stress that being overweight places on the vertebrae.

EKG (electrocardiogram): recorded measurement of the spontaneous electric activity of the heart, using multiple leads to assess the heart from a variety of directions. This study is commonly obtained before surgery to give a baseline in the event of operative or postoperative cardiac complications, such as pulmonary embolus or cardiac arrest.

EEG (electroencephalogram): recorded measurement of the spontaneous electric activity of the brain, using multiple leads placed on the head and ears. This study is obtained to detect certain seizures and brain disorders and the lack of activity when there has been severe damage leading to brain death.

6

Casts, splints, dressings, and in-house traction

In presenting the various methods of care for fractures, dislocations, and postoperative management of patients, it is most appropriate to begin with the role of the orthopaedic nurses and technicians, to whom this realm of responsibility is generally delegated.

Although some orthopaedists in private practice do immobilization procedures themselves, in group practice and larger institutions, the orthopaedic nurses and technicians assist in providing these services. These qualified individuals work in the hospital clinics, wings (wards), emergency rooms, and depending on educational background and training and hospital policies, may "scrub in" on orthopaedic surgical procedures in the operating room or may assist with minor procedures in the physician's office.

The orthopaedic nurse, in addition to basic nursing skills, specializes in musculoskeletal pathology and care of patients requiring fracture management, who have had or will require surgical procedures, and who do not require surgery but have other musculoskeletal problems. This includes the responsibility of proper application of traction, weights, and various equipment used in patient rehabilitation. Under the supervision of the nursing staff, the technician assists in setting up traction appliances, circ-O-lectric (special mechanical) beds, and similar devices of care. Administrative tasks are shared in ordering supplies and equipment for the plaster room, examining rooms, wings, and the clinic and conferring with suppliers regarding supply catalog items.

The orthopaedic technician is skilled in the art of cast application, utilizing the many types of casts for specific injuries or conditions—that is, plaster of Paris, plastics, and fiberglass—and instructing patients on cast care and prevention of complications. In the clinical setting technicians must maintain and prepare the plaster room for specific procedures as well as the cleanup duties that follow.

In addition, these individuals may assist the physician in measuring, fitting, and altering braces, splints, and orthoses for patients. They may teach patients the use of these devices, and assist them in learning crutch-assisted walking, how to ascend and descend stairs, and various home exercises following immobilization.

The orthopaedic specialty is so diversified and changing that there is a need for continuing medical education for the nursing staff and technicians. Many opportunities are offered through AAOS instructional courses throughout the country and within the organizations of orthopaedics.

The National Association of Orthopaedic Nurses (NAON), founded in 1980, is the professional organization designed to assist the orthopaedic nurse in further developing skills in the management and care of orthopaedic patients. The NAON provides support and educational opportunities through its sponsored activities.

The National Association of Orthopaedic Technologists (NAOT) is the professional organization for the technician. The NAOT offers a certifying exam given by the National Board of Orthopaedic

Technologists (NBOT). These organizations within the orthopaedic community seek to promote the highest standards of care and are an integral part of the orthopaedic team.

This chapter discusses and defines the materials applied and prescribed by an orthopaedist or assigned individual in the direct care of patients and the teamwork necessary for this care.

• • •

The techniques used in cast immobilization, splints, dressings, and traction devices are designed to provide an external means of support or protective covering while healing proceeds under optimal conditions. The purpose of any type of casting is to immobilize a part in order to maintain or obtain a correction of deformity, promote alignment following surgery, and to give support to damaged soft tissues in the healing process of fractures, dislocations, and sprains.

In traditional usage the term *cast* applies to a circumferentially wrapped plaster of Paris-impregnated bandage or encasement applied to a portion of the body. Technology has provided additional materials, such as fiberglass and plastics, that are sometimes used instead of plaster of Paris.

The term *splint* applies to a rigid or semirigid, noncircumferential material used to reinforce a soft dressing or to provide additional support for or immobilization of the body part being treated. The splint may be made of plaster of Paris, metal, wood, plastic, or, in an emergency, newspapers or magazines.

The term *dressing* applies to those materials used to cover a wound or surgical incision, a fabric with or without accessory medications or self-adhesive properties.

The term *bandage* applies to a nonrigid, usually cotton material that may be used to hold a dressing in place or act as the dressing by itself. It may be applied to provide padding over a body prominence under a cast. A bandage can provide elastic support for a joint or soft tissue in controlling circulation; this is called an elastic bandage.

Traction devices refer to any adjustable external appliances used in early treatment of fractures that suspend or deliver pull to any given part of the body.

Casting materials have changed considerably over the past 10 years. However, plaster of Paris casts are still widely used and familiar to all practitioners. These rolled crinoline bandages are impregnated with gypsum powder (calcium salt) that, when exposed to water, crystallizes. The reaction then slows to a maturation process (hardening) that takes approximately 24 hours to dry. The heat felt by the patient is the crystallization process that takes place within the cast material. Fabricating and molding plaster of Paris bandages is considered an art, and the technician soon learns the numerous techniques of application.

Fiberglass casts have become a popular form of treatment. They are lightweight, radiolucent, easier to apply, can tolerate moisture, and harden within 30 minutes, allowing for immediate weight-bearing. This type consists of fiberglass and resin, fiberglass and plastic polymer, and polyurethane that also crystallize on exposure to water. The polyurethane type differs in that the reaction time for hardening is within 30 minutes to maturity. Most fiberglass casts are long-wearing.

CAST MATERIALS

cast padding: a synthetic fiber rolled padding used with fiberglass casts.

cotton roll: material made from cotton that can be rolled as a bandage and acts as a buffer between the skin and plaster material. Also called *Webril*.

felt padding: thick felt or feltlike material added to the undersurface of a cast on local areas of bony prominences or pressure areas.

fiberglass cast: lightweight fiberglass material that is "cured" after being wrapped and exposed to ultraviolet light or water, which makes the material firm. Also called *light cast*.

moleskin: adhesive, thin, velvetlike material used to smooth edges of casts or to buffer areas of excessive skin wear.

plaster rolls: gauze roll impregnated with plaster of Paris, which when dipped in warm water can be applied, rolled smoothly, and molded, becoming hard within minutes.

Scotchcast: composed of lightweight plastic material that becomes rigid when applied.

sheet wadding: strong, cotton material that clings to part being applied and molded to contour of that part. Contraindicated where swelling is great (after an operation).

stockinette: a cloth stocking roll used in many cast applications; comes in many sizes; can be covered by padding followed by firm cast material.

CAST IMMOBILIZATION

Cast immobilization may involve the following anatomic areas: upper extremity, lower extremity, cervical region, spinal (vertebrae), or hip and shoulder joint areas (called *spica*), which incorporates the limb and a portion of the trunk. The various types are described by the portion of anatomy involved.

Body casts

A body cast, a circumferential cast enclosing the trunk of the body, may extend from the head or upper chest to the groin or thigh. This type of cast immobilization is used in treating diseases of the cervical, thoracic, and lumbar spines such as fractures and scoliosis, or it may be applied following some types of surgery on the spine. There are several types of body casts.

flexion body cast: a chest-groin cast in which the patient is positioned so that the trunk is flexed forward; usually used in treatment of painful lower back conditions.

extension body cast: a chest-groin cast in which the patient is positioned so that the trunk is extended backward; usually applied for specific fractures.

scoliosis cast: a special modification of the body cast, used in preoperative and postoperative treatment of scoliosis (curvature of the spine). Modifications of this type are:

Cotrel cast: modified scoliosis cast applied following Cotrel traction.

turnbuckle cast: a special modification to allow changes in angle by use of turnbuckles on either side of the cast.

Risser localizer: specialized body cast with localizer pressing over convex side of curve.

halo cast: for cervical fractures: a thoracic to pelvic level cast incorporating the necessary extensions used to support the posts that are attached to a metal halo skeletally affixed to the head.

Minerva jacket: cast immobilization extending upward along the side and in back of the head and neck, incorporating a plaster of Paris headband; used in fractures of the neck and in certain scoliosis problems.

Spica cast

A spica cast is used to immobilize an appendage by incorporating a part of the body proximal to that appendage. The most common spica casts are hip, thumb, and shoulder spicas. They are listed by anatomy in the following sections.

Upper limb casts

arm cylinder cast: a long-arm cast with the elbow flexed and the wrist free.

banjo cast: cast with a large ring extension that goes past the fingers and then holds the fingers in extension by the use of rubber bands or string; was originally used for distal radial fractures and is now used for finger and toe injuries.

Dehne cast (three-finger spica): cast incorporating the thumb with a separate extension incorporating the index and middle fingers; used to treat fractures of the navicula.

figure 8 cast: a cast applied around both shoulders, crossing at the back in the form of an 8; used in treatment of clavicular fractures. It is now more common to use a soft dressing.

gauntlet cast: a short cast extending from slightly above or proximal to the wrist to some point in the palm; usually has some outrigger to control one or more digits; used for metacarpal and phalangeal fractures or dislocations.

hanging arm cast: a long-arm cast that, through suspension from a sling around the neck, brings about traction of fracture fragments, of the humerus.

long-arm cast (LAC): cast extending from the palm and wrist to the axilla, preventing movement at the elbow; used in treatment of fractures of the forearm, elbow, and humerus. *Cottonloader position cast* is a special long-arm cast used for certain distal forearm fractures.

short-arm cast (SAC): any of a number of casts extending from the elbow to the palm or digits; commonly used for distal forearm and wrist fractures.

shoulder spica (airplane cast): a cast that incorporates the upper torso and envelopes a part or all of the extremity in a position of abduction; used for proximal humeral fractures and rotator cuff tears.

thumb spica: short- or long-arm cast that incorporates the thumb; used in treatment of navicular fractures.

Lower limb casts

hip spica: cast incorporating the lower torso and extending to one or both lower extremities. Various types are the following:

single hip spica: a cast incorporating the lower torso and entire position of only one leg; commonly used for femoral fractures.

1½ spica: a cast that incorporates the lower torso, the entire affected limb, and the opposite limb to just above the knee; used for proximal femoral fractures and some pelvic fractures.

double hip spica: a cast incorporating both the lower torso and lower limbs, usually because of bilateral fractures of the hips, femur, and/or tibia.

Petrie spica cast (broom-stick): a specially applied cast for abduction to assist in ambulation for Legg-Perthes disease.

long-leg cast (LLC): a non-weight-bearing cast extending from the upper thigh to the toes; most commonly used for fractures of the tibia and fibula or ligamentous injuries of the knee.

long-leg walking cast (LLWC): a cast from the upper thigh to the toes, with an attached rubber sole device called a walker.

Quengle cast: for flexion contracture of the knee, a two-part cast hinged at the knee level, with the lower end of the cast ending at the ankle or foot, and the above-knee portion ending at the upper thigh.

well-leg cast: casts applied to both lower extremities and then attached together; used in some rare instances for treatment of femoral fractures.

cylinder cast: cast from proximal thigh to just above the ankle, most commonly used for injuries of the knee.

short-leg cast (SLC): a non-weight-bearing cast extending from just below the knee to the toes; used in injuries of the ankle and foot.

short-leg walking cast (SLWC): cast with an attached rubber walker or reinforced to accept a cast shoe used for ankle and foot injuries.

patellar tendon weight-bearing cast (PTB): also known as a *Sarmiento cast;* a short-leg cast with a walker; a special feature is the molding about the knee; used for management of tibial fractures.

slipper cast: cast incorporating the foot up to the ankle; used as a rigid postoperative dressing following forefoot procedures.

toe spica: cast specifically designed to incorporate all of the great toe and a portion or all of the foot; usually used after bunion surgery.

gel cast: a semirigid paste cast, usually applied to the lower leg and foot for ankle injuries or swelling. Also called *Unna boot.*

Other cast terms

bivalve cast: a cast that is split in half by cuts made on opposite sides of the cast to release pressure or allow removal and reapplication of the cast such as would be needed for physical therapy treatments.

Boston bivalve: cast split in half with a step cut rather than a straight line; most often used when the cast is going to be removed often for physical therapy and then reapplied.

univalve cast: a cast split on one side to relieve pressure.

cast boot: rubber and canvas device that looks like a large shoe, which can fit over the end of a cast for walking. Also called cast shoe, plaster boot.

collar and cuff: a design of sling with a soft portion wrapped around the neck, and a cufflike device wrapped around to support the distal forearm; often used in humeral fractures treated with a coaptation splint.

corrective cast: a cast used to correct deformity

by nonsurgical technique; commonly applied to clubfeet.

petaling edges: to eliminate abrasion from the edge of a cast, small vertical slits are made at the edges of the cast, and then the edges (petals) are folded out and held in place by adhesive tape, moleskin, or other material.

serial casts: any sequence of casts used in the progressive correction of deformity.

walker (walking heel): hard rubber wedge directly incorporated into the sole of a cast to allow walking or resting the leg on the ground.

wedge: circumferential cutting of the cast and reapplication of plaster over the same cast after a manipulation has been performed to change bony position.

closing wedge: removal of a segment of plaster, with closing of that wedge by manipulation and reapplication of plaster.

opening wedge: circular cut cast that is opened by manipulation and then covered with a new layer of plaster.

window: removal of a piece of cast, usually square or rectangular, to allow inspection of a wound or relieve pressure at a specific point. Also said, to "fenestrate."

DEVICES APPLIED TO CASTS

abduction bar: to help maintain hip abduction, any bar placed between two long-leg casts.

cast brace: modifications of standard casts often applied to facilitate early motion. The cast brace is designed with normal physiology in mind while still protecting the fracture site; it is molded in the manner of prosthetic-type devices. In addition, it is usually hinged at the joints to allow free motion of joints and to improve muscle recovery.

electrical stimulation: direct electric current applied to bone fractures that are immobilized in a cast, whereby current is delivered by a battery device contained outside or buried within the skin; designed to aid in fracture healing, inducing early callus formation.

magnets: electromagnetic coils applied on templates that have been placed on the surface of the cast, allowing placement of the magnets directly over the fracture site. Pulsating electromagnetic fields (PEMF) are being used to stimulate bone formation, particularly in cases of delayed bone formation or delayed union.

CAST COMPLICATIONS

There are numerous complications due to cast treatment. The related terms are listed here in conjunction with the description of cast treatment and application.

burns: applying casting material with water temperature too warm, added to the crystallization process that produces heat, can produce skin burns.

constrictive edema: disruption of normal venous drainage with resulting fluid accumulation in soft tissue and swelling distal to the point of constriction caused by circulatory impairment.

decubitus ulcer: an area of pressure necrosis caused by patient lying in same position; also results from continuous or uneven pressure applied with continued immobility; commonly occurs at the rims of cast and heel. Also called *pressure sore*.

dropfoot: when referring to a complication of cast treatment, applies to paralysis of the peroneal nerve resulting from pressure over the fibula head with inability to dorsiflex the ankle.

pin tract infection: direct bacterial contamination of area where pins have been used for external traction or skeletal fixation; could potentially lead to osteomyelitis.

pressure sore: breakdown of skin and/or subcutaneous tissue because of direct pressure of displaced or bunched cotton padding under cast creating pressure lasting usually in excess of 4 hours; often caused by patient inserting object in cast to reach an area that is itching from plaster dust in cast. Also called *decubitus ulcer*.

superior mesenteric artery syndrome: disruption of circulation to the bowel, commonly occurring following application of body cast, resulting in abdominal pain, diarrhea, and, if unrecognized, severe problems. Also called *cast syndrome*.

SPLINTS AND ACCESSORIES

This section will be restricted to discussion of those splints applied in the early treatment of injury or management of postoperative conditions and their accessories.

Splints

airplane splint: a removable cast or metal device used to hold the arm in abduction.

aluminum foam splint: a straight, metallic foam, padded splint of various widths from ½ inch to 2 inches; can be used by themselves or in association with casts and are used for hand and finger injuries.

baseball splint: a prefabricated metallic splint applied to the volar forearm and hand; the palm portion of the splint positions the hand as if it were holding a baseball.

Bohler splint: for spiral phalangeal fractures of the fingers, a device designed to maintain proper position and continous traction.

coaptation splint: two slabs of plaster that are placed on either side of the limb and held together by some outer dressing; commonly used in limb injuries.

dynamic splint: any splint device that incorporates springs, elastic bands, and other materials that produce a constant active force that helps reduce a deformity or counteract deforming forces.

frog splint: an aluminum foam splint used for finger injuries; before application the splint has a frog-shaped appearance.

gutter splint: a semicircular or U-shaped splint fashioned around the injured part, usually in metacarpal and phalangeal fractures on the ulnar side of the hand.

hairpin splint: a spring-assisted splint to help gain extension in a finger injury affecting the joint.

half shell: usually refers to spica casts; this term is not a medical one but is often used to signify the section of cast that remains after it has been bivalved and a portion removed.

long-arm splint: a splint applied from the axilla to wrist or distal palm posteriorly; holds the elbow and wrist in any given position.

long-leg splint: a splint extending from the thigh to the lower calf or distally to the toes.

night splint: any splint or similar device used only at night.

short-arm splint: a splint extending from distal elbow to palm; used for advanced fracture healing or nondisplaced fractures.

short-leg splint: splint extending from the upper calf to toes and used in the prevention of *dropfoot;* has recently become commercially available.

sugar tong splint: a long slab of plaster applied to the affected extremity in the fashion of a sugar tong and held together with outer dressing; most commonly used for injuries to the shoulder, arm, and forearm. Also called *sugar tong cast.*

Velcro splint: a commercial name becoming generic referring to splints that have two straps or surfaces which adhere to each other; these surfaces may be approximated and separated as many times as needed, and there is no loss of the original strength of the adhesion of the two surfaces; can be used for any part of the body.

volar splint: specifies a splint applied to the anterior forearm.

universal gutter splint: a wire mesh splint for lower extremity fractures.

wraparound splint: various commercially available splints that can be wrapped around a limb but are easily removable for physical therapy or wound care.

Accessories

Commonly taken for granted in the area of casts, splints, and dressing are the following important aids to patient management.

orthoses: provide required stability while allowing selective joint motion when properly fitted to lower limbs; also used to relieve weight-bearing.

canes: for a painful hip; the patient is instructed to hold cane in hand opposite affected hip to transmit load through cane at the same moment that weight-bearing takes place on affected extremity. Proper use decreases one body weight of weight-bearing.

crutches: used where a three-point gait is needed to relieve weight-bearing on affected side; used in fractures, sprains, and after surgery. A three-point gait is where both crutches are placed on the ground simultaneously with the affected limb, decreasing body weight from three to one.

walkers: assistive lightweight metallic devices (usually four legged) that allow patient to apply weight-bearing bilaterally when there is instability in walking.

DRESSINGS

The term *dressing* may apply to any material used to cover a wound; however, when considerable swelling without a wound is present, a dressing is used to apply pressure.

General types of dressings

Adaptic dressing: nonadhesive mesh dressing for the direct covering of wounds.

Betadine dressing: any dressing that has been impregnated with povidone-iodine (Betadine) and then applied directly to the wound.

compression dressing: any dressing intended to apply pressure to reduce or prevent swelling.

dry dressing: dressing that has not been impregnated with any solution.

figure 8 dressing: a dressing applied in the shape of an 8, as is often done for clavicular fractures; commmercially prefabricated dressings, referred to as clavicle straps, are available.

gauze dressing: any dressing made of cheese-cloth-type material, for example, Kling, Kerlix, 4 x 4.

Iodoform dressing: a narrow gauze strip impregnated with an iodine compound; usually used for the treatment of open wounds.

Kerlix dressing: a broad elastic gauze dressing often used as a part of a compression dressing.

Kling dressing: a narrow gauze elastic bandage used for compression.

Koch-Mason dressing: a warm occlusive saline dressing used over a limb with cellulitis.

occlusive dressing: any dressing used to protect a wound from outside contamination.

packing: term used to describe that portion of a dressing which is placed inside an open wound.

pressure dressing: dressing designed to apply pressure to a specific location.

protective dressing: any dressing used to keep a wound protected from trauma.

saline dressing: any dressing impregnated with normal saline; used in treatment of open wounds.

sterile dressing: dressing that, when applied, is free from bacteria.

telfa dressing: sterile nonadherent dressing, often used on fresh wounds or incisions.

wet-to-dry dressing: dressing that is impregnated with normal saline and allowed to dry; used as a part of open wound treatment.

Xeroform dressing: a nonadherent mesh dressing commonly applied to fresh wounds or incisions.

Other dressing materials

Ace bandage: a nonadhesive, elastic material that is used as a direct compressive wrap or to hold other dressings or splints in place. The trade name is now used generically.

adhesive tape: a sticky nonpermeable tape used to secure local dressing.

bandage adhesive: a sticky material applied to the skin to help in the application of various forms of tape; commonly used adhesive is tincture of benzoin.

pads: a variety of bulky materials (rectangular or square) used to cover large wounds; often referred to as ABD (abdominal) pads.

Specialized dressings

Esmarch bandage: special rubber, rolled bandages used to expel blood from a limb before surgery. Also called Martin bandage.

Gibney bandage: strips of adhesive tape applied in alternate directions about the ankle; used for ligamentous and other injuries.

high Dye dressing: a method of noncircumferential ankle taping designed to support the ankle following an inversion injury.

Kenny-Howard splint (A/C harness): for acromioclavicular separations, a sling that supports wrist and elbow with a counterforce strap to push the clavicle down and a chest strap to hold the device in place.

Low Dye: a taping technique for plantar faciitis.

Robert Jones bandage: a layered bulky dressing applied to the lower limbs for a variety of injuries, but specifically following knee surgery or injury. Also called *Shanz dressing*.

Shanz dressing: composed of two layers of cast padding and two layers of elastic bandage applied to the leg and foot; used for ankle sprains and nondisplaced fractures of the metatarsals.

universal hand dressing: used for compression or extensive injuries involving the hand and fingers; a bulky, even-pressured hand dressing composed of cotton or gauze fluffs and wrapped with gauze or other circular dressing material, leaving the fingertips exposed. Over this dressing a cockup splint is applied to hold the wrist in 15 degree extension. Some of these dressings are incorporated into a stockinette sling for elevation.

Velpeau dressing: bandage applied to the arm and torso such that the elbow is at the side in flexion and the hand is pressed against the upper chest.

TRACTION DEVICES

Traction devices are adjustable appliances that may be used in conjunction with casts or splints. They may be used to suspend or deliver pull to any part of the body by means of pulleys, bars, weights, and other supports which may be attached to beds, chairs, or doors. These devices may be used in the home or in the hospital in the treatment of patients with fractures or scoliosis, or preoperatively and postoperatively.

Many of the parts of various suspensions and traction devices are known by the originator's name. To relate where devices are used in con-junction with each other they are listed by placement, each with its component.

New techniques and methods of traction can be found in suppliers' catalogs, but the user should find this section helpful in deciphering why such devices are used in the care of patients.

Suspension

Suspension is the means by which a limb or part thereof is held suspended by some external device. Traction often accompanies the suspension.

balanced suspension (Fig. 6-1): suspension device that allows the patient to move the affected limb without changing the fracture position of that limb; preferred for treatment of long bone injuries of the lower limbs. There are two components:

Arizona universal leg support: for lower limb fracture, a balanced suspension device with adjustable anterior thigh pad and suspension support by two parallel lines from the knee and foot.

Thomas splint: originally designed to help splint fresh fractures; composed of a full ring around the thigh and two metal rods that extend down either side of the limb and are joined distally to the foot. The *half-ring Thomas splint* is the most commonly used. Most are adjustable for length and are thus called *adjustable Thomas splints*.

Pearson attachment: attached to a Thomas splint; consists of two metal rods joined distally, allowing flexion of the knee.

overhead suspension: the forearm is suspended

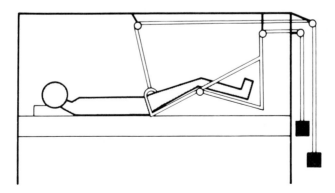

Fig. 6-1. Balanced suspension. (Used with permission of Carol L Wills.)

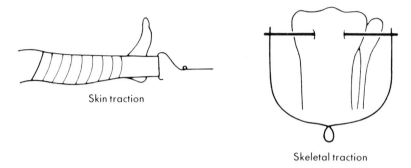

Skin traction

Skeletal traction

Fig. 6-2. Traction. (Used with permission of Carol L. Wills.)

overhead with the elbow bent; used in treatment of forearm and elbow fractures.

Traction

Traction means that there is some pull on a limb or part of a limb (Fig. 6-2). Traction can be accomplished by a bandage pulling on the skin or with the use of wire inserted through bone. *Skin traction* is used when light traction is required, whereas *skeletal traction* is used for longer periods and heavier weights. Not all of the following are traction devices, but all are commonly used in conjunction with traction.

Böhler-Braun frame: metallic adjustable frame for support of the thigh and leg; used most commonly for leg elevation and often in severe ankle fractures where os calcis traction is applied.

Bryant traction (Fig. 6-3): for infants only, an overhead suspension of leg and thigh such that the knees are extended and the thighs flexed to 90 degrees.

Buck traction: originally designed as skin traction incorporating the entire lower limb, but now used to describe skin traction of the leg only; generally used in knee injuries but also a temporary measure applied in hip fractures.

Cotrel traction: combination of a sling cervical and pelvic traction used in scoliosis before surgery or casting to help straighten the back.

cervical traction: a cloth, halterlike sling for traction of the neck; applied when patient is sitting or lying down, continuously or intermittently; head halter traction.

Crutchfield tongs: a type of cranial skeletal tongs used for traction of the cervical spine.

Dunlop traction: commonly used for elbow fractures; the arm is held suspended by skin or a combination of skin and skeletal traction, with a weight applied to the lower arm.

halo-femoral traction: a bed-type traction using a ring-shaped device directly affixed to the bone of the skull in conjunction with femoral skeletal traction; used in scoliosis or injury distraction.

halo-pelvic traction: an ambulatory-type traction using a ring-shaped device directly affixed to the bone of the skull in conjunction with pelvic skeletal pins. These are interconnected to hold the spine rigid when the patient is ambulatory.

Kirschner wire (K-wire) skeletal traction: small wires are placed across bone(s) so that some traction device can be placed externally; applied to some pediatric and hand fractures.

Lyman-Smith traction: use of olecranon pin and overhead traction for supracondylar (elbow) fractures.

Neufeld roller traction: for fractured femur, a cast for the calf and thigh is hinged at the knee and suspended by a line to the anterior mid-thigh looped around a pully and to a spring attached to the anterior mid-leg. The pulley for this loop is then supported by an overhead suspension with weight and a second pulley.

pelvic sling: sling encircling the hip and pelvic region in treatment of pelvic injuries; sling is suspended overhead.

pelvic traction: a cloth, girdle-type device with

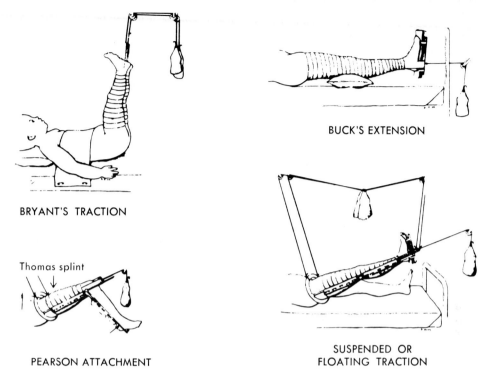

BRYANT'S TRACTION

BUCK'S EXTENSION

Thomas splint

PEARSON ATTACHMENT

SUSPENDED OR
FLOATING TRACTION

Fig. 6-3. Various traction devices. (From the American Orthopaedic Assocation: Manual of orthopaedic surgery, ed 5, Chicago, 1979, The Association.)

traction directed at the foot of the bed; used often for lower back disorders such as herniated disks.

Quigley traction: for lateral malleolar and tri-malleolar fractures, a stockinette is placed around the leg and ankle with the ankle being suspended by the stockinette attached to an over-head frame.

Russell traction: skin traction on the lower limb from thigh to ankle or knee to ankle, attached to a sling that suspends the distal thigh. This may be done with a continuous rope and a number of pulleys (simple) or with two different weights for one leg and knee suspension portion (split). Russell traction is often used in the elderly as a temporizing treatment for fractured hips or in the very young in treatment of femoral fractures.

semi-Fowler position: semisitting position with knees flexed; used in lower back and lumbar disk disorders.

skeletal traction: any traction using a pin through the bone to deliver traction; most commonly used in the tibia, femur, olecranon, os calcis, and metacarpal.

Steinmann pin: a wide-diameter pin used for heavy skeletal traction such as in the tibia or femur.

traction bow: U-shaped piece of metal for placement onto a K-wire or Steinmann pin in skeletal traction.

Vinke tongs: special set of skeletal traction tongs used for skull traction in neck injuries.

well-leg traction: bilateral casting of lower limbs with an interconnecting metal bar that allows traction on one leg to be supported by the other; used for femoral fractures and has the advantage that a patient can be moved out of bed.

90-90 traction: usually skeletal; the patient is placed supine, with hips and knees flexed to 90 degrees such that the calf is suspended; used for femoral fractures.

Frames

Frames are specialty units for an entire bed or additions to a bed.

Balkan frame: upright metal bars based at the corners of a bed and connected by overhead metal bars that hold suspension and traction pulleys.

Bradford frame: canvas bed suspended from rectangular poles with opening for the buttocks; split Bradford.

claw-type basic frame: traction frame that is attached to the bed by a clawlike clamp device.

Foster frame: a special bed composed of two stretcherlike parts that, when connected, hold the patient sandwiched firmly between them, allowing the patient to be completely turned without injury to the spine; used for tuberculosis and spinal fractures or for patients with scoliosis following a Harrington instrumentation and fusion. A *Stryker frame* is a similarly constructed device.

Heffington frame: a device that attaches to a standard operating table to allow prone position of a patient for lumbar spine surgery. The table end is dropped 90 degrees with patient's hips flexed over the edge and the patient further flexed to reverse the lumbar lordosis.

IV-type basic frame: traction frame that is attached to the bed by a device similar to that used for holding intravenous (IV) poles.

Jones abduction frame: a special frame used on standard beds to assist in gaining hip abduction in tuberculosis, acute arthritis, and other diseases of the hip.

Whitman frame: specially constructed frame to assist in gaining spine extension; may be used when cast application is necessary.

EMERGENCY DEVICES FOR STABILIZATION

The use of emergency measures in trauma situations has saved many lives and limbs. There are many new types of equipment made for stabilization of the injured. These "temporary" measures of tamponade, fracture immobilization, and tissue protection are generally performed by trained emergency medical technicians (EMTs) and paramedics acting under the guidance of emergency room physicians. The various types of air splints should be used only by those trained in their use. The following emergency equipment may be used before the patient reaches the hospital.

air pressure splints: double-walled plastic tubes that, in the deflated state, are placed around the injured limb and are then inflated (by mouth) to bring about even pressure and immobilization.

Gardner-Wells tongs: a device for immobilization of cervical spine injuries in which two sharp metal pins are screwed into the superficial layer of the skull. They are then connected to hanging weights or other traction devices for stabilization of the spine. They may also be used for definitive treatment of spine injuries.

Hare traction: a metallic splint with multiple straps and a special distal traction device for use in transporting unstable lower-limb-injured patients.

inflatable splint: sometimes referred to as an *airsplint*, it is a first-aid device used at the onset of injury; when blown up, this balloonlike splint provides good immobilization with even pressure. It is usually applied to the lower leg and foot, but other inflatable splints incorporate the entire arm or entire lower limb.

Mast (medical antishock trousers): pressure suit encompassing lower limbs and abdomen to provide sufficient pressure to force blood to the central portion of the body. This provides some stabilization of shock and provides stability for pelvic, hip, and femoral fractures and aids in preventing further tissue damage. In addition to tamponading sites of bleeding, they sometimes act by increasing pulse and blood pressure. Their use is controversial, and when *improperly* applied, can cause injury. MAST are inflated by a foot operated pump.

Neal-Robertson litter: a modified spine board for transporting trauma patients with spinal injuries to the emergency room.

posterior splint: for emergency immobilization, rigid devices used for initial stabilization of upper and lower limb fractures.

Sager traction splint: for femoral fractures, emergency traction splint that has a unit that measures the force of traction at the ankle. Used for children and adults, this device maintains fracture position and alignment without excessive pressure around the ankle or sciatic nerve injury.

spinal board: a rigid board with multiple slots for straps, designed to transport patient with head and thoracolumbar restraints in a relatively immobile state.

Thomas splint: can be used in several ways, but when used as an emergency device, is a temporary application of a full or half thigh ring splint with two long metal extensions for either side of the leg. Traction is provided with a twisted cloth or elastic strap applied to the ankle and end of the splint. (Also called *traction splint*.)

7

Prosthetics and orthotics

Prosthetists and orthotists are allied health professionals who measure, design, fabricate, and fit prostheses (artificial limbs) and orthoses (braces).

Prosthetics is the science that deals with functional and/or cosmetic restoration for all or part of a missing limb, following the directive of a physician's prescription.

Orthotics is the science that deals with orthoses designed to provide external control, correction, and support for the patient in need of nonoperative management of musculoskeletal disorders. Service in this area is also provided on a prescription basis.

The words *prosthetics* and *orthotics* may be used as nouns to describe the body of knowledge each pertains to, as in the preceding two paragraphs. The devices themselves are called prostheses and orthoses. When referring to a specific device, the words *prosthetic* and *orthotic* are adjectives needing an appropriate noun.

Specialists in these areas are certified by the American Board for Certification (ABC) and titled certified prosthetist (CP) and certified orthotist (CO). A CPO has demonstrated proficiency in both fields during examinations by the board. Supportive personnel are assistants and technicians, with varying responsibilities and duties.

Many major institutions have ongoing prosthetic and orthotic clinics or conferences, which meet as often as the patient load requires. Members of the clinic team consist of a chief physician, physical and occupational therapists, prosthetist, orthotist, rehabilitation nurse, and social worker. The clinic team approach is oriented toward management of the total patient, so although the rationale for prescription of an appropriate prosthetic or orthotic system is a prerequisite, the complete rehabilitation program is the long-range goal and responsibility of the team. Factors such as vocational retraining, if necessary, financial considerations of various phases of management, the necessity and duration of physical or occupational therapy, and a possible need for psychologic counseling are all taken into account. Perhaps most important, the patient must be made to feel comfortable in the clinical setting and be assured that the result will be as satisfactory as is realistic and attainable for the individual.

The prosthetist or orthotist is responsible for assisting with the prescription regarding components, elements of design, definitive and proper fitting of the system, and follow-up and adjustments as indicated at future visits to the clinic.

If the prosthetic and orthotic practitioner is to serve patients at the highest professional level, he or she must maintain a program of further education to remain informed of new techniques, components, and concepts. Such programs are available through the American Academy of Orthotists and Prosthetists (AAOP).

PROSTHESES

Prosthetic systems, or artificial limbs, are designed to replace function and/or cosmesis of a missing body part. Internal prostheses are surgi-

This chapter contributed in part by Wilton H. Bunch, MD, PhD, Dean, College of Medicine, Professor, Department of Orthopaedic Surgery, University of South Florida, Tampa, Florida; and Stephen Kramer, CPO, President, Universal Orthopedic Laboratories, Chicago, Illinois.

cally implanted devices, such as the artificial hip, and are described in Chapter 8.

Upper limb

An upper limb prosthesis is any external system designed for the amputee from the partial hand level distally to the interscapulothoracic forequarter level proximally.

partial hand amputation: distal to or through one or more of the phalanges or metacarpals or re-section at any level of the thumb. Restore function with cosmetic individual finger replacements with fillers and/or opposition-type posts. Slightly more proximal amputation sites necessitate cosmetic gloves and wired finger fillers and/or more intricately designed opposition posts to restore function.

wrist disarticulation (WD): amputation through the wrist joint. Correct with wrist disarticulation prosthesis designed to fit over the sometimes bulbous distal end of the residual limb, retaining as much pronation and supination as possible; trimmed anteriorly to allow maximum flexion; used with cable and figure 8 harness control, flexible elbow hinges, wrist unit, and terminal device.

below-elbow (BE) amputation: proximal to wrist but distal to elbow joint. Correct with below-elbow prosthesis designed to fit the residual limb, retaining pronation and supination in the longer levels and allowing maximum flexion; used with cable and figure 8 harness control, flexible or rigid elbow hinges, wrist unit, and terminal device. Münster or Hepp-Kuhn prosthetic sockets make the system applicable for short to very short below-elbow amputations; they are carefully fitted proximal to the epicondyles at the elbow to provide adequate suspension without the aid of additional devices; sometimes limit forearm flexion because of restriction of tissue at cubital fold; used with cable and figure 8 harness control, wrist unit, and terminal device.

elbow disarticulation (ED): amputation through the elbow joint. Correct with elbow disarticulation prosthesis with socket encompassing the residual limb and trimmed proximally at the shoulder to allow good range of motion; used with cable and figure 8 harness control, external elbow hinges with lock, wrist unit, and terminal device.

above-elbow (AE) amputation: proximal to elbow joint but distal to shoulder. Correct with above-elbow prosthesis with socket extending over the acromion to support axial loading and carefully fitted at axilla; used with cable and figure 8 harness, internal locking elbow, forearm lift assist, wrist unit, and terminal device.

shoulder disarticulation (SD): amputation through the glenohumeral joint. Correct with shoulder disarticulation prosthesis with larger socket extending from the spine posteriorly to near the xiphoid process anteriorly and fitted closely at the neck; used with cable and modified chest strap-type harness, shoulder joint or bulkhead (spacer) to allow abduction and adduction, passive positioning, and flexion and extension, internal locking elbow, forearm lift assist, wrist unit, and terminal device.

interscapulothoracic forequarter amputation: through the midsection, including resection of the scapula. Correct with cosmetic shoulder cap to restore normal appearance for clothing or forequarter prosthesis with socket similar to that used for shoulder disarticulations but differing in that an extension is usually employed going around and over the sound shoulder to provide additional suspension; used with cable, modified chest strap, and waist belt-type harnessing, excursion amplifier, shoulder joint similar to that used in shoulder disarticulations, internal locking elbow, forearm lift assist, wrist unit, and terminal device.

Upper limb prosthetic components

The components of an upper limb prosthesis comprise any device that is a supportive or integral part of the prosthesis, including terminal devices.

shoulder harness, chest straps, and waist belts: an infinite variety of Dacron, cloth, and leather materials is used to fabricate these components, which provide suspension as well as control through their attachment to cables that operate

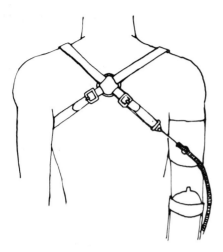

Fig. 7-1. Cross point of harness connected by stainless steel ring. (From Below and above elbow harness and control system, Evanston, Ill, 1966, Northwestern University Prosthetic-Orthotic Center.)

locks for various joints and provide function for the terminal device. The figure 8 ring harness is one of the most common (Fig. 7-1).

control cables: steel cable traveling inside housing, used to move and lock mechanical joints, for example, flexion and locking of the elbow joint; also provide prehension to the terminal device. The housing is sometimes Teflon lined to reduce friction and thereby increase efficiency. Cable systems are generally lightweight, as for small children, with standard ⅛-inch or heavy-duty cable. Common examples are Bowden single, dual, and triple control cables (Fig. 7-2).

elbow hinges: mechanical types of hinges to provide specific strength or allow controlled mobility. The following are commonly used; single pivot, providing mediolateral control, suspension polycentric, multiple action, sliding action step-up, and stump-activated locking. These are all designed in one way or another to provide additional forearm flexion for the very short below-elbow amputee or the patient with flexion contracture.

flexible hinges: hinges made of Dacron tape or metal spirals to provide suspension while allowing

retention of available pronation and supination.

outside locking hinge: commonly used on the elbow disarticulation system because of length of residual limb. Outside locking elbow and internal positive locking elbow hinges with nine locking positions are most commonly used for above-elbow, shoulder disarticulation, and forequarter systems.

forearm lift assist: adjustable spring-loaded device attached to the elbow to provide initial forearm flexion; especially applicable for those with higher level amputations such as shorter above-elbow amputation and shoulder disarticulation.

nudge control: a mechanical unit that can be pressed by the chin to lock or unlock one or more joints of the prosthesis; most commonly seen in forequarter systems.

excursion amplifier sleeve: pulley and cable system used to increase efficiency in patients with limited excursion; generally used in shoulder disarticulation and forequarter systems.

wrist units: integral components at the distal end of the prosthesis that allow attachment, interchangeability, and pronation and supination of the terminal devices; common types are standard constant friction and quick change; units are oval or round and available in different diameters.

wrist flexion unit: allows prepositioning of terminal device closer to the midline of the body; generally used for the bilateral patient.

terminal devices: hooks or hands affixed to the wrist unit, affording function and/or cosmesis.

   hooks: lyre-shaped fingers that open in opposition to one another, achieved by forces exerted through the harness and cable systems, and close voluntarily by means of dynamic rubber bands or springs. Hooks are available in numerous sizes, generally in aluminum with plastisol covering for children, aluminum or stainless steel with neoprene lining, stainless steel with serrated inner surface such as the model 5X, and for heavy-duty tasks the 7 or 7LO types, designed to hold devices such as shovels or rakes. Although certain hooks differ, such as the Trautman Locktite and the APRL (Army Prosthetics Research Laboratory) types, most employ rubber bands or

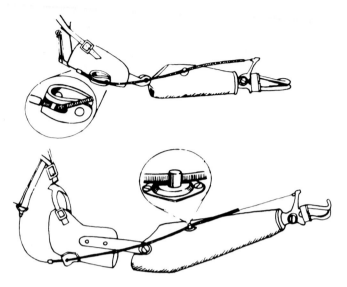

Fig. 7-2. Control cable housing. (From Below and above harness and control system, Evanston, Ill, 1966, Northwestern University Prosthetic-Orthotic Center.)

springs to close, and prehension is directly proportional to the strength and number used.

hands: there are a number of both functional and passive hands available. The mechanically functional hand provides prehension by means of springs attached to its internal parts; a cosmetic glove matched to the patient's skin color is applied externally. Passive hands, although nonfunctional, generally provide increased cosmesis.

myoelectric control: sophisticated prosthesis available for the patient with wrist disarticulation or below-elbow amputation; uses electrodes placed over the flexor and extensor muscle groups to pick up the milliamperes of electricity emitted by a muscle during contraction. This electric stimulus is then used to operate a motor in a mechanical hand. Prosthetic sockets are generally self-suspended, thereby eliminating the need for any harness.

electric switch control: prosthesis for the patient with shoulder disarticulation or above-elbow or forequarter amputation; uses switches to control current from a battery that operates an electric elbow and/or hand. The switches are placed in strategic positions within the harness system,

and by opening these switches the patient is able to operate the electric elbow and/or hand. This type of system is most feasible for patients with limited excursion from causes such as contractures, higher levels of amputation, or bilateral limbs, since each position in the switch is $\frac{1}{16}$ inch excursion—considerably less than that required to operate the standard system.

Lower limb

Lower limb prostheses are any external system designed for the amputee from the partial foot level distally to the hemipelvectomy level proximally.

Lisfranc amputation: through the medial metatarsophalangeal joint. Correct with extended steel shank in shoe to provide a place to push off and toe filler or foot plate with toe filler.

Chopart amputation: distal to the ankle joint. Correct with distal weight-bearing socket with partial foot replacement.

Syme amputation: through the ankle joint. Correct with prosthesis that distributes weight between the weight-bearing distal end and patellar tendon, that is, a prosthetic leg.

below-knee (BK) amputation: proximal to the ankle but distal to the knee. Correct with PTB (patellar tendon-bearing) prosthesis, designed to apply greatest portion of weight through the patellar tendon of the knee; use soft- or hard-socket condylar cuff suspension and prosthetic foot. Self-suspended variations of the PTB, which eliminate the need for additional suspension components, include the following.

PTB supracondylar (SC) suprapatellar (SP): hard socket, built-in medial wedge, prosthetic foot.

PTB-SC-SP: soft insert, built-in medial wedge, prosthetic foot.

PTB-SC: hard socket, removable medial wedge, prosthetic foot. For the patient with mediolateral instability of the knee, very short below-knee amputation, or residual limb incapable of supporting total body weight because of conditions such as burns and skin-adherent tissue, the following is often prescribed; PTB-type or conventional wooden socket, external mechanical knee joints, thigh corset, fork strap, waist belt, and prosthetic foot.

knee disarticulation (K/B, knee bearing): amputation through the knee joint. Correct with leather or plastic prosthetic socket designed to provide distal weight-bearing, with external hinges, fork strap, waist belt, and prosthetic foot.

above-knee (AK) amputation: proximal to the knee joint but distal to the hip joint. Correct with above-knee wooden or plastic quadrilateral socket designed to transpose weight through the ischial tuberosity, hip joint, pelvic band, and control belt, or with a suction socket, and mechanical knee joint and prosthetic foot.

hip disarticulation (HD): amputation at the hip level but with the ischial tuberosity intact. Correct with plastic socket designed to transpose weight through the ischial tuberosity and related gluteal musculature, mechanical hip and knee joints, and prosthetic foot.

hemipelvectomy: amputation at hip level with ablation of the ischial tuberosity. Correct with plastic socket designed to distribute weight using remaining musculature, rib margin, cosmetic socket buildup, mechanical hip and knee joints, and prosthetic foot.

foot and ankle components: allow normal gait patterns.

SACH foot: solid ankle cushioned heel.

SAFE foot: stationary attachment flexible endoskeletal.

single axis: allows anteroposterior motion and controlled plantar flexion with dorsiflexion stop.

multiaxial: allows anteroposterior and mediolateral motion.

knee components: designed to prevent sudden flexion gait or assist in making gait smooth.

single axis: constant friction.

safety: constant friction and adjustable braking feature when knee is in slight initial flexion.

four-bar linkage: a polycentric system providing knee stability.

manual locking: ability to lock knee in complete extension.

external: most common application in knee bearing; no controlled friction.

hydraulic: provides swing phase control to eliminate excessive heel rise; types include Dupaco, Dynaplex, Hydracadence.

Henschke-Mauch S'n'S: provides stance as well as swing phase control.

pneumatic: provides swing phase control.

below-knee suspension: used to support below-knee prostheses.

condylar cuff: mediolateral attachment to prosthesis with strap proximal to femoral condyles.

billet: connects supracondylar cuff to waist belt.

fork strap: anterolateral attachment to prosthesis with capability of waist belt connection.

waist belt: webbing wrapped circumferentially at pelvis with connection to billet or fork strap.

knee disarticulation suspension: fork strap and waist belt.

above-knee suspension: used to support above-knee prostheses.

hip joint: mechanical free-motion joint positioned anatomically on lateral wall of socket.

pelvic band: metal band contoured to pelvis and attached to upright of hip joint.

control belt: leather wrapped circumferentially at pelvis and attached to pelvic band.

suction: provides suspension through vacuum in socket, achieved by means of a valve insertion distally.

shoulder harness or suspenders: webbing straps traversing shoulders with roller and cord or various attachments to socket.

Silesian bandage or belt: webbing over hip on sound side with one lateral and two anterior socket attachments; most commonly used in conjunction with the suction socket.

modified Silesian bandage or belt: One lateral and one anterior socket attachment or similar variation.

CAT-CAM: conversion of quadrilateral socket to a *c*ontoured *a*dducted *t*rochanteric-*c*ontrolled *a*lignment *m*ethod device that gives a more even proximal distribution of prosthetic forces.

hip disarticulation or hemipelvectomy suspension: webbing over shoulder on sound side with anteroposterior socket attachments.

Other components, materials, and techniques

stump sock: wool or cotton sock worn over residual limb to provide a cushion for friction between skin and socket interface.

stockinette: tubular open-ended cotton or nylon material used to don suction socket, sometimes used with or in place of stump socks; especially applicable for the new above-knee amputee during volume reduction of the residual limb.

cast sock: used to take negative plaster impressions; sometimes used with or in place of stump socks; especially applicable for the new below-knee amputee during volume reduction of the residual limb.

soft cosmetic cover: rubberized material matched to patient's skin tone.

extension aid: elastic placed between pelvic control belt and shin to assist knee extension in the above-knee prosthesis.

rotator or **torsion unit:** component in the prosthesis designed to compensate for shear forces, thereby reducing torque and friction between the residual limb and interface of the socket.

socket: custom-designed receptacle into which the residual limb fits.

soft socket insert: foam/rubber inner liner for PTB.

silicone gel socket insert: inner liner made of a leather and gel composition designed to absorb shear as well as direct forces and used primarily for problem fitting of below-knee amputees.

total contact: intimacy between socket and residual limb.

distal pad: injection of Silastic or an equivalent foam socket of below- or above-knee systems, providing total contact distally to reduce possibility of edema.

check socket: a disposable socket used to ensure integral fit before definitive fabrication.

pylon: adjustable tubular section connecting socket and prosthetic foot.

rigid dressing: plaster socket worn on residual limb to reduce volume.

stump shrinker: elastic sleeve worn on residual limb to reduce volume.

Specialized systems

modular (endoskeletal): selectively applicable for below-knee or any level of proximal amputations; use socket according to prescription with adjustable pylon and foot and socket attachment plates; exterior surface is made of custom-shaped foam and covered with cosmetic material.

immediate postsurgical fitting (IPSF): procedure performed immediately after surgery; patient is fitted with plaster-type socket, adjustable pylon, and prosthetic foot. Advantages include early ambulation, more rapid stump maturity, and psychologic benefits.

intermediate (temporary): thermoplastic-type socket with adjustable pylon and prosthetic foot; intermediate phase of management used to expedite fitting, establish early ambulation, and reduce volume of residual limb prior to definitive fitting.

ORTHOSES

An orthosis is an externally applied system designed to provide control, correction, and support.

The lack of standardization of nomenclature has long presented a communication problem. Although trade and other descriptive names are still used, work done by the Task Force on Standardization of Prosthetic-Orthotic Terminology of the Committee on Prosthetic-Orthotic Education (CPOE), National Research Council, and the American Orthotic and Prosthetic Association (AOPA) has been largely responsible for the implementation of the terminology generally in use today. In an effort to enhance communication between the prescribing physician and the orthotist the following descriptive guideline has been adopted. The standardization is based on indicating those joints and regions that the orthosis is to encompass or control.

FO: foot orthosis.
AO: ankle orthosis.
AFO: ankle-foot orthosis.
KO: knee orthosis.
KAFO: knee-ankle-foot orthosis.
HO: hip orthosis.
HKAFO: hip-knee-ankle-foot orthosis.
HO: hand orthosis.
WHO: wrist-hand orthosis.
EO: elbow orthosis.
EWHO: elbow-wrist-hand orthosis.
SO: shoulder orthosis.
SEWHO: shoulder-elbow-wrist-hand orthosis.
SIO: sacroiliac orthosis.
TO: thoracic orthosis.
TLSO: thoracolumbosacral orthosis.
CO: cervical orthosis.
CTLSO: cervicothoracolumbosacral orthosis.

Use of the foregoing terms leaves the materials, design, and components to the discretion of the orthotist unless otherwise indicated by prescription, as demonstrated in the following typical examples.

Prescription: AFO to provide dorsiflexion assist. (This simple prescription leaves orthotic management regarding materials for the system to be determined by the orthotist according to patient evaluation.)

Prescription: AFO to provide dorsiflexion assist; double uprights, Klenzac ankle, calf band, Velcro closure, and shoe attachments.

Prescription: AFO to provide dorsiflexion assist; thermoplastic fabrication.

As demonstrated this format provides the prescribing physician with various controls over the patient's management.*

Lower limbs (Fig. 7-3, *A, B*)

Since all orthoses currently in use are too numerous to discuss, we will confine our list to those most commonly prescribed.

Foot orthoses

flexible orthosis: leather, foam, or equivalent, providing longitudinal arch and/or metatarsal support; orthosis is removable from shoe.

rigid orthosis: stainless steel, Monel, or equivalent; designed to provide arch support for pes planus or other related problem; orthosis is removable from shoe. Also called *Whitman plate, Schaeffer type,* and modifications thereof.

UCB orthosis (developed at the University of California, Berkeley)**:** similar to the rigid type, but fabricated of thermoplastic or thermoset resin.

hallux valgus orthosis: Designed for day and night use; reduces bunion pain by decreasing valgus deformity (pulls toe to midline of body).

Denis Browne bar: consists of a rigid bar riveted or clamped to shoes at either end. The bar provides hip abduction, with ratchet adjustments controlling rotation; generally prescribed for treatment of clubfoot, equinovarus, pes planus, or tibial torsion. When this system is used with an extra-long bar to treat congenital hip dislocation, an A-frame orthosis is sometimes incorporated to control the tendency for genu valgum (knock-knee), which may occur because of extensive hip abduction. The A-frame consists of a metal component fitted medially from the bar up both legs with calf and thigh bands and valgus control pads.

Fillauer bar: a clamp-on bar to place on feet to hold leg in internal or external rotation. Attaches to shoes by a clip-on device.

---

*Those individuals in need of further information in the area of orthotics would benefit from American Academy of Orthopaedic Surgeons: Atlas of orthotics, biomechanical principles and applications, St. Louis, 1975, The C.V. Mosby Co.

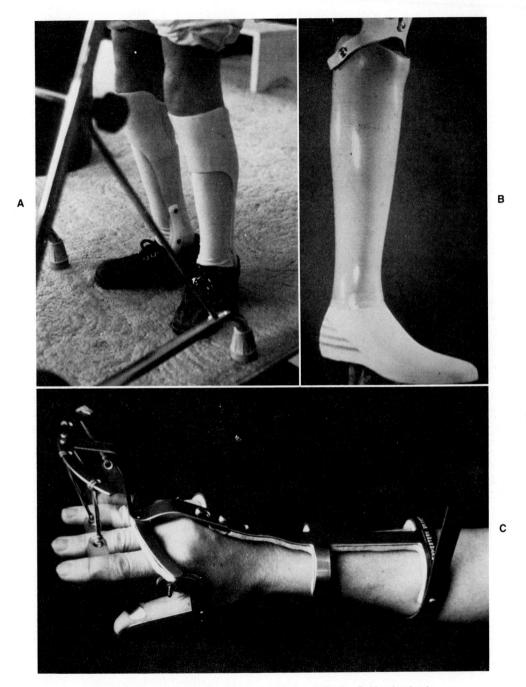

Fig. 7-3. A, Lower limb orthosis. **B,** Lower limb prosthesis. **C,** Hand orthosis.

Ankle orthoses

elastic orthosis: provides minimal support; helps control swelling.

rigid orthosis: leather, canvas, or equivalent material provides substantial immobilization of the ankle to alleviate pain caused by motion.

Ankle-foot orthoses

functional orthosis: a support usually made from acrylic constructed from a mold of the foot, which controls the motions of the foot during gait. Device commonly used for flatfoot.

standard orthosis: fitted ¾ inch distal to head of fibula and is an integral part of the shoe; examples are single or double upright jointed ankle, free motion, limited motion, and dorsiflexion assist; used with calf band, buckle, or Velcro closure and stirrup with shoe attachments.

spring wire orthosis: medial and lateral spring wire uprights attached to calf band proximally and the shoe distally; designed to provide dynamic dorsiflexion assist.

thermoplastic orthosis: terminates at or near the apex of the gastrocnemius muscle proximally, with molded foot plate fitted into shoe distally; ambulatory, nocturnal, or combination of both; designed to control and correct specific problems of the foot-ankle complex.

Some specific thermoplastic orthoses include:

IRM spiral	Seattle
PSA	Teufel
Rancho	TIRR

plastic floor reaction orthosis (saltiel): terminates just proximal to the patellar tendon and is fitted around knee; molded foot plate and solid ankle; designed with full anterior PTB-type section at knee, using floor reaction force to influence knee extension; posterior opening with or without Velcro closure.

patellar tendon bearing (PTB) orthosis: weight-bearing terminates just proximal to the patellar tendon and is fitted around the knee similar to the below-knee prosthetic socket; used with molded foot plate or ankle joints and stirrup with shoe attachments; designed to transmit body weight through the patellar tendon and medial femoral condyle to achieve controlled unloading of weight on the tibia and ankle-foot complex; anteroposteriorly sectioned proximally.

Knee orthoses

elastic knee cage: elastic sleeve encompassing the knee; provides minimal support and stabilization. Variations are the following.

with medial and lateral contoured knee joints: similar, with the addition of joints providing some increased stabilization. Other options include medial and lateral condylar pads, adjustable anterior laces, and additional spiral control straps.

Swedish knee cage: metal and leather system allowing flexion but preventing hyperextension of the knee.

static orthosis: leather, thermoplastic, or equivalent; immobilizes knee in desired attitude of flexion or extension.

dynamic orthosis: similar to static with the addition of external knee joints with or without locks to allow controlled motion.

Lenox Hill orthosis: metal, rubber, and elastic system designed to control medial and lateral instability as well as hyperextension.

Knee-ankle-foot orthoses

standard orthosis: fitted approximately 1½ inch inferior to the perineum and is an integral part of the shoe; single or double upright jointed ankle, free motion, limited motion, or dorsiflexion assist calf, distal and proximal thigh bands, buckle or Velcro closures, jointed knee with or without lock, stirrup, and shoe attachments.

thermoplastic orthosis: similar to the standard orthosis but fabricated of plastic material with molded foot plate fitted into shoe distally. This type of system has found increased acceptance because of its lighter weight and total contact fitting capabilities.

Legg-Perthes disease orthoses: the following are specialized systems designed for the treatment of Legg-Perthes disease.

trilateral orthosis (Tachdjian): plastic quadrilateral socket fitted at the level of the ischium similar to that of the above-knee prosthetic socket; single upright with shoe attachments; designed to provide weight unloading, hip abduction, and internal rotation.

Atlanta brace: a hip abduction brace that allows ambulation without crutch assistance.

Toronto orthosis: bilateral proximal thigh cuffs, center tubular column with universal multiaxial joints at base, outriggers with angled mounting blocks at either end to receive attachment of shoes; ambulatory system providing hip abduction and controlled rotation.

Newington orthosis: bilateral and similar in design to the Toronto o.; differs in that flat bars are used, and no joints are incorporated.

A-frame orthosis: see Foot orthoses, Denis Browne.

Salter sling: sling device that holds hip in abduction and internal rotation while the knee is held flexed.

Other specialized knee-ankle foot orthoses include those designed to manage patients with cerebral palsy and fractures, using plaster or plastic with polycentric knee joints, and other sophisticated components.

Hip orthoses

The following are specialized hip orthoses designed for treatment of congenital hip dysplasia or Legg-Perthes disease.

pillow (Frejka) orthosis: soft splint fitted between the thighs to provide hip abduction with straps over the shoulders to maintain positioning.

abduction orthosis (Ilfeld splint): bilateral thigh cuffs of plastic, covered metal, or equivalent with adjustable bar to provide hip abduction and waist belt and/or thoracic section to maintain positioning. Some systems have additional adjustment for hip flexion control.

Pavlik harness: a series of straps passing over the shoulders both anteriorly and posteriorly, transversing the chest and leading to the feet where they are attached to plastic booties; designed to provide hip flexion, abduction, and external rotation.

Von Rosen splint: malleable aluminum system fitted around the thighs, crossing posteriorly and going over the shoulders; designed to provide hip flexion, abduction, and external rotation.

plastic orthosis: custom-fabricated system designed to maintain the hips in degrees of flexion, abduction, and rotation, as prescribed.

Scottish Rite orthosis: pelvic band, bilateral free-motion hip joints, proximal thigh cuffs, adjustable tubular spreader bar with universal joints at inferior medial aspect of cuffs; ambulatory system providing hip abduction for treatment of Legg-Perthes disease.

Hip-knee-ankle-foot orthoses

The following orthoses, except for the standing frame type, are described in a unilateral application, although they can be fitted bilaterally.

standard orthosis: thermoplastic or combination of materials used in any of the knee-ankle-foot orthoses to which has been added a pelvic band that is static or with a mechanical hip joint for dynamic control of the pelvis.

elastic twister orthosis: pelvic belt with elastic straps wrapped around leg and attached to a hook in the shoe; provides dynamic control of hip rotation and tibial torsion.

cable twister orthosis: pelvic belt, free-motion hip and ankle joint, plastic-covered cable, connecting joints, stirrup, and shoe attachments; calf and thigh bands are incorporated as necessary; adjustable at hip and ankle to provide dynamic control of hip rotation and tibial torsion.

standing frame (parapodium) orthosis: thoracic region reaches to floor, pelvic band, lateral uprights attached to platform base, which has cutouts to accept patient's shoes, uprights are generally overlapped to allow growth adjustment. Some type of control is employed for knee extension. Joints are optional at hips and knees. This system is used to achieve standing and increase awareness in the child with afflictions such as spina bifida.

Components and descriptions applicable to lower limb orthoses

upright: metal, plastic, or equivalent used to connect various other components.

calf band: metal covered with leather or equivalent fitted to the calf area on ankle-foot or knee-ankle-foot orthoses.

distal thigh band: lower thigh band on knee-ankle-foot orthoses.

proximal thigh band: higher thigh band on knee-ankle-foot orthoses.

stirrup: attaches orthosis to upper shoe sections; has receptacles for ankle joints.

extended steel shank: inserted in sole of shoe to or past metatarsal heads to more effectively use floor reaction force.

Klenzak orthosis: dorsiflexion or plantar flexion assist for ankle joint; spring-loaded dynamic assistive control of the foot.

limited- or free-motion ankle joint: permanently adjustable to allow motion as desired.

double-action ankle joint: anterior and posterior compartments provide infinite adjustment for solid, limited, or dynamic assist.

split stirrup: component mounted on various shoes to allow interchangeability of the orthosis.

NYU (New York University) insert: plastic foot plate with ankle joints attached as receptacles for orthosis; provides correction of the foot and allows various shoes to be worn.

metal foot plate: similar to NYU insert but fabricated of stainless steel, Monel, or equivalent.

spreader bar: attached medially to both stirrups of bilateral knee-ankle-foot orthoses to prevent uncontrolled abduction.

varus or valgus corrective ankle straps: soft, padded leather or equivalent component that wraps around the opposite side.

patellar pad: leather or equivalent; fits over patella with straps around uprights to maintain knee extension.

suprapatellar and infrapatellar straps: small straps above and below knee, continuing around uprights to maintain knee extension.

varus or valgus knee control pads: leather or equivalent component that wraps around an opposing upright to correct deformity.

overlapped uprights: uprights placed on top of one another to accommodate growth in children.

drop-lock ring: fitted into place at knee joint to maintain extension; may be unlocked for sitting.

ankle, knee, or hip joint: mechanical axis placed anatomically to allow or control motion.

lateral spring-loaded lock: spring-loaded ring lock with lever that dynamically locks at full extension.

dial lock: may be set in varying degrees of flexion or extension to accommodate and/or reduce contractures; other comparable types.

Bail knee lock: posterior spring-loaded ring extending from medial to lateral knee joints with capability of automatic locking.

ischial weight-bearing ring or band: metal or equivalent component covered with soft material and fitted at the level of the ischial tuberosity; designed to unload weight from the lower limb; Thomas ring.

quadrilateral brim: similar to ischial weight-bearing ring but fabricated of plastic.

Upper limb

Physiology in design considerations for hand and wrist-hand orthotic systems include the following:

1. Maintain thumb in opposition for prehension.
2. Allow for thumb abduction as may be required.
3. Maintain skeletal integrity.
4. Avoid restrictions in use of the orthosis.
5. Prevent or correct contractures.
6. Maintain wrist in the functional 25 to 35 degrees of dorsiflexion.

Because of infinite and intricate variety of systems, only a few common examples will be given.

Wrist-hand and hand orthoses (Fig. 7-3,C)

Bennett basic hand splint: for muscle weakness in the hand, a dorsal splint that wraps around the ulnar, distal, and volar side of the hand and held in place with a strap around the distal wrist.

cock-up splint: one plastic section providing wrist

dorsiflexion with incorporation of a C bar for prehension.

Engen palmar basic wrist splint: easily removable volar wrist splint that has molded palmar extension that helps hold thumb in functional position.

Engen reciprocal finger prehension orthosis: for severe paralysis of forearm and hand, this orthosis allows patients to use their good hand to adjust and set the fixed position of fingers.

long opponens orthosis: identical to short opponens with forearm extension for wrist control.

Rancho flexor hinge tenodesis orthosis: for nerve paralysis, wrist-hand orthosis with connected hinge at wrist and MP joint located such that extension of wrist brings about finger flexion.

safety pin orthosis: fitted to individual fingers to dynamically influence flexion or extension of a joint.

short opponens orthosis: consists of radial extension, opponens bar, palmar arch, ulnar extension, and dorsal extension; fabricated of plastic or metal. Positions hand and thumb for opposition.

Warm Springs rachet flexor tenodesis splint: complex wrist-hand orthosis to help give power to grasp in a partially paralyzed forearm and hand.

wrist-driven flexor hinge orthosis: similar to long opponens with jointed radial side and a rod or connection between hand and forearm sections and thumb post. Wrist dorsiflexion produces a prehension pattern using the mechanical axis.

Elbow orthoses

Elbow orthoses may be static with humeral and forearm sections for immobilization, as in hand orthoses, and external joints to allow motion. Some are designed with turnbuckles or the equivalent to reduce contracture and may be static or dynamic.

Elbow-wrist-hand orthoses

These are static systems to provide immobilization. A torsion bar may be incorporated to assist in pronation or supination.

Shoulder orthoses

Generally these are static or passive jointed systems used for positioning.

Shoulder-elbow-wrist-hand orthoses

static orthosis: provides controlled positioning.

airplane splint: jointed elbow and shoulder, allowing controlled flexion and rotation; glenohumeral joint permits controlled abduction; used for muscle injuries, humeral fractures, dislocations, surgery involving the glenohumeral joint, and nerve injuries such as brachial plexus.

Components and descriptions applicable to upper limb orthoses

opponens bars: exerts a static holding force on saddle joint of thumb. Keeps thumb in palmar abduction, an optimal position for opposition.

spring swivel thumb: wire spring attached to radial aspect of orthosis and in turn connected to thumb ring. Patient flexes against this dynamic resistance; in a relaxed state the thumb is held in the open position.

first dorsal interosseous assist: principle similar to that of the spring swivel thumb; designed to hold the metacarpophalangeal (MP) joint of the index finger in abduction to provide opposition with the thumb.

thumb interphalangeal (IP) extension assist: principle similar to the first dorsal interosseous assist; designed to return IP of the thumb to neutral after flexion and during prehension.

thumb post: static control for prehension achieved by rigid member encompassing thumb.

joint stabilizer: rigid component extending proximally and distally to a joint of a digit; provides stability or realignment for subluxation.

outrigger: MP, proximal interphalangeal (PIP), or distal interphalangeal (DIP) extension assist; MP stop (lumbrical bar) positioned just proximal to the IP joints; holds MP joints in approximately 15 degrees of flexion.

C bar: component attached to or an integral part of the palmar arch, designed to maintain the web space between the thumb and hand.

turnbuckle: adjustable component used to reduce contractures.

flail-elbow hinge: used to overcome muscle deficit at the elbow. Spring assist provides flexion and locks in position for a chosen activity.

Specialized systems for upper limb

For those patients with severe involvement, external power sources are at times employed. Electrically powered or CO_2-operated artificial muscle systems are available.

Spine
Sacroiliac orthoses

cloth binder: material encompassing appropriate region with Velcro closure.

sacroiliac belt: adjustable corset with posterior pad.

Lumbosacral orthoses

lumbosacral corset: custom-fitted corset, generally having rigid paraspinal uprights.

surgical corset: garment encasing the torso and hips and having circumferential adjustability. Adjustments may be made anteriorly, posteriorly, laterally, or a combination. In general the following statements apply.

function: serves as a reminder to restrict anteroposterior and mediolateral motions; minimal unweighting of vertebral bodies and disks; restricts some rotary and twisting motions; creates intracavitary pressure system, lending support to the spinal column.

materials: nylon, cotton, canvas, elastic, or a combination.

fabrication: single or multiple layers.

anterior height: superior border 1 inch below xiphoid process or above lower ribs; inferior border ½ to 1 inch above symphysis pubis.

posterior height: superior border 1 inch below inferior ankle of scapula; inferior border extends to the sacrococcygeal junction or approximately the gluteal fold.

modification possibilities: posterior semirigid or rigid paraspinal uprights, posterior semirigid or rigid plate, posterior inflatable control pads,

additional abdominal reinforcements with flexible stays, thoracic extension with shoulder straps and axillary loops, separate frame posteriorly, one-piece garment, special control pads for ptosis (prolapse of any organ), hernia pads, perineal straps, thigh skirt.

chairback orthosis (anteroposterior and mediolateral control): posterior frame with lateral and posterior uprights and apron front anteriorly; control restrictions include anterior flexion, extension, and lateral flexion; used for lower back pathologic conditions, severe strain, arthritis.

Williams orthosis (posterior and mediolateral control): posterior frame; lateral sliding uprights with apron front anteriorly; control restrictions: extension and lateral flexion; permits free anterior flexion; used for herniated disks, severe lordosis, and situations where desirable to increase intervertebral space posteriorly.

Thoracic orthoses

rib-belt: foam padded or elastic with Velcro closure; minimal control, reducing muscle strain; used for fractures and costochondritis.

clavicle orthosis: figure 8 harness under the axilla and over the shoulder, crossing posteriorly; control restrictions: glenohumeral flexion; used for clavicular fractures.

Thoracolumbosacral orthoses (TLSO)

anterior control (Jewett, hyperextension) orthosis: anterior frame with superior and inferior pads; three-point fixation provided by additional posterior pad; control restrictions: maintains hyperextension and tends to increase lumbar lordosis; used for spondylitis, compression fractures, osteoporosis (reduction in the quality of bone or skeletal atrophy; remaining bone is normally mineralized), arthritis, spinal fusion, adolescent epiphysitis, and osteochondritis.

anteroposterior and mediolateral control (Knight-Taylor) orthosis: chairback-Taylor combination; posterior and lateral uprights with corset front; control restrictions: anterior flexion, extension, and lateral flexion; used for high-spinal fusion, lordosis, and osteoporosis.

anteroposterior control (Taylor) orthosis: posterior uprights with shoulder straps and apron front; control restrictions: anterior flexion and extension; used for kyphosis, fractures, arthritis, lordosis, carcinoma (any of the various types of malignant neoplasms derived from epithelial tissue), and after spinal surgery.

Arnold brace: brace primarily molded over the sacroiliac area with posterior support and rigid scapular thoracic support harness.

body jacket: anteroposterior sectioned, posterior or anterior opening; thermoplastic fabrication; control restrictions: general immobilization and intracavitary pressure; may be designed to provide some distraction; used for conditions such as postsurgical management of fusion, spina bifida, and muscular dystrophy.

Boston brace: molded brace used in scoliosis and other special disorders, for example, osteoarthritis of the dorsal and lumbar spine.

C.A.S.H. orthosis: a hyperextension TLSO that allows more freedom of chest movement.

dorsal lumbar corset: high corset with shoulder straps and paraspinal uprights; control restrictions: forward flexion, used for problems related to higher levels of amputation; see Thoracolumbosacral anterior control.

Gillette orthosis: for treatment of scoliosis, a prefabricated TLSO.

Lexan jacket: for scoliosis treatment, a prefabricated TLSO.

New York Orthopedic front-opening orthosis: for scoliosis treatment, a prefabricated TLSO.

Prenyl jacket: for scoliosis treatment, a prefabricated TLSO.

underarm orthosis: custom-fabricated or modular system; thermoplastic, generally with posterior opening; used for scoliosis. Application is most effective when apex of curve is inferior to T-10.

Wilmington jacket: used in scoliosis in circumstances in which control through the cervical spine is not essential.

Cervical orthoses (Fig. 7-4)

Cervical orthoses are employed when immobilization is necessary due to whiplash-type injuries, fractures, and surgical fusion. The following provide minimal restrictions.

Florida brace: two-poster cervical brace with chest and waist circular support.

four-poster orthosis: same as two-poster o., but employs two bars anteriorly and two posteriorly.

halo extension: fitted bands at forehead and back of head in conjunction with a two- or four-poster device attached to a thoracolumbar or thoracolumbosacral orthosis.

halo traction: skeletal immobilization traction using a pelvic plaster cast or plastic girdle; outriggers to metal ring encircling head; pins are then inserted into skull and outriggers adjusted for distraction.

hard (plastic) collar (Mayo Thomas): overlapping plastic sections with Velcro closures; wraps around neck and contacts chin.

molded Thomas collar: custom-fabricated leather or plastic over modified cast.

When optimum control and restriction are required, the following are prescribed.

Plastazote collar: unicellular foam, contoured to fit chin and making contact with occiput; Velcro closure.

SOMI (*s*ternal *o*cciput *m*andibular *i*mmobilization) orthosis: chin and occiput sections and sternal and posterior sections; may be fitted while patient is supine.

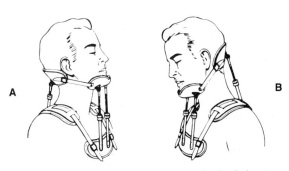

Fig. 7-4. Cervical flexion-extension control orthosis (poster appliance). **A,** Cervical spine in slight extension with head erect. **B,** Cervical spine in flexion with chin depressed. (From American Academy of Orthopaedic Surgeons: Atlas of orthotics, St Louis, 1975, The CV Mosby Co.)

soft collar: foam with Velcro closure; wraps around neck.

two- or four-poster orthosis with extension to waist: body length orthosis for greater neck stability and control.

two- or four-poster orthosis with thoracic extension: anterior and posterior bands incorporated into the cervical orthosis.

two-poster orthosis: chin and occiput pieces and sternal and posterior section, with one adjustable bar between each; straps connect the components.

wire frame collar: rounded, rectangular ring that fits under chin and onto chest, held in place by two straps supported by expansion of material on posterior neck.

Cervicothoracolumbosacral orthoses

Milwaukee orthosis: leather or thermoplastic pelvic girdle, throat mold, occiput pads, neck ring, and full, connecting superstructure with control pads as necessary; used for spinal scoliosis or kyphosis.

Components and descriptions applicable to spinal systems

rotary control: modification of rigid spinal orthosis with lateral extensions or sternal plate fitted bilaterally into the deltopectoral grooves to restrict rotation.

thoracic extension: component parts attached to cervical orthosis and fitted to the chest and back regions to provide increased control.

uprights: see Components and descriptions applicable to lower limb orthoses.

corset front: cloth anteriorly attached to lateral uprights of spinal orthosis.

sternal attachment: component fitted to chest.

perineal loops: straps passing between legs to reduce migration of spinal orthosis superiorly.

Milwaukee cervicothoracolumbosacral orthoses:

pelvic girdle: custom-fitted section serving as foundation for orthosis.

superstructure: two posterior and one anterior metal component connecting pelvic girdle and neck ring.

neck ring: metal ring at neck that opens posteriorly for donning and doffing and serves as attachment for throat mold and occiput pads.

throat mold: plastic or equivalent material, attached to neck ring and fitted to within 0.5 cm of throat and just below chin; limits anteroposterior motion.

occiput pads: plastic or metal oblong disks fitted bilaterally to the inferior angle of the occiput bones of the head; aligned to provide slight distraction.

thoracic pad: floating pad attached to anterior and posterior uprights on same side as thoracic curve.

lumbar pad: firm foam or metal and leather incorporated into or attached near posterosuperior edge of girdle on same side as thoracic curve.

axillary sling: axillary pad with webbing used to maintain alignment of neck ring.

shoulder ring: component fitted to axilla and over acromion; attached to the orthosis and used to depress an elevated shoulder.

SHOE MODIFICATIONS

Shoe modifications are various alterations made in a shoe to complement the orthosis. On occasion a shoe modification is prescribed by itself to correct a specific problem; for example, leg length discrepancy is treated by a shoe elevation on the shorter side, and valgus ankles may on occasion be treated with medial sole and heel wedging or medially flared heel.

orthopaedic oxford: a hard leather shoe with a leather or rubber sole; sometimes such a shoe has a steel shank (portion of shoe that lies between the floor of the shoe and the sole), with firmly constructed sides that support the foot in an upright position. This type of shoe is constructed uniformly, allowing for the addition of assistive devices.

surgical shoe or boot: a hard shoe that is constructed of thick walls, usually leather, with lacing designed to allow the shoe to be firmly tightened around the foot; generally used as part of an orthosis.

space shoes: specially and individually constructed shoes designed to fit a patient with multiple foot deformities, as occur with rheumatoid arthritis.

Devices commonly used for flatfeet

Thomas heel: a heel with a curved extension for the arch side of the foot.

extended counter: a piece of leather extending from the inner back side of the shoe to the level of the arch, giving arch support.

scaphoid (navicular) pads: better known as *shoe cookies* or tarsal supports; inserted directly under the arch of the foot in the shoe.

medial heel wedge: small wedge of extra leather or rubber placed on the arch side of the heel.

plantar arch support: an interchangeable pad that helps support the tarsal arch.

combined arch support: an interchangeable arch support that has both a tarsal (arch) component and a forward pad to support the metatarsal arch.

Metatarsal supports

metatarsal pads: pads permanently placed in shoe just proximal to the ball of the foot.

metatarsal supports: interchangeable supports that have a raised areas just proximal to the ball of the foot.

metatarsal bars: an extra piece of rubber applied externally to the sole, providing support proximal to the metatarsal heads; used in treatment of callosities on the ball of the foot.

Devices used in treatment of callosities

sole inserts: known by a variety of trade names, these inserts are made of foam rubber or other material and are designed to cushion the entire walking surface of the foot.

heel pad: any soft pad inserted into the shoe to cushion the heel; used for tendinitis, heel spurs, Achilles bursitis, and other problems.

calcaneal spur pad: a heel with a special cutout center designed to redistribute the weight from a painful area of the heel.

Special shoes for infants and children

reverse last shoes: shoes that look as if the left shoe were made for the right foot and vice versa; the side where the arch would normally be is curved out; used in treatment of clubfeet and metatarus varus.

straight last shoes: shoes that look as if they could be worn on either foot, with a straight sole; used in treating mild forefoot problems such as metatarsus varus.

normal last shoes: constructed with normal sole; term used to distinguish this from a reverse or straight last shoe.

tarsal pronator shoes: used in treatment of clubfoot condition.

equinovarus outflare shoes: used in treatment of clubfoot condition.

torque heels: specially designed heels to make the foot turn in or out, depending on the direction of rubber slits that are arranged to cause torsion on weight-bearing.

8

Anatomy and surgical intervention

Orthopaedic surgery is a means of attempting to alter normal or abnormal anatomic structures of the musculoskeletal system. Therefore, anatomy and the surgical procedures performed on specific tissues are considered here by region or tissue type. Associated surgical terms are included at the end of the chapter. Table 2 is presented to indicate the procedures normally performed on specific tissues.

OSTEO- (BONE)
ANATOMY OF BONE (Fig. 8-1)

Osteology reveals bone to be living, hard connective tissue composed of submicroscopic laminations of protein and crystal layers, nearly all of which are within reach of the living cell. If all the mineral were removed from a bone, the resulting structure would be firm, pliable, and have the exact shape of the mineralized bone. The process of *calcification* is not restricted to bones; it may occur in an amorphous form in tendons, bursae, and other tissue. *Ossification* is actual formation of bone tissue, which then calcifies by addition of hydroxyapatite crystals composed of calcium, phosphate, and hydroxyl ions. The following terms relate to the shape, structure, and microanatomy of bone.

apophysis: that portion of bone which contributes to its growth but is the point of strong tendinous insertion rather than a part of the joint.

articular cartilage: epiphyseal covering; thin layer of hyaline cartilage covering articular surface (ends) of bone to respond to shear forces.

bone marrow: red bone marrow is an "organ," whose function is the manufacture (hemopoiesis) of the formed elements of blood, that is, red cells, white cells, and platelets, the most important material in the body. It is found in the proximal epiphysis of the humeri and femora, ribs and sternum, and cancellous bone of vertebrae. Yellow bone marrow is found in the medullary cavity (in adults) and contains fatty marrow.

calcium: a necessary mineral in combination with phosphorus to form calcium phosphate (apatite crystals), the dense, hard material of bones (and teeth); it is the most abundant mineral in the body and found in all organized tissues. Calcium is important in the function of muscles, nerves, blood coagulation, and heartbeat. Bones are a storage center for calcium.

condyle: the bony projection at the end of a long bone.

cortical bone: the thick outer portion of bone, sometimes called *compact bone.*

cut-back zone: in growing bone, the zone just proximal to the epiphyseal growth plate, where the diameter of the bone is being cut back.

diaphysis: the thick, compact long shaft of bone providing strong support.

endosteum: a condensed layer of bone marrow in and lining the medullary canal.

epiphyseal plate: the cartilage between the apophysis or epiphysis and the shaft of the bone. This cartilage is responsible for most of the longitudinal growth of the bone. Although the epiphyseal cartilage is called the growth plate, as in the previous definition, the term *epiphyseal cartilage* may also refer to the cartilage lining the joint. Also called *growth plate, physis.*

Table 2. Orthopaedic procedures*

Prefixes/roots: tissue types	Suffixes: procedures
Osteo- (bone) 2, 4, 5, 6, 7, 8	1. -centesis: surgical puncture; perforation or tapping with aspirator, trocar, or needle
Myo- (muscle) 2, 3, 4, 5, 6, 7	2. -clasis: surgical fracture or refracture of bones and other tissue by crushing; refracture of bone in malposition
Tendo- or teno- (tendon) 3, 4, 5, 6, 7, 10	3. -desis: binding, fixation by means of suture (tendon) or fusion (joints); not to include spine
Desmo- (ligament) 5	4. -ectomy: excision of organ or part
Syndesmo- (ligament) 6, 7	5. orrhaphy: to suture, or sew
Fascio- or fascia- (fibrous bands) 4, 5, 6, 7, 9	6. -otomy: surgical incision into a part or organ; cut into
Burs- (bursa, sac, pouch) 1, 4, 6, 9	7. -plasty; to form, mold, or shape; surgical shaping or formation
Spondylo- (spine) 3, 6	8. -synthesis: putting together, composition, surgical fastening of ends of fractured bones by sutures, rings, plates, or other mechanical means
Myelo- (spinal cord, meninges, bone marrow) 1, 5, 6, 9	9. -gram: injection of contrast media for x-ray examination
Lamin- (lamina) 4, 6	10. -lysis: dissolution of tissue; decomposition, freeing of scar or adhesions
Rachio- (spine) 1, 6	11. -oscopy: to view by a scope
Neuro- (nerves) 4, 5, 6, 7, 10	
Arthro- (joint) 1, 2, 3, 4, 6, 7, 9, 10, 11	
Chondro- (cartilage) 2, 4, 6	
Synov- (synovium) 4	
Capsul- (capsule) 3, 4, 5, 6, 7	
Condyl- (condyle) 4, 6	
Aponeur- (fascial bands) 4, 5, 6	

*The left column (prefixes/roots) indicates the anatomy, with corresponding numbers to the right column (suffixes) that describe the types of surgery performed on those tissues.

epiphysis: the bulbous end of a long bone, usually wider than the shaft and entirely cartilaginous or separated from the shaft by a cartilaginous disk. The epiphysis is a part of the bone formed from a secondary center of ossification, commonly found at the ends of long bones, margins of flat bones, and at the tubercles and processes. During growth the epiphyses are separated from the main portion of bone by cartilage, properly termed the *physis* or *epiphyseal plate*.

facet: a flat, platelike surface that acts as part of a joint; facets are seen in the vertebrae and in the subtalar joint of the ankle.

haversian canal: canals running lengthwise in os-

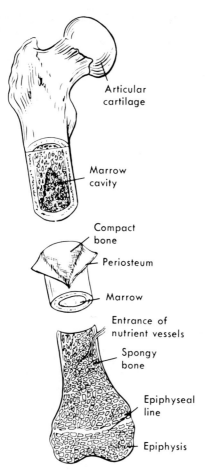

Articular cartilage

Marrow cavity

Compact bone

Periosteum

Marrow

Entrance of nutrient vessels

Spongy bone

Epiphyseal line

Epiphysis

Fig. 8-1. Composition of bone. (From Young, CG and Barger JD: Learning medical terminology step by step, ed 3, St. Louis, 1975, The CV Mosby Co.)

teonal bone where the blood vessels are centrally enclosed and protected, an important system in transporting blood-borne material to widely separated bone cells. This transport system is comprised of the haversian canals, surrounding lamellae, connecting canaliculi, and lacunae. The lateral branches of these vessels are called *Volkmann canals.*

isthmus: narrow portion of the canal in the shaft of the bone.

lamellar bone: description of bone that, under a microscope, reveals a pattern of lamination.

line: a less prominent ridge on bone, for example,

iliopectineal line; while a crest is a ridge (iliac crest).

medullary canal: round canal in center of a shaft of bone containing soft marrow elements.

metaphysis: the portion of a long bone between the shaft and the wide parts of the ends.

ossification: process of forming bone (ossifying, adj.). Other related terms are the following:
osseous: general term referring to bony matter.
ossiferous: implies that bone is being produced.
ossific: refers to the presence of bone.
osteoid: the uncalcified bony matrix (young bone).

osteoblast: bone-forming cell.

osteoclast: cell that removes bone.

osteocyte: bone cell.

osteonal bone: a microscopic description of bone that is seen in mature adults and is composed of little tubes that look like stubby pieces of chalk, having an arteriole running down the middle. There are circular laminations of bone concentric with the artery. An *osteon* is a single unit and is barely visible to the eye.

periosteum: firm, thin, two-layered fibrous outer covering of bone; outer layer contains blood vessels; inner layer contains connective tissue cells and elastic fibers. The periosteum is important for circumferential bone growth and in bone repair because of its bone-forming cells and blood vessels that supply the osteogenic layer. The nerve endings in periosteum are responsible for the sensitivity of bone in trauma.

sesamoid: denoting a small round bone found in tendons (and some muscles), with the function of increasing movement in a joint by improving angle of approach of tendon into its insertion. The patella is the largest sesamoid bone in the body.

subchondral bone: bone directly under any cartilaginous surface.

trabecula: type of bone that is in small spicules, normally referred to as trabecular bone *(cancellous bone);* predominantly makes up the ends of long bones.

trabecular pattern: refers to the arrangement of the trabeculae of bone such that, when seen on x-ray film or in cross-section, there is a pattern of arches or other designs, like the spokes of a bicycle, providing the structural needs of the bone.

tubercle (small), tuberosity (large): rounded elevated projection of bone giving attachment to a muscle or ligament; for example, ischial tuberosity or lister's tubercle (dorsal, of radius).

Volkmann canals: found in osteonal bone, a passageway for transporting bone-forming cells (osteoblasts) to the haversian canals, central in the osteone.

woven bone: immature bone seen in very early growth and development, fracture healing, and some disease states. Also known as *wormian bone*.

General surgery of bone

bone marrow biopsy: surgical or local needle aspiration of bone marrow for microscopic inspection to determine the presence of disease affecting bone; that is, decreased cellular production or abnormal white blood cells (leukemia); usually drawn from superior iliac crest.

bone marrow transplant: a special procedure done (occasionally) in an effort to treat certain disease conditions of bone marrow. Diseased marrow is chemically destroyed and replaced (transfused) with healthy donor marrow of the same blood type. The transfused cells eventually matriculate to recipient's bone marrow where, if the transplant takes, they become established.

closed reduction: nonsurgical manipulation of the fractured part, with return to proper position (called apposition) and alignment.

condylectomy: excision of a condyle at the joint; more specifically, removal of the round bony prominence of the articular end of bone.

condylotomy: surgical incision or division of a condyle or condyles.

corticotomy: complete transection of the cortex of a bone without transection of the intramedullary structures. This procedure is basically an osteotomy with care taken to preserve the intramedullary vessels.

diaphysectomy: removal of the shaft of bone, leaving the distal and proximal ends of bone intact.

diaplasis: reduction of a fracture or dislocation.

ebonation: removal of fragments of bone from a wound.

epiphyseodesis: fusion of an epiphysis to the metaphysis of a bone by disruption of the growth plate (epiphyseolysis) or by metallic fixation between the epiphysis and metaphysis of bone. An epiphyseolysis may also occur traumatically.

fenestration: cutting a window in bone to allow drainage or access to an object covered by the bone, such as a tumor or foreign body.

open reduction: the surgical incision and correction of a bone fracture in the operating room under anesthesia; may or may not include internal fixation.

ostectomy: removal of a portion of bone.

osteoarthrotomy: the excision of the articular end of bone.

osteoclasis: surgical fracture or refracture of bone to bring about a change in alignment in cases of nonunion.

osteoplasty: surgical correction by shaping or formation of bone (osteorrhaphy).

osteosynthesis: surgical fixation of bone by the use of any internal mechanical means; usually done in the treatment of fractures.

periosteotomy (periostomy): incision through the membranous covering of bone.

sequestrectomy: removal of a portion of dead bone.

synostosis: surgical fusion of any two or more bones that would otherwise be separated; may occur in a natural state as well.

Osteotomy

An osteotomy is a surgical procedure that changes the alignment of bone with or without removal of a portion of that bone. It may be considered for correction of a malaligned fracture, osteoarthritis, or other joint conditions. The following are types of osteotomies.

Abbott and Gill procedure: for bone growth asymmetry in lower limbs; a distal femoral and proximal tibial epiphyseodesis done through a medial approach. Also, proximal tibial and fibular epiphyseodesis through a lateral approach.

Amspacher and Messenbaugh: for cubitus varus

with rotatory deformity of the elbow, correction of both deformities is with a distal humeral osteotomy.

Amstutz and Wilson osteotomy: for congenital coxa vara.

Bailey and Dubow procedure: for deformities of the femoral shaft, multiple osteotomies held by a telescoping intramedullary rod.

Baker and Hill osteotomy: of the calcaneus.

ball-and-socket osteotomy: dome-shaped osteotomy.

Bellemore and Barrett (modified French): for varus deformity of elbow, lateral closing wedge osteotomy of distal humerus.

Blount displacement osteotomy: for hips osteoarthritis.

Blount procedure: for bone growth asymmetry in the lower limbs; epiphyseal growth is arrested using staples across the growth plate.

Blundell Jones varus osteotomy: varus osteotomy of the hip for paralysis.

Borden, Spencer, and Herndon osteotomy: for coxa vara.

Brackett osteotomy: ball-and-socket type for the hip.

Brett osteotomy: of proximal tibia for genu recurvatum.

closed wedge osteotomy: wedge cut out of bone, the open space closed, leaving a straight line.

Cole osteotomy: anterior tarsal wedge for cavus deformity.

Cotton osteotomy: for correction of a distal tibial deformity.

Coventry osteotomy: a proximal tibial osteotomy for varus or valgus knees.

Crego osteotomy: for femoral anteversion.

cuneiform osteotomy: a cuneiform-shaped wedge cut in bone allowing for correction of deformities in two planes.

derotation osteotomy: correction of rotational misalignment of a long bone.

dial osteotomy: dome- or circular-shaped osteotomy.

Dickson osteotomy: for malunion of the femoral neck.

Dimon osteotomy: for intertrochanteric fractures.

Dwyer osteotomy: for clubfoot and pes cavus deformities.

Ferguson-Thompson-King osteotomy: two-stage procedure for tibial bowing.

Fish osteotomy: for fixed slipped capital femoral epiphysis deformity, a cuneiform osteotomy at the base of the femoral head.

French osteotomy: for cubitus varus (elbow); a closed-wedge osteotomy.

Gant osteotomy: open-wedge osteotomy for the hip.

Ghormley osteotomy: part of a hip fusion procedure.

Hass osteotomy: for dislocation of the hip.

Ingram procedure: for fusion of growth plate because of trauma; opening wedge osteotomy with concurrent insertion of fat at growth plate area.

innominate osteotomy: of the pelvis for dislocation of the hip; two common types are *Pemberton* and *Salter*.

Irwin osteotomy: for pelvic obliquity.

Kramer, Craig, and Noel osteotomy: for fixed slipped capital femoral epiphysis deformity, osteotomy at base of femoral neck.

Langenskiöld procedure: for fusion of growth plate, an excision of bony bridge across the epiphysis with insertion of fat. Also called coxa vara procedure.

Lorenz osteotomy: for dislocation of the hip.

Lucas and Cottrell osteotomy: notched rotation type of the proximal tibia.

Macewen and Shands osteotomy: for congenital coxa vara.

Martin osteotomy: for fixed slipped capital femoral epiphysis deformity, a closing wedge osteotomy at base of femoral head and superior neck.

McMurray osteotomy: for nonunion of the femoral neck.

Moore osteotomy: two-stage procedure for a midshaft long bone deformity.

Müller osteotomy: for osteoarthritis of the hip.

open-wedge osteotomy: straight cut made across the bone, creating angulation, and leaving an open wedge-shaped gap.

Osgood osteotomy: for correction of malrotation of the femur.

Pauwels osteotomy: for nonunion fracture of the femoral neck.

Pauwels-Y osteotomy: for congenital coxa vara.

Phemister procedure: for bone growth asymmetry in the lower limbs; a block of bone is fashioned at the growth plate and then rotated 90 degrees.

Platou osteotomy: for femoral anteversion.

Pott eversion osteotomy: for correction of a distal tibial deformity.

Sarmiento osteotomy: for intertrochanteric fractures.

Sofield osteotomy: multiple osteotomies of the tibia or femur for bowing deformities or nonunions.

Southwick osteotomy: for slipped capital femoral epiphysis.

Speed osteotomy: for malunion of the distal radius.

spike osteotomy: creation of a bony spike in a long bone to help hold the fixation of position.

Sugiuka osteotomy: for avascular necrosis of femoral head, the femoral head and neck are rotated in order to transpose the avascular area away from the weight-bearing portion of the joint.

Thompson telescoping V osteotomy: used in distal femoral deformities.

Whitman osteotomy: closed-wedge procedure for the hip.

Y-osteotomy: for cavus deformity of the foot. Also referred to as *Japas osteotomy.*

Bone grafts

This section on bone grafts was contributed by Gary E. Friedlaender.*

Bone grafts are used several hundred thousand times annually in the United States to aid in repair or reconstruction of the skeleton. The scope of applications is associated with congenital (skeletal hypoplasia, pseudarthrosis), developmental (scoliosis), traumatic (fractures, segmental loss), de-

---

*Gary E. Friedlaender, MD, Professor and Chairman, Department of Orthopaedics and Rehabilitation, Yale University School of Medicine, New Haven, Connecticut.

generative (osteoarthritis), and neoplastic (benign, malignant) disorders. Most bone grafts are autogenous, and their advantages include maximal biologic potential, histocompatibility, and no potential of transfer of disease from donor to recipient.

In general, bone grafts are removed from one site and transferred to another without direct reestablishment of the blood supply. Consequently, osteogenic cells fail to survive unless they receive sufficient nutrition by diffusion, a circumstance met only by those cells very close to the bone surface. These few surviving cells play an important role in initiation or augmentation of the early phase of bone graft incorporation.

Bone graft repair depends on local factors at and emanating from the recipient site, including ingrowth of new blood vessels and both specialized and multipotential cells required for resorption and new bone formation. The exception to dependence on local tissues occurs with immediate reanastomosis of the blood supply to the graft, often requiring microvascular techniques.

General terminology

histocompatibility: immunologic similarity or identity with respect to cell surface antigens determined by genes of the major histocompatibility complex. There can be varying degrees of histocompatibility, some consistent with successful transplantation and some incompatible with this approach unless accomplished with immunosuppression.

major histocompatibility complex: a sequence of genes that control expression of cell surface glycoproteins that are recognized as foreign when transferred into a genetically dissimilar host. Different terms are used to identify this gene complex, depending on the species, for example, HLA in humans, H-2 in mice, RLA in rabbits.

immunosuppression: a term applied to any effort directed at lowering the body's natural immune response to foreign substances. Specifically, in transplant physiology, the use of specific chemicals to decrease the body's reaction to transplanted tissues from sources outside the body.

Nonspecific immunosuppression reduces host responses to most or all antigens and is usually caused by a systemic drug or chemical agent. Total body (or lymphoid) irradiation is another approach to nonspecific immunosuppression, useful in conjunction with bone marrow transplantation in humans and for a variety of investigational approaches in laboratory animals. Specific immunosuppression is targeted at a specific antigen or small group of related antigens, leaving responsiveness to most other foreign proteins intact. The use of monoclonal antibodies or induction of tolerance are forms of this selective approach.

implant: a synthetic device or the act of transferring into a host a synthetic device. Some include implants to reflect biologic material without cell viability.

transplant: a tissue or organ transferred from one site to another or the act of accomplishing this transfer. Some use this term to denote the transfer of viable tissue only (versus implant), and others use it in reference to any biologic material.

Classification by species source

allograft (allogeneic, formerly homograft): a tissue or organ transferred between genetically dissimilar members of the same species.

autograft (autogenous, autochthonous): a tissue or organ removed from one site and placed in another within the same individual.

isograft (isogeneic): a tissue or organ transplanted between genetically identical members of the same species. Synonymous with *syngraft* (syngeneic).

xenograft (xenogeneic, formerly heterograft): a tissue or organ transferred between species, for example, cow to human, rat to dog.

    boplant: a commercially prepared xenograft acquired from young calves and treated by extraction with a detergent, a fat solvent, sterilized by betapropiolactone and then freeze-dried. (This product is no longer available in the United States because of its lack of clinical efficacy.)

    Kiel bone: a commercially prepared, partially deproteinized xenogeneic tissue of calf origin extracted with hydrogen peroxide, dried with acetone, and sterilized with ethylene oxide. (Available in Europe only.)

Special procedures for preserving bone grafts

Most grafts are subject to some form of long-term preservation. The most common approaches to storage include deep-freezing, freeze-drying (lyophilization), chemosterilization and clinical extraction of proteins, or combinations of these techniques. The methods applied to long-term preservation have some impact on biologic, immunologic, and biomechanical properties, but these changes are predictable and often compatible with clinical success. Storage permits time for careful assessment of the donor graft material for potentially harmful transmissable diseases. Some bone recovery methods are:

AAA bone: a chemosterilized, autolysed antigen-extracted and partially demineralized allogeneic preparation.

chemosterilized grafts: graft material rendered free of microbial organisms by exposure to a chemical, such as ethylene oxide, although thimerosal and alcohol have been used for bacteriostatic properties.

demineralized bone graft: one that has undergone extraction of minerals (superficially or completely) usually by exposure to hydrochloric acid.

freeze-dried grafts: the removal of water from tissue in a frozen state, the same as lyophilized. With respect to bone, usually reflects residual moisture being reduced to approximately 3% or less by weight. Tissues can be stored indefinitely at room temperature in evacuated, sealed containers until required for use. Moisture is then reconstituted by submerging the tissue in water (saline).

irradiation sterilized grafts: exposure of tissues to high-dose ionizing irradiation for the purpose of killing potential pathogens, requiring a dose between 1.5 and 5.0 megarad.

lyophilized grafts: same as freeze-dried grafts.

Revascularization of grafts

The application of immediately revascularized *autografts* is limited by expendability of bone at the donor site, a discrete blood supply to the graft, vessels of sufficient caliber for repair (the fibula, ribs and iliac crest represent the practical limitations), as well as microvascular expertise. This approach is especially well suited for recipient sites compromised by prior irradiation or infection, or where rapid repair is mandatory.

The incorporation of devitalized grafts occurs by a lengthy process analogous to "creeping substitution," in which the sequence of events includes revascularization of the bone, followed by resorption and new-bone formation. Autografts transferred on a vascular pedicle or in which the blood flow is reestablished immediately by vascular anastomoses are incorporated rapidly by a process analogous to fracture repair.

In cases of bone *allografts*, immediate reanastomosis of blood supply is not clinically feasible because it engenders the same immunologic considerations encountered with viable solid organ transplantations, adding the requirement for substantial immunosuppression of the recipient. The following are related terms.

creeping substitution: the process by which a devascularized segment of bone in situ or a transferred bone without immediate reanastomosis of its blood supply, undergoes repair, beginning with vascular invasion, followed by bone resorption and subsequent new-bone formation (incorporation). This is a lengthy process that may take large cortical segments several years to incorporate, and even then, substantial portions of the graft may escape remodeling.

incorporation: a process by which recipient site factors grow into and remodel an initially devascularized bone graft. This includes invasion by blood vessels, resorption and new-bone formation. Often used interchangeably with creeping substitution with reference to grafts.

free-revascularized autograft: tissue transferred to a distant site along with its discrete blood supply such that direct reanastomosis of circulation can be accomplished immediately.

Classification by type of bone

cancellous graft: a bone transplant consisting of cancellous (or medullary) tissue as opposed to cortical bone.

composite graft: a transfer of more than one type of tissue simultaneously, such as bone and muscle transferred at the same time, or bone, muscle, and skin transferred simultaneously, and must be accomplished in conjunction with reanastomosis of its blood supply at the recipient site. This provides the potential advantage of repairing both bone and soft tissue defects simultaneously.

cortical graft: a transferred bone composed of the cortical (outer) tissue.

strut graft: cortical bone graft used to give mechanical support in the area of a cancellous bone graft.

corticocancellous graft: transferred bony tissue with both cortical and cancellous elements.

free graft: a bone graft freed of its vascular supply and soft tissue that would encumber its transfer from one location to another. This includes free revascularized autografts as well as other bone graft preparations.

intercalary graft: a segment of transferred bone without an articular surface; usually a portion of diaphysis or diaphysis plus metaphysis, with bone intercalated into bone to reestablish continuity.

intramedullary graft: one taken from medullary canal. Also called medullary graft.

osteoarticular graft: bone graft containing an articular surface.

osteochondral graft: a transplant composed of both bone and cartilage (articular surface).

osteoperiosteal graft: bone graft taken complete with periosteal membrane coverings.

pedicle graft: tissue transferred to another site while retaining (at least temporarily) its required blood supply at the donor site, consequently limiting the distance over which a pedicle can be transferred. The recipient site vascularity can be transsected or interrupted following reestablishment of sufficient vascularity at the recipient site.

segmental graft: a portion of transferred tissue representing less than the entire anatomic part being replaced.

Classification by shape and bone grafted

bone block: a bone graft that is inserted next to a joint to prevent a given direction of motion in that joint; also, a bone graft that is shaped in the form of a block and used for fusion of a joint.

chip graft: bone graft broken up into chips.

clothespin graft: coarsely shaped graft used in the spine; resembles a clothespin.

hemicylindric graft: graft cut into the shape of half a cylinder.

inlay graft: any grafted place in a bone that has been cut in a fusion procedure to receive the shape of that graft.

  diamond inlay graft: graft cut in a diamond shape with recipient site cut to receive that shape.

  sliding inlay graft: a slot of bone cut and moved across the graft site, usually a fracture of a large bone.

massive sliding graft: large graft designed to slide when two portions of recipient bone are compressed.

onlay graft: graft laid directly onto the surface of recipient bone.

dual onlay graft: two strips of bone laid down on either side of the shaft.

peg graft: cylindric bone graft to be inserted into or through the medullary canal of a bone.

Eponymic bone graft terms

Albee	Hey-Grooves-Kirk
Banks	Hoaglund
Boyd	Huntington
Campbell	Inclan
Codivilla	McMaster
Flanagan and Burem	Nicoli
Gillies	Phemister
Haldeman	Ryerson
Henderson	Soto-Hall
Henry	Wilson

Osteosyntheses: internal fixation devices

Osteosynthesis is a surgical procedure that uses internal fixation devices, especially in the treatment of fractures. This procedure is referred to in context as open reduction and internal fixation (ORIF). It cannot be overemphasized how the orthopaedic surgeon must apply the principles of engineering to biology. The surgeon must be adept in using metal plates, nails, rods, pins, bands, screws, bolts, and staples in the correction of skeletal defects (Fig. 8-2). Pegging, pistoning, reefing, shelving, shaving down, shucking, doweling, and saucerization are a few of the engineering procedures applied within biologic principles. The following internal fixation devices are used in orthopaedic surgery.

AO: abbreviation for designer of a variety of implant devices. The letters stand for *Arbeitsgemeinschaft Fur Osteosynthesefragen.*

ASIF: abbreviation for group that studies internal fixation systems and engineering. The letters stand for *Association for the Study of Internal Fixation.*

biodegradable fixation: a variety of screws, pins, plates, and other fixation devices made of material that will be absorbed by the body. Such

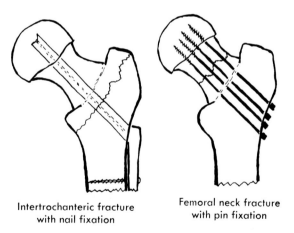

Intertrochanteric fracture with nail fixation

Femoral neck fracture with pin fixation

Fig. 8-2. Two internal fixation devices for hip fractures.

materials include *polyactide-glycolide copolymer (polyglactin 910)*.

blade plate: general class of plate fixation devices that has a right-angle or nearly right-angle flange.

Blount plate: a blade plate commonly used in distal femurs.

Blount staple: type of staple used around the knee.

bollard: a short, flat-headed, nail-like device that is slotted along a portion of the shaft, used in fixation of ligaments into bone.

Brooker-Wills nail: for unstable femoral fractures, a femoral nail with distal locking screws.

Calandruccio nail: for hip fractures, a sliding compression screw and plate associated with two smaller threaded pins through the plate and into the femoral head.

cancellous screw: used for trabecular problems near the joints, especially the hip.

cannulated nail: general class of nail with a hole in the center.

cloverleaf nail: used in femoral fractures.

cruciate screw: screw with cross-shaped head.

Derby nail: for femoral shaft fracture, an intramedullary nail with wings that can be extended at the distal tip, and an antirotation washer at the proximal end.

Eggers plate and screw: used in long-bone fractures.

elastic stable intramedullary nailing (ESIN): for fixation of femoral fractures in children, insertion of a highly elastic intramedullary nail that allows early protected weight-bearing.

Elliott plate: a type of blade plate used mostly in distal femoral procedures.

encirclage: wiring or banding of bony fragments in the shaft of a bone.

Ender nail: intramedullary nail that is curved and can be used to fix intertrochanteric hip fractures through a small incision just above the knee joint.

Gore AO screw: AO cortical bone screw modified to affix a ligament replacement implant.

Gouffon pin: threaded pin used in the fixation of cervical fractures of the hip.

grommet: a short, flat, hollow cylinder with a head. The device fits over a screw that is considerably narrower than the inner portion of the grommet. Used for fixation of ligaments into bone.

Gross-Kemph nail: for unstable femoral shaft fractures; a locking nail system.

Hagie pin: used for hip fractures.

Hansen-Street nail: used for larger bony fractures.

Harrington rod: used in spinal fixation for scoliosis and some fractures.

Harris nail: intramedullary nail system for intertrochanteric fractures.

Henderson lag screw: used for hip fractures.

Herbert screw: for wrist scaphoid fixation, a short screw threaded at both ends.

Hessel/Nystrom pins: threaded pin for internal fixation of femoral neck fractures.

hex screw: hexagon head screw.

hook-pin fixation: for femoral neck fractures, a hollow nail has internal hooked pins that can be deployed into the femoral head after introduction of the nail.

Huckstep nail: for osteotomy of femur with limb lengthening; a nail with holes for cross-screw fixation.

intramedullary nail: class of nails placed in medullary canal of long bones for midshaft fractures; includes Hansen-Street, Küntscher, Lottes, and Schneider.

Inyo nail: for fractures of the distal fibula, a tapered V-shaped nail made of malleable stainless steel.

Jewett nail: nail plate used in hip fractures.

Ken nail: 135-degree sliding nail plate used for hip fractures.

Kirschner wire (K-wire): small wire used for fixation or traction.

Knowles pin: used for hip fractures.

Küntscher nail (rod): used in femoral fractures.

Kurosaka screw: special screw designed for fixation of tendon attached to bone transplants in ligament reconstruction.

lag screw: screw with threads at the tip only, used for compression.

Lane plate: plate for long bone fixation.

Leinbach screw: long flexible screw, used often for olecranon fractures.

Lewis nail: intramedullary nail for metacarpal bone fixation.

Lorenzo screw: bone fixation screw.

Lottes nail (pin): used for tibial fractures.

Martin screw: used in hip fractures.

Massie nail: 155-degree sliding nail used in hip fractures.

McLaughlin plate, screw: used in hip surgery.

medullary rod (pin): metallic device used in central shaft of bone.

Moore plate (pin): used in hip surgery.

Müller plate: type of blade plate used in hip surgery.

nested nails: a general term for two nails placed side by side in the medullary canal of long bones.

Neufeld nail: a plate with nail spike for the greater trochanter, used to encircle shafts of long bones.

Ogden plate: for fixation of long bone fractures associated with preexisting intramedullary devices such as rods or the stem of a prosthesis. Long metal plates are designed with slots that are designed to accept encircling bands in locations where screws cannot be easily used.

Parham band: for oblique long bone fractures, a metal band that can be tightened around the shaft of the bone to achieve fixation by compression.

Partridge band: for oblique long bone fracture, a band with ribbed undersurface so that when band is tightened there might be less interference with periosteal and cortical blood flow.

PGP nail: a flexible nail used in intramedullary fixation of femoral fractures.

Phillips screw: any screw with a Phillips head.

Pugh nail: 155-degree sliding nail used for hip fractures.

Rush nail, rod, pin: used for major long bone fractures.

Russell Taylor nail: intramedullary nail for femur with slots for cross-screw fixation.

Rydell nails: for femoral neck fractures, a four-flanged spring-nail.

Sage rod: diamond-shaped rod used in forearm fractures.

Schneider nail, rod: used in femoral fractures.

Sherman plate: used for long bone fractures.

slide plate: used for long bone fractures.

Smillie nail: small pin used for attachment of the osteochondral fragments in the knee.

Smith-Petersen nail: used in hip surgery.

Steinmann pin: used in skeletal traction; of larger caliber than a K-wire.

Street medullary pin: used for large long bone fractures.

Thornton nail: for femoral neck fractures, a three-flanged spring-nail.

tibial bolt: used for proximal and distal tibial fractures.

toggle: a small metallic cylinder with each end slightly larger than the center. Used by tying sutures around it to affix ligaments or tendons to bone.

von Bahr screw: for femoral neck fracture, a pin threaded at the tip for multiple screw fixation.

Weiss spring: spring device used in some spinal fusions, particularly spondylolisthesis.

Wilson plate: for spinal fusions.

Zickle nail: a curved 75- and 60-degree nail and screw device for a femoral supracondylar fracture; or an intramedullary rod with transfixing nail for subtrochanteric fractures.

Zuelzer hook plate: commonly used in ankle fractures.

External skeleton fixation

The use of external wires transfixed through bone to hold the position of a fracture is not new. Pins in plaster have been the usual method for holding bone fragments in proper position during the healing process. Recently there has been increased use of multiple pins placed through one cortex or both cortices of bone and held by one external device. These external fixation devices are also known as *fixateurs* or *fixators*. This allows easy access to wounds, adjustment during the course of healing, and more functional use of limb involved. The devices used have increased in number and include the following.

Type by configuration

unilateral	triangular
bilateral	semicircular
quadrilateral	circular

Types by design and manufacturer

Ace-Colles	Kronner-ring
Ace-Fischer	Monticelli-Spinelli
Calandruccio	Rezaian
Denham	Roger Anderson
four-bar	Sukhtian-Hughes
Hoffman	Videl-Adrey
Hoffman-Vital	Volkov-Oganesyan
Ikuta	Wagner
Ilizarov	Wasserstein

Electric and magnetic stimulation of fracture healing

The use of direct electric currents and magnetic impulses in the treatment of fractures has been studied for the effect on fracture healing. In the past the presence of nonunion (extended failure of fracture healing) has often required extensive surgical attention, including bone grafts. However, electric and magnetic stimulation in treating fractures has been approved by the Food and Drug Administration for established nonunion of long bones.

electric stimulation: a procedure involving small voltage and amperage electric currents passed through electrodes placed immediately at the fracture site. The source of current is a battery placed external to the body or under the fat, similar to a cardiac pacemaker. For the external battery devices, the electrodes can be placed directly through the skin, eliminating the need for an incision. The limb involved is usually held in a cast.

magnetic stimulation: large magnetic coils applied externally and connected to a specific pulsating current. The home treatment device, used to control the magnetic field, is a small boxlike apparatus that is plugged into a standard 110-volt outlet; can be used up to 12 hours a day. As in electric stimulation, the affected limb is immobilized in a cast during the treatment period. Chapter 12, Musculoskeletal research, pro-

vides more specific information on this modality of treatment.

INTERNAL PROSTHESES

Numerous devices composed mostly of alloys and plastic have been developed to aid in joint replacement efforts. Prosthetic replacements are now available for almost every joint in the body, and even a spinal segment can now be replaced. This field continues to rapidly expand, with a constant influx of new components and the outdating of others. Therefore some of the prostheses listed here may already be or soon will be obsolete. They are mentioned because they will still be found in some patients in the future. Chapter 12 discusses research efforts in internal prostheses.

The advent of a polymer called *methylmethacrylate* led to the development of new types of devices held firmly in place by polymers (glue). It is a cementlike substance that forms no chemical bonds but instead holds components to bones by space filling and locking effects. When applied, methylmethacrylate is soft and pliable, but it becomes very hard and firm within 15 minutes. Problems encountered with this method prompted further research and improvement in the development of joint resurfacing techniques. Although the use of methylmethacrylate is currently the preferred concept for joint replacement, new materials and methods are still being researched. The various types of internal prostheses are presented here according to anatomic structure and part most subjected to the need for these devices.

Hip prostheses
Straight stem femoral components

These are now obsolete. The original effort to replace the hip joint was centered around femoral head replacement. One of the first femoral head components was made of acrylic attached to a metal stem (Judet). These became loose fairly rapidly, and as bone remodeling and response to stress became better understood, the devices were no longer used.

Single femoral component with intramedullary stem

It was found that there was longer fixation of the femoral head replacement if the stem was in the medullary canal. Although the cartilage on the acetabular side would often disappear over time, many of these prostheses lasted for years. Additionally, they were fairly easy to replace. These prostheses are still used in some cases for femoral head replacement in hip fractures.

Austin-Moore   Matchett-Brown
d'Aubigne   McBride
Dubinet   Naden-Rieth
Eftekhar   Thompson
Eicher   Valls

Acetabular side of the hip
Cup arthroplasty

A purposeful effort was made to stimulate the body to make new cartilage at the femoral head

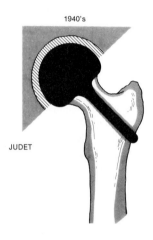

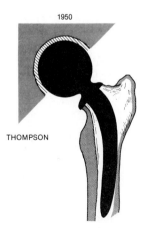

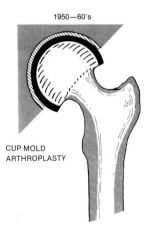

Fig. 8-3. Development of the total hip prosthesis with improvements in fixation and biological acceptance over a period of four decades. Lined areas are cartilage, grossly stippled areas are cement (methacrylate), finely stippled areas are plastic, and solid black areas are metal. (Drawing by Frances Langley, USUHS.)

region. By removing the osteoarthritic surface of the femoral head and acetabulum, the cup would allow the raw exposed bony surface to form a covering of cartilage. This required extensive rehabilitative time and patient participation. It met with success in many instances.

Aufranc   Crawford-Adams   Smith-Petersen

Total hip replacement (THR) (Fig. 8-3)

The evolution of total hip replacement is a compliment to the efforts of biologists, clinicians, and engineers. As the concepts were tested and used, a very rapid evolution of new developments produced the subcategories of the total hip replacement. Both components held by cement.

Metal on metal

Most original total hip replacements were made of metal. Fixation was secured by the use of methylmethacrylate to cement the two components in place. These prostheses had general success, but there were problems of stress fracture in the pelvis, loosening of the acetabular component, and metal fatigue.

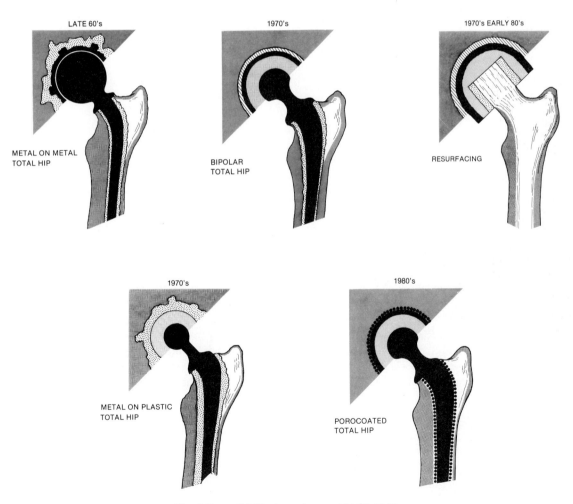

Fig. 8-3, cont'd. For legend, see opposite page.

Mckee-Farrar   Scarborough
Ring   Stanmore

Plastic on metal

Metal wear was found to be one of the problems of the metal on metal total joint replacements. The introduction of plastic to replace the metal cup was found to give better wear characteristics. The incidence of stress fractures of the pelvis was less. Methylmethacrylate is used to secure the two components to bone.

Amstutz
Amstutz (TR-28)
Aufranc-Turner
Charnley
Charnley-Muller
CHD
Calandruccio
Contour
DF-80
Freeman
Harris
Harris (HD 2)
Howse
Ling (Exeter)
Matchett-Brown
Müller
Sarmiento (STH-2)
Trapezoidal (T-28)
Wilson-Burstein

Metal-backed plastic on metal

The problems encountered with plastic on metal acetabular components included loosening of the acetabular component. Backing the plastic with metal seemed to protect against some of the abnormal forces and thus reduce the incidence of loosening. These metal on plastic components still require methylmethacrylate to achieve fixation.

Iowa   TPL-6

Resurfacing procedures

The purpose of research into resurfacing rather than replacement was to leave as much bone stock as possible. The effort that is required to remove a preexisting total hip prosthesis often destroys a fair amount of surrounding bone. The advantage of the resurfacing procedure was that it did not require removal of the femoral head and placement of a stem with methylmethacrylate down the femoral canal. However, the acetabular cap was held with methylmethacrylate and the portion placed over the reshaped femoral head was also held with methylmethacrylate. The problem with this procedure has been an eventual loss of the femoral component because of absorption of bone. If the method did fail, replacement with other total hip devices was easier, with more bone available for fixation. Some of the techniques used are:

Amstutz
bicentric
Freeman
Gerard
ICLH (Imperial College, London Hospital) double cup arthroplasty
Indiana conservative
Paltrinieri-Trentani
Salzer (uncemented ceramic double cup)
Sharrard-Trentani
TARA (*total articular replacement arthroplasty*)
THARIES (*total hip articular replacement by internal eccentric shells*)
Tillman
Wagner

Bipolar total hip replacement

The bipolar total hip was designed to allow for some regeneration of the acetabular cartilage and two components of motion: one at the acetabular-prosthetic interface, and the other between the acetabular and femoral components. Although the femoral component is often fixed with methylmethacrylate, the acetabular component is not, making this a more conservative approach than the firmly fixed acetabular components. On the acetabular side, there is a plastic cup inserted into a metal cup.

Bateman   Hastings
Christiansen   Monk
Giliberty   Varikopf

"Cementless" total hip replacements

The effort of removing a "cemented" prosthesis can often be prodigious. Some of the early efforts involved complex metal acetabular components. With the advent of metal-backed plastic components, there has been a sudden influx of different designs. The obvious advantage is the relative ease in removal of the two components and the involvement of less bone in the removal process.

In some of the prostheses a portion of the stem and metal cup may have a coat of scintered metallic beads or threads that produce a rough surface into which bone may grow. This is called *porocoating*.

Press fit	Porous coated
Averill (normalize)	Engh (AML)
Capello	Harris-Galante
Jaffee	Lunceford
Judet	PCA
Lord (Madreporic)	Pilliar
Oh (Biofit)	
Osteonics	
Phoenix	
Ring UPM	
self-bearing ceramic	
Sivash	
TTAP (threaded titanium acetabular prosthesis)	

Other "cementless" total hips

Combination of tight-fitting femoral and acetabular components of metal, plastic, and ceramics have been devised.

Judet	Self-bearing ceramic	Sivash

KNEE PROSTHESES

Knee prostheses are designed to replace portions or all of the knee joint. The original attempts involved solid metal to replace one side or the other of the joint. Metal with plastic interfacing, better joint mechanical design, and superior attention to detail in surgical applications have improved the relative success of knee joint replacements.

The total knee devices are listed in categories based on the degree of constraint of knee motion, that is, stability.

Unicompartmental replacement: The unicompartmental design has evolved into a metal unicondylar component for the femur making contact with a plastic or plastic on metal tibial component. There are few patients for whom this limited procedure is appropriate. Some unicompartmental devices include:

Charnley	MacIntosh
Compartmental II	Modular
Geomedic (unilateral)	Oxford
Gunston-Hult	PCA (unicompartmental)
Lotus	Sevastano
Lund prototype	St. George sledge

Bicompartmental replacement: The medial and lateral side of the joint is replaced but there is no patellar resurfacing. The breakdown of the patellar mechanism resulted in a disuse of this design.

Tricompartmental: Most knee replacements entail a design that replaces both tibial-femoral surfaces as well as the patella. There are three basic categories: constrained, semiconstrained, and unconstrained.

fully constrained: The prostheses are not necessarily totally constrained. They include pure hinges, some rotating hinges, and nonhinged linked prostheses. The term *fully constrained* implies no motion and actually denotes a block of anteroposterior shifting on lateral motion. Because there is restriction in at least one plane of motion, there are forces that produce high stresses on the bone. These devices are more likely to become loose as the bone breaks down or the prosthesis itself fails. Some "fully" constrained prostheses include:

Attenborough	Noiles
Guepar	St George
Herbert	Sheehan
Kenematic	Shiers
Lacey	Spherocentric
Stanmore	Walldius

semiconstrained: the degree of constraint is from minimal to nearly full in any given plane. This is the design of many of the current prostheses.

Cintor	Stabilocondylar
Insall/Burstein	Total Condylar (HSS)
Kinematic II	Whiteside
Robert Brigham	

unconstrained: the most minimally constrained prosthetics with the maximal freedom of motion of the knee joint. These devices require good soft tissue stability.

Anametric	Liverpool
Buckholz	Lubinus
Cloutier	Marmor
Cruciate Condylar	Modular
Deane	PCA
Duocondylar	Polycentric
Duopatellar	RAM
Eriksson	RMC
Freeman-Swanson	Ring
Geomedic	Sevastano
Geotibial retainer	SKI
Gunston	TCCK
Gustuilo	Townley
Herbert	UCI (Waugh)
ICLH	Wright
LAI (Charney)	YIS

Ankle prostheses

The forces acting on the ankle are biplanar, yet by design, the prosthetics are monoplanar. With the highly active forces that exist across the ankle joint, there are fewer occasions for replacement of that joint. Prosthetic fixation is not as secure as for the lower limb joint replacements, with loosening a continuing problem. Some replacements include the following:

Conaxial	Oregon
Conoidal	Oregon Poly II
ICLH	St. George-Buckholz
Mayo	Smith
Newton	TPR
Odland	

Upper limb prostheses

Because of the special problems of fixation and the minimal occurrence of severe dysfunction in the upper limbs, there are fewer varieties of upper limb devices. However, there are total joint replacements for the shoulder (glenohumeral), elbow, wrist (including some individual carpal bones), and the fingers, including the metacarpophalangeal and interphalangeal joints. Following are the upper limb prostheses:

Bechtol prosthesis: for replacement of the glenohumeral joint.

Biometric prosthesis: for replacement of interphalangeal and metacarpophalangeal joints.

Calnan-Nicole prosthesis: for metaphalangeal and interphalangeal joints.

Coonrad prosthesis: for wrist joints.

Dana total shoulder: a plastic component for glenoid associated with metallic-stemmed prosthesis for humerus.

Eaton prosthesis: for trapezium bone replacement.

Flatt prosthesis: for metacarpophalangeal and interphalangeal joint replacements.

Gristina and Webb prosthesis: nonarticulated, semiconstrained shoulder prosthesis.

Hamas prosthesis: with Silastic interface of the wrist.

Hunter rod: two-stage tendon graft procedure using a Silastic rod tendon prosthesis to preform canal for eventual transfer of tendon.

Kessler prosthesis: for carpometacarpal joint with a silicone arthroplasty.

Michael Reese prosthesis: replacement for shoulder joint involving an interlocking device.

Neer prosthesis: shoulder replacement prosthesis.

Niebauer prosthesis: for the interphalangeal and metacarpophalangeal joint replacement.

Smith prosthesis: Silastic prosthesis for interphalangeal and thumb joint replacement.

Swanson prosthesis: a silicone prosthesis used in the fingers, wrist, and radial head of the elbow; specifically, for the interphalangeal and metacarpophalangeal joints, the multangular, scaphoid, lunate, radial head, and great toe.

Volz prosthesis: a single prong metal on plastic wrist prosthesis.

Elbow prostheses

The classification of elbow prostheses is similar to that used for knee prostheses. They are generally categorized as constrained, semiconstrained, or unconstrained.

Unconstrained

anatomic surface prosthesis	Lowe-Miller
capitellocondylar (Ewald)	London
Ishizuki	Souter
Kudo	Wadsworth

Semiconstrained

AHSC (Arizona Health Science Center-Volz)	Pritchard-Walker
Coonrad	Schlein
Mayo	Tri-Axial

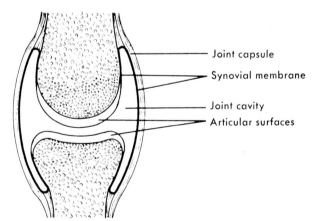

Fig. 8-4. Typical structure of diarthrotic joint. (From Hilt NE, and Cogburn SB: Manual of orthopedics, St Louis, 1980, The CV Mosby Co.)

Constrained

Dee	McKee
GSB (Gschwind, Scheir, and Bahler)	Stanmore
Mazas	

ARTHRO- (JOINTS)
Anatomy of joints

Joints are the places of union between two or more bones. All joints are not alike in structure and fall into the following categories according to function.

ball-and-socket joints: main points of articulation; femur to acetabulum of hip, humerus to glenoid of shoulder.

hinge joints: located in the elbows and knees.

immovable joints: for orthopaedic concern, in the symphysis pubis region.

synovial joint: two bones connected by fibrous tissue (capsules) with space between them and lined with synovial membrane.

weight-bearing joints: located in the lower spine, hips, knees, and ankles.

Basic parts of a joint (Fig. 8-4)

bursa sac: helps tendons and muscles to glide easily over bones at the joint outside the synovial fluid.

capsule: the general fibrous and ligamentous tissues that act as encasements and enclose the immediate joint area.

cartilage: the strong smooth covering at the ends of the articular surface of bone. In highly mobile joints like the wrist, fingers, and elbows this cartilage is called *hyaline*. In less mobile segments, such as the intervertebral disks, *fibrocartilage* is present.

meniscus: a crescent-shaped fibrocartilaginous disk between the two joint surfaces. There are three groups of menisci in the body. The medial and lateral menisci of the knee receive the most surgical attention.

subchondral bone: named for the bone immediately next to the joint cartilage. Also called subchondral plate.

synovium: inner lining of a joint, which is a one- or two-layer membrane *(synovial membrane)* on a bed of fat. The synovial membrane normally produces and absorbs a clear synovial fluid, which lubricates and feeds cartilage surfaces.

General surgery of joints

arthrectomy: excision of a joint.

arthrocentesis: needle puncture and aspiration of fluid from a joint.

arthroclasis: surgical breaking down of an ankylosis to secure free movement of a joint.

arthrodesis: a procedure to remove the cartilage of any joint to encourage bones of that joint to fuse, or grow together, where motion is not desired, for example, the spine. Also, an external fusion of a joint by means of a bone graft. The many types of arthrodeses are listed separately.

arthroereisis: a procedure to limit abnormal motion in a joint. Could be in any joint, but frequently referred to in the foot.

arthrogram: x-ray examination of the joint performed with radiopaque solution; commonly done on the shoulder, hip, and knee joints.

arthrokleisis: ankylosis of a joint by closure; production of such ankylosis.

arthrolysis: loosening adhesions in an ankylosed joint to restore mobility.

arthroplasty: reconstructive surgery of a joint or joints to restore motion because of ankylosis or trauma or to prevent excessive motion. This repair and reconstruction may use silicone, metallic, or other implants.

arthroscopy (arthroendoscopy): surgical examination of the interior of a joint and evaluation of joint disease by the insertion of an optic device capable of providing an external view of the internal joint area. This technique represents a major advance in orthopaedic technology during the past decade. The optical system is fiberoptic, giving the surgeon a high resolution view of a joint, anywhere from a direct forward view to a view at 70 degrees to the end of the microscope,

allowing the surgeon literally to see around corners. The arthroscopes vary in diameter from 2.7 to 5.0 mm. Miniature television cameras are attached directly to the arthroscope, allowing all operating room personnel to view the interior joint.

With the advancement of arthroscopic surgery, a wide variety of instruments has made it possible to remove synovium and plicas, repair peripheral tears, excise meniscal tissue, remove loose bodies, shave cartilage, and do many other procedures. The knee receives the most attention in arthroscopic procedures; however, the arthroscope is often used in ankle and shoulder surgery.

arthrotomy: surgical incision into a joint for exploration and removal of joint material; usually refers to knee exploration but can apply to any joint.

arthroxesis: scraping of diseased tissue from the articular surface of bone.

Arthrodeses
Three basic categories of arthrodeses

extraarticular arthrodesis: fusion of the joint outside the joint capsule; rarely used.

intraarticular arthrodesis: fusion of a joint all within its capsule, with or without intraarticular bone grafts.

compression arthrodesis: a general class of arthrodeses in which the pins on either side of the joint have some external compression device; the appliance is removed after fusion takes place.

Specific arthrodeses

Abbott-Fisher-Lucas arthrodesis: two-stage hip fusion that includes a delayed femoral osteotomy.

Baciu and Filibiu arthrodesis: intraarticular ankle fusion using dowel bone graft taken from the joint to include the medial and a portion of the lateral malleolus. The graft is rotated 90 degrees and reinserted.

Badgley arthrodesis: intraarticular and extraarticular hip fusion, using anterior iliac crest of bone.

Blair arthrodesis: a tibiotalar fusion, using an anterior sliding tibial graft.

Bosworth arthrodesis: a method of fusing the hip following tuberculosis infection.

Brett arthrodesis: extraarticular shoulder fusion, using tibial graft.

Brittain arthrodesis: four procedures have this name: (1) *intraarticular knee fusion* using anterior tibial grafts, (2) *extraarticular hip fusion* requiring a subtrochanteric osteotomy and tibial bone graft, (3) *extraarticular graft* to the medial side of the humerus of shoulder, and (4) *intraarticular fusion of the elbow,* using two crossed intraosseous grafts.

Campbell arthrodesis: extraarticular fusion of the ankle and subtalar joint.

Chandler arthrodesis: intraarticular and extraarticular hip fusion, using the deep portion of the greater trochanter.

Charnley arthrodesis: intraarticular type of ankle or knee fusion, using a temporary metallic external compression clamp.

Charnley and Henderson arthrodesis: intraarticular and extraarticular fusion of the shoulder, using the glenoid and acromial surface abutting a split humeral head.

Chuinard and Petersen arthrodesis: of the ankle, using a wedge of iliac bone.

Compere and Thompson fusion: intraarticular hip fusion, using iliac crest and wing for bone graft.

Davis arthrodesis: intraarticular and extraarticular hip fusion, accomplished by using a live pedicle of iliac crest.

Ghormley arthrodesis: intraarticular and extraarticular hip fusion, using anterior iliac crest graft.

Gill arthrodesis: extraarticular and intraarticular fusion, using acromion bone graft from and to the shoulder.

Henderson arthrodesis: intraarticular and extraarticular hip fusion, using detached iliac cortical bone graft.

Hibbs arthrodesis: intraarticular and extraarticular hip fusion, using greater trochanter as a graft.

Horwitz and Adams arthrodesis: ankle fusion, using the distal fibula as a graft.

Key arthrodesis: knee fusion, using anterior inlay bone graft.

Kickaldy and Willis arthrodesis: intraarticular and extraarticular hip fusion, using iliac crest bone from the ischium to the inferior neck.

King procedure: intraarticular hip fusion, using iliac and tibial bone grafts.

Kuntscher modified arthrodesis: knee arthrodesis, using a bridging intramedullary rod.

Lucas and Murray arthrodesis: knee fusion, using patella for bone graft and held by an internal plate.

Marcus, Balourdas, Heiple arthrodesis: chevron-shaped tibiotalar fusion, using inlay graft taken from medial and lateral malleolus.

Muller arthrodesis: intraarticular shoulder fusion, using bent plates for fixation.

Potter arthrodesis: knee fusion, using a retrograde tibial rod and graft from the distal tibia.

Putti arthrodesis: knee fusion, using anterior tibial graft.

Putti arthrodesis: extraarticular, using the acromion of the scapula; also an intraarticular fusion of the shoulder.

Schneider arthrodesis: intraarticular hip fusion, using innominant osteotomy with greater trochanter for a bone graft.

sliding arthrodesis: anterior ankle fusion, using tibial bone.

Smith-Petersen: technique for fusion of the sacroiliac joint.

Stamm procedure: intraarticular hip fusion, using free iliac crest bone grafts.

Staples arthrodesis: intraosseous and extraosseous elbow fusion.

Steindler arthrodesis: intraarticular fusion of the shoulder or the elbow, using posterior bone graft.

Stewart and Harley procedure: for fusion of ankle, using lateral and medial malleoli as grafts.

Stone arthrodesis: intraarticular hip fusion, using a split acetabulum and bent plate from the ilium to the femoral neck.

Trumble arthrodesis: extraarticular hip fusion, using a tibial graft from the ischium to the femur.

Watson-Jones arthrodesis: intraarticular and extraarticular hip fusion, using a nail and iliac crest graft; also, a shoulder fusion, using a piece of acromion.

White arthrodesis: intraarticular hip arthrodesis, using posterolateral approach and iliac bone graft.

Wilson procedure: extraarticular fusion of the elbow.

John C. Wilson arthrodesis: intraarticular and extraarticular hip fusion, using an iliac side graft.

Chondro- (cartilage)

Cartilage is a fine, glistening, resilient tissue that absorbs shock and facilitates the mechanics of joint motion. All mobile joint surfaces contain cartilage. *Perichondrium* is a connective tissue that covers cartilage in some places. Cartilage cells are widely separated and found in tiny spaces surrounded by joint fluid, better known as a ground substance, composed of collagen and mucopolysaccharides. Cartilage cannot be seen on x-ray examinations; if open space is apparent between two bones on x-ray film, cartilage is present. However, if an x-ray film shows two bones touching at a joint, such as the femur on the tibia, osteoarthritis and dissolution of the cartilage in that joint may have occurred.

Surgical procedures on cartilage

chondrectomy: surgical removal of cartilage.

chondroplasty: plastic surgery on cartilage by repair of lacerated or displaced cartilage.

chondrosternoplasty: surgical correction of funnel chest.

chondrotomy: dissection or surgical division of cartilage.

synchondrotomy: incision and division of an articulation that has no appreciable mobility and in which cartilage is the intervening connective tissue.

Capsulo- (capsule)

A capsule is the circumferential sleeve surrounding a joint composed of a tough band of fibrous and ligamentous tissues. It may be referred to as a joint capsule or a capsular ligament.

Surgical procedures on the capsule

capsulectomy: excision of a joint capsule; most commonly done on the hip.

capsuloplasty: plastic operation on a joint capsule.

capsulorrhaphy: suturing of a joint capsule. If used by itself, the term implies a procedure on the shoulder (glenohumeral joint) because this joint commonly has soft tissue reconstructions.

capsulotomy: incision into a joint capsule; capsotomy.

Bursae

A bursa (sac or saclike cavity) is filled with viscid fluid and situated in places in tissue where friction would otherwise develop. Bursae act as cushions, relieving pressure between moving parts. A bursal sac is easily recognized during a surgical operation and is involved in only three procedures.

bursectomy: excision of a bursa.

bursocentesis: puncture and removal of fluid from a bursa.

bursotomy: incision into a bursa.

OTHER SPECIFIC TISSUE(S)

The entire musculoskeletal system is made up of connective tissues, that is, cell elements that establish structure and shape. Bones and joints receive the most attention in orthopaedic surgery and therefore are listed separately.

All connective tissues have, to some degree, cohesion that is supplied by a protein structure called *collagen*. Collagen, in its most familiar form, is a household product, gelatin. However, when combined with other chemical and cell elements, it is the basic molecule matrix of bone, cartilage, tendons, and many other tissues. The connective tissue cells are the following.

adipose tissue: fatty tissue.

chondroblasts: cells that form cartilage.

chondroclasts: cells that remove cartilage.

chondrocytes: cartilage cells.

fibroblasts: cells that predominantly form collagen.

fibrocytes: cells seen in tendons, ligaments, and similar structures.

histiocytes: cells involved in removal of cellular or chemical debris; a type of phagocyte.

myoblasts: muscle-forming cells.

myocytes: muscle cells, voluntary (striated) and involuntary (nonstriated).

Myo- (muscle) (Fig. 8-5)

Muscle is the contractile tissue essential for skeletal support and movement. The anatomy of muscles with associated tissues, and surgery is presented here.

Muscle fibers are composed of small bundles of cells combined to form distinct muscular units. Terms often related to muscle include actin, myocin, sarcomere, nerve spindle, motor unit, neuromuscular junction, and spindle cell.

Surgical procedures on muscles

myectomy: excision of a portion of muscle.

myoclasis: intentional crushing of muscle; rare.

myomectomy (myomatectomy): surgical removal of tumors with muscular tissue components (myoma).

myoneurectomy: surgical interruption of nerve fibers supplying specific muscles; used for patients with cerebral palsy.

myoplasty: plastic surgery on muscle in which portions of partly detached muscle are used for correction of defects or deformities.

myorrhaphy (myosuture): muscle repair by suturation of divided muscle.

myotenontoplasty: surgical fixation of muscles and tendons.

myotenotomy: surgical division of a tendon of muscle.

myotomy: incision or dissection of muscle or muscular tissue.

Aponeuroses

Aponeurosis is the name given to the end of a muscle that becomes a tendon. This muscular component is a white, flattened tendinous expansion that connects muscle with the parts it moves.

Surgical procedures on aponeuroses

aponeurectomy: excision of the aponeurosis.

aponeurorrhaphy: repair and suture of muscle and tendon. Also called *fasciorrhaphy*.

aponeurotomy: surgical incision into the aponeurosis.

Teno- (tendons)

The extension of muscle into a firm, fibrous cord that attaches into a bone or other firm structure is a tendon. Some muscles have a tendon at both ends, some have direct attachment to bone at one end, and a few attach directly to bone at both ends and have no tendon.

Surgical procedures on tendons

The nomenclature of surgical procedures on tendons has a certain amount of overlap, since several prefixes are used—teno-, tendo-, and tendino-. Therefore the same surgical procedure may have several forms of spelling. The preferred term for a surgical procedure is listed first, with the related term appearing after the definition.

tendon release: surgical transection of a tendon, with or without repair.

tenectomy: excision of a lesion (ganglion or xanthoma) of a tendon or of a tendon sheath.

tenodesis: tendon fixation by suturing proximal end of a tendon to the bone or by reattachment of the tendon to another site.

tenolysis: surgically freeing a tendon from adhesions. Also called *tendolysis*.

tenomyoplasty: procedure involving repair of tendon and muscle. Also called tenontomyoplasty.

tenomyotomy: lateral excision of a portion of tendon and muscle.

tenonectomy: excision of a portion of tendon to shorten it.

tenontomyotomy: incision into the principal ten-

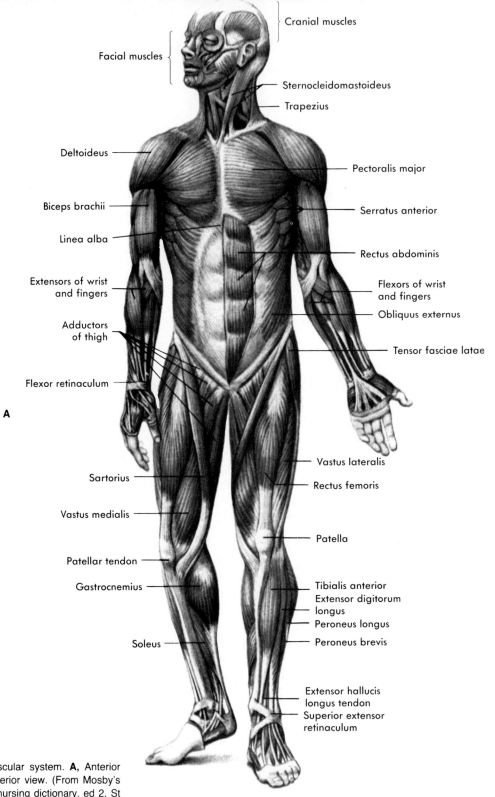

Cranial muscles

Facial muscles

Sternocleidomastoideus

Trapezius

Deltoideus

Pectoralis major

Biceps brachii

Serratus anterior

Linea alba

Rectus abdominis

Extensors of wrist
and fingers

Flexors of wrist
and fingers

Obliquus externus

Adductors
of thigh

Tensor fasciae latae

Flexor retinaculum

A

Vastus lateralis

Sartorius

Rectus femoris

Vastus medialis

Patella

Patellar tendon

Gastrocnemius

Tibialis anterior

Extensor digitorum
longus

Peroneus longus

Peroneus brevis

Soleus

Extensor hallucis
longus tendon

Superior extensor
retinaculum

Fig. 8-5. Muscular system. **A,** Anterior
view. **B,** Posterior view. (From Mosby's
medical and nursing dictionary, ed 2, St
Louis, 1986, The CV Mosby Co.)

ANTERIOR VIEW

Sternocleidomastoideus

Seventh cervical vertebra

Deltoideus

Teres minor

Teres major

Triceps

Latissimus dorsi

Extensors
of the wrist
and fingers

Semitendinosus

Biceps femoris

Semimembranosus

Gastrocnemius

Peroneus longus

Peroneus brevis

Splenius capitis

Trapezius

Infraspinatus

Portion of rhomboideus

Obliquus externus

Gluteus maximus

Adductor magnus

Gracilis

Iliotibial tract

Plantaris

Gastrocnemius tendon
(Achilles tendon)

Soleus

Superior peroneal retinaculum

B

Fig. 8-5, cont'd. For legend, see opposite page.

POSTERIOR VIEW

don of a muscle, with partial or complete excision of that muscle.

tenoplasty: surgical repair of a ruptured tendon. Also called *tendoplasty, tendinoplasty, tenontoplasty.*

tenorrhaphy: union of a divided tendon by a suture. Also called *tenosuture, tendinosuture.*

tenosuspension: surgical repair that fashions a soft tissue sling to hold the tendon in a specific place.

tenosynovectomy: resection or excision of a tendon sheath.

tenotomy: incomplete or complete division of a tendon, as in clubfoot. Also called *tendotomy.*

Desmo- (ligaments)

Ligaments are bands of fibrous tissue connecting bones primarily at the joint, tying bones together. For this reason the prefix *syn-* (together) is used when referring to ligamentous surgery.

Surgical procedures on ligaments

desmotomy: surgical division of a ligament or ligaments.

syndesmectomy: excision of a ligament or portion thereof.

syndesmopexy: surgical fixation of a dislocation by using the ligaments of a joint.

syndesmoplasty: ligaments sutured together.

syndesmorrhaphy: suture or repair of ligaments.

syndesmotomy: dissection or cutting of ligaments.

Fasciae

Fasciae (pronounced fash-e-e) (fascia, sing.) are sheets of dense connective fibrous tissue that act as a restricting envelope for muscular components and bind groups of muscles, blood vessels, and nerves into bundles. Generally the fascia does not play any role in the movement of joints and bones. The exception to this is the fascia lata of the outer thigh; this fascia has its own muscle (tensor fascia lata) that, when tightened, will pull through the fascia to points across the knee.

Surgical procedures on fasciae

fasciaplasty: plastic surgery of fascia. Also called fascioplasty.

fasciectomy: excision of strips of fascia.

fasciodesis: suturing a fascia to another fascia or tendon.

fasciogram: a nonsurgical procedure in which air is injected into the fascia layers for x-ray examination.

fasciorrhaphy: suturing and repair of lacerated fascia. Also called aponeurorrhaphy.

fasciotomy: surgical incision or transection of fascia, commonly done for forearm and leg injuries.

Neuro- (nerves)

Nerves are cordlike structures that convey impulses between a part of the central nervous system and some other region of the body. Structural components of the nerves include epineurium, perineurium, nerve sheath, axon, Schwann cell, and myelin.

Orthopaedic surgical procedures on nerves

neurectomy: resection of a segment of a nerve.

neurolysis: destruction of a perineural adhesion by a longitudinal incision to release the nerve sheath.

neuroplasty: plastic repair of a nerve.

neurorrhaphy: suture of a severed nerve; repair.

neurotomy: division of a nerve or nerves.

neurotripsy: surgical crushing of a nerve.

rhizotomy (radicotomy, radiculectomy): procedure dividing the nerve roots close to their origin from the spinal cord; rhizo- meaning root of the spinal cord.

VASCULAR (BLOOD VESSELS) SYSTEM (Fig. 8-6)

This section on the vascular system was contributed by James M. Salander.*

There are thousands of miles of blood vessels in the human body and approximately 2000 gallons of blood per day coursing through these vessels, likened to a road map with its major arteries, trib-

---

*James M. Salander, MD, FACS (COL, MC, USA), Associate Professor of Surgery, Uniformed Services University of the Health Sciences, Bethesda, Maryland.

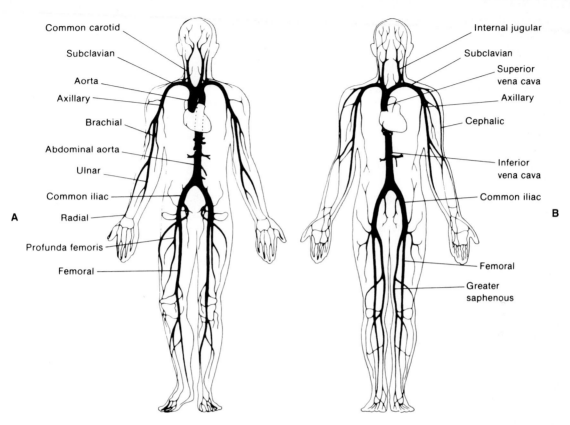

Fig. 8-6. A, The major named arteries of the body distribute oxygenated blood from the heart to the principal organs of the body. The name of each artery corresponds to the organ or region served. **B,** The major veins are named to correspond to the regions of the body they drain: Blood is returned by these veins to the heart, which pumps it through the lungs for oxygenation. (From American Academy of Orthopaedic Surgeons: Emergency care and transportation of the sick and injured, Chicago, 1981, The Academy.)

utaries, and branches. The *arteries* are the major pipelines that distribute oxygenated blood from the heart to the various organs. In each group, the main artery resembles a tree trunk that gives off numerous branches and these rebranch forming smaller vessels called *arterioles*, which branch again forming microscopic vessels called *capillaries*.

The *veins* are an extension of the capillaries in that capillaries unite into vessels of increasing size to form *venules* and eventually *veins*. Their function is to carry deoxygenated blood from the various organs back to the heart. Veins differ from arteries in that they have *valves* which create a

unidirectional flow. Arteries and veins often have the same name for their location in the body, for example, femoral artery and femoral vein. The following general terms relate to blood vessels.

adventitia: loose outside lining of a blood vessel; outermost wall of artery.

artery: blood vessel that carries oxygenated blood away from heart on its way to various organs and tissues in the body.

arterioles: smallest vessels considered arteries (.2 mm diameter) made mostly of smooth muscle; blood flows through arterioles and moves to capillaries.

capillaries: tiny network of blood vessels supplying oxygen directly to cells of body. At this level, oxygen and other nutrients are delivered to cells, and carbon dioxide and waste materials are passed from the tissues back to the bloodstream.

cardiovascular: pertaining to blood vessels (arteries and veins) and the heart.

cerebrovascular: pertaining to blood vessel circulation of the brain and to the brain.

collateral circulation: named and unnamed secondary vessels supplying blood to an organ or extremity through indirect channels. These collateral vessels become particularly important when the main artery is damaged (occluded), for example, genicular arteries around the knee in support of an occluded popliteal artery.

diastole: filling or relaxation phase of the heart cycle.

intima: the innermost lining of the arterial wall.

lipid: one of many chemical compounds normally found in blood that are considered fats and have a relationship between the amount and kinds of lipids in the blood and hardening of the arteries.

lumen: the space inside a blood vessel, duct, or hollow viscus.

patency: refers to an open blood vessel (artery or vein) where blood is flowing.

systole: contraction phase of cardiac cycle.

vascular: pertaining to vessels. Can also refer to amount of blood supply to an organ, such as a very vascular tumor, that is, good blood supply.

vein: blood vessel that carries blood from the various organs in the body back to the heart. Veins usually have valves creating a unidirectional flow, whereas arteries do not. Small veins are then called *venules*.

Vascular surgical procedures (arteries/veins)

Peripheral vascular surgery procedures center around the treatment of disorders of the blood vessels, that is, the arteries and veins (not including the heart), and may be performed in conjunction with orthopaedic procedures, such as the repair of a disrupted popliteal artery following a knee dislocation. An understanding of peripheral vascular surgery is also necessary in diagnosing patients with vascular disease who come to the orthopaedic surgeon. For example, a patient may see an orthopaedic surgeon for a painful foot believing it to be a bony problem, only to find it is "rest pain" from occluded arteries in the thigh and calf. In this case, the patient is referred to the vascular surgeon for further evaluation and treatment. Since these two specialties overlap in diagnosis, treatment, and surgery, vascular procedures are included for reference.

Most peripheral vascular surgical procedures performed today are done to correct the problem of arteriosclerosis (hardening of the arteries). In this regard, the problems can usually be corrected by a bypass, by replacing the artery, or by cleaning it out (endarterectomy). The terms relating to blood vessel surgery follow.

aortofemoral bypass (AFB): surgical procedure whereby the narrowing or occlusion of the abdominal aorta and iliac arteries (from arteriosclerosis) is bypassed with a graft (usually Dacron) going from just below the renal arteries down to the femoral arteries in the groins. Considered one of the bigger vascular procedures requiring opening the abdomen (taking from 3 to 6 hours). Separate bypass grafts may be taken off the main aortofemoral graft to increase the blood supply to the kidneys, intestines, or pelvic viscera to include the male genitalia.

aortoiliac bypass: a bypass graft going from just below the renal artery down to the iliac arteries. This procedure is usually performed for abdominal aortic aneurysms (AAA).

aneurysmorrhaphy: a repair of an aneurysm in which it is left in place, but disconnected from the circulation, and a graft is sewn in its place. Following this, the aneurysm wall can either be wrapped around the graft or left in place. (Totally removing the aneurysm is rarely done since it may jeopardize adjacent organs.)

arthrectomy catheter (Simpson): a vascular procedure for a localized endarterectomy where a device is passed percutaneously or intraoperatively to an area of stenosis, using a small circular knife blade.

autogenous saphenous vein graft (ASVG): the greater saphenous vein of the lower extremity is removed and used to either bypass or replace a diseased segment of artery or vein elsewhere in the body. When the vein is removed and placed in a different location, care must be taken to ensure that the valves of the vein are either destroyed or that the vein is put in a reversed fashion so that the arterial blood will flow unimpeded.

axillofemoral bypass (AxFem): an extraanatomic bypass whereby either Dacron or PTFE graft is used to carry blood from the axillary artery (under the arm) down to one or both common femoral arteries. This procedure is usually performed in lieu of an aortofemoral bypass because the abdomen is inaccessible resulting from infection in the abdomen, for example, infected aortofemoral graft, severe cardiac disease, or severe pulmonary disease. The patency rate for these grafts is not nearly as good as a usual aortofemoral bypass graft.

balloon angioplasty: a relatively new procedure usually performed by a radiologist or cardiologist, using radiologic techniques whereby a balloon catheter is passed up to an area of stenosis, a balloon is inflated, and the area of the stenosis (stricture) is dilated. This procedure is applicable only for a short segment isolated stenosis in large vessels, such as the common iliac or renal arteries. It is also utilized in the coronary arteries as well. The long-term benefit of this procedure is becoming more acceptable. Also called percutaneous transluminal angioplasty (PTLA).

carotid endarterectomy: an opening up and cleaning out of the common carotid and internal carotid artery in the neck. During this procedure, the diseased intima and portions of the media are removed to open and smooth out the channel of blood flow to the brain. The procedure removes the roughened irregular buildup of atherosclerosis and is done to prevent transient ischemic attacks (TIA) and strokes.

carotid subclavian bypass: a procedure involving either vein or prosthetic material whereby a bypass graft is placed between the carotid artery and subclavian artery. It is done to improve the blood flow in the subclavian artery to the arm and hand, by bringing blood up the carotid artery and down into the subclavian, bypassing a "narrowing" at the origin of the subclavian artery. (See also subclavian-carotid bypass.)

coronary artery bypass graft (CABG): a procedure on the blood vessels of the heart whereby narrowed areas in the arteries leading to the heart muscle itself are bypassed with a vein graft going directly from the aorta to more distal portions of the coronary (heart) arteries. This procedure, performed by cardiac surgeons, is done while the patient is on a cardiac bypass machine.

distal bypass: procedure performed with either synthetic material or vein whereby blood is brought from either the common femoral or superficial femoral artery down to the small named blood vessels below the knee. The procedure is usually performed to prevent amputation of an extremity from severe ischemia. The patient frequently has severe pain and skin breakdown before the operation.

endarterectomy: an opening up and cleaning out of blood vessels diseased by hardening of the arteries, which begin in the intima and progress down through the media. In this procedure, the diseased intima and much of the media is removed; the roughened irregular surface of the blood vessel can produce a surface on which blood clots will collect and break off—moving downstream, or a surface on which more clot can form and occlude (close off) the artery.

end-to-end anastomosis: a joining of two vascular structures—arteries, graft and arteries, or vein and arteries—to bypass an occluded or damaged segment; the end of one structure is sewn to the end of the other.

end-to-side anastomosis: a joining of the end of an artery or vein or prosthetic material to the side of another vein, artery or prosthetic material to bypass an occluded or damaged segment.

extraanatomic bypass: bypass graft in which prosthetic material or vein is used to route blood between the two arteries or two veins. The route of the graft is other than a usual anatomic position, such as axillofemoral or femoral-femoral bypass.

extracranial/intracranial bypass (ECIC): a procedure performed by neurosurgeons whereby severely narrowed or occluded blood vessels within the brain are bypassed. The usual procedure is to take the superficial temporal artery, which is a branch on the scalp, make a bone flap in the skull, and move the distal end of this artery down into the brain to supply blood flow directly into the brain.

femoral-femoral bypass (fem-fem bypass): a bypass procedure using a synthetic or vein graft material whereby one femoral artery is used to supply the blood to both lower extremities. This could be done to bypass an infection, or to provide blood flow from one undiseased iliac femoral system to another femoral system. It is considered an extraanatomic bypass.

femoral popliteal bypass (FPB): bypass graft from the femoral artery to the popliteal artery. The distal end of the graft can go to a portion of the popliteal artery above the knee or the popliteal artery below the knee. May be performed with vein or prosthetic material. It is done to correct an occluded superficial femoral artery. Indications for this procedure are claudication, rest pain, or threatened limb loss.

in situ bypass: a procedure whereby instead of removing the greater saphenous vein and reversing it, it is left in place and the valve destroyed through a variety of techniques. The proximal end is sutured into the inflow artery, and the distal end of the vein is sutured into the recipient artery. The side branches of the vein are ligated in distal artery of leg. This technique provides better patency than taking the vein out and reversing its course.

laparotomy: a procedure whereby the abdomen is opened for exploration or to conduct another surgical procedure.

laser endarterectomy: a technique of using a laser beam to disobliterate plaque from an artery. It can either be done intraoperatively or, in some instances, percutaneously.

limb salvage: a general category of procedures performed on the lower extremity to improve the blood supply and prevent amputation. Skin ulceration and gangrene are often present.

patch angioplasty: a local procedure whereby the artery is opened, the inside of the vessel is cleaned out and a patch of vein or prosthetic material is used to widen that area of the artery. This procedure is also done in the repair of traumatic injuries.

polytetrafluoralethylene (PTFE): (Gor-tex) a new plastic graft that has gained tremendous popularity in bypassing and replacing occluded arteries throughout the body.

reversed vein bypass graft: a technique where a vein, usually the greater saphenous, is removed and used as a bypass. The small end of vein is sutured to proximal artery (inflow) and distal (large) end of vein is sutured to outflow artery. The vein must be turned around in this fashion to obviate the function of valves.

subclavian carotid bypass: bypass procedure between the subclavian artery and carotid artery to correct a severe narrowing at the origin of the common carotid artery. This allows blood to flow up the subclavian artery, along the graft, into the carotid artery, and into the brain without interrupting blood flow to the arm or hand.

thrombolytic therapy: a dissolution of thrombus in an artery or vein with urokinase or streptokinase. Has been most useful in recent thromboses, but some contraindications must be considered.

Specific anatomy and surgery by location
THE SHOULDER

Shoulder separations and shoulder dislocations are very distinct injuries and involve two different joints. Palpating the collarbone (clavicle) and working the fingers laterally, a distinct bump is felt—the acromioclavicular (A/C) joint, which is the junction between the collarbone and shoulder blade (Fig. 8-7). The acromion is the part of the shoulder blade that connects with the collarbone. Injury of this joint is often called a shoulder separation. On the other hand, a person dislocating the shoulder has disrupted the ball-and-socket joint between the arm and the shoulder blade (gleno-

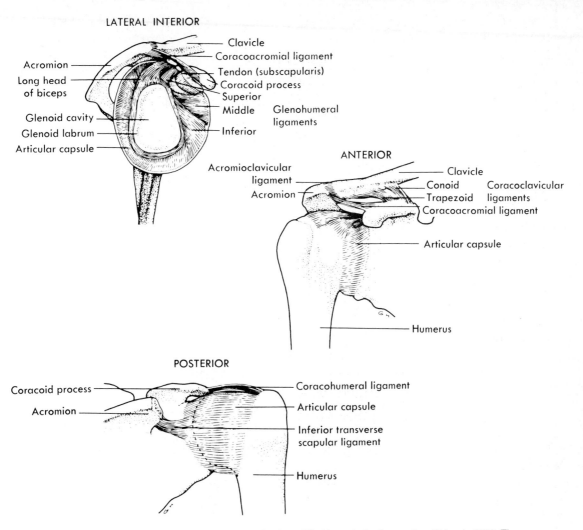

LATERAL INTERIOR

Clavicle
Coracoacromial ligament
Acromion
Tendon (subscapularis)
Long head of biceps
Coracoid process
Superior
Middle — Glenohumeral ligaments
Glenoid cavity
Glenoid labrum
Inferior
Articular capsule

ANTERIOR

Acromioclavicular ligament
Clavicle
Conoid — Coracoclavicular ligaments
Acromion
Trapezoid
Coracoacromial ligament
Articular capsule
Humerus

POSTERIOR

Coracoid process
Coracohumeral ligament
Acromion
Articular capsule
Inferior transverse scapular ligament
Humerus

Fig. 8-7. Shoulder joints. (From Hilt NE, and Cogburn SB: Manual of orthopaedics, St Louis 1980, The CV Mosby Co.)

humeral joint). The orthopaedist may not be able to feel this joint dislocation under the numerous muscles, but its presence is apparent through pain and an inability to place the arm behind the back or raise it over the head.

Anatomy of the shoulder

axilla: armpit.

scapula: shoulder blade.

coracoid: knob of bone attached to the anterior scapula just medial to the shoulder.

spine: outcropping portion of the posterosuperior scapula.

glenoid fossa: saucer-shaped depression of the scapula that has direct contact with the humerus and glenohumeral joint.

acromion process: outermost tip of the shoulder.

clavicle (cleido-): collarbone.

acromioclavicular joint: between clavicle and scapula.

sternoclavicular joint: at the junction of the clavicle and breast bones.

rhomboid fossa: an inconsistent feature on the medial side of the clavicle. It is the attachment of the costoclavicular or rhomboid ligament and has importance only because it may be mistaken for a tumor.

humerus: arm bone between the shoulder and elbow.

biceps groove: groove for the long head of the biceps muscle.

greater and lesser tuberosity: points of attachment for the rotator cuff.

surgical neck: most common point of fracture of the humerus.

anatomic neck: point of attachment of shoulder capsule (humerus).

humeral head: half circle-shaped portion of the humerus for the shoulder joint.

rotator cuff (Fig. 8-6): arrangement of four muscles from the scapula to the humerus, which with the capsule and glenoid (labrum), a cartilaginous margin of the joint, hold the shoulder together. The muscles of the rotator cuff are supraspinatus, infraspinatus, teres minor, and subscapularis.

Muscles around the shoulder

sternocleidomastoid
levator scapulae
trapezius
deltoid
coracobrachialis
pectoralis major and minor
rhomboideus major and minor
teres major and minor
latissimus dorsi
serratus anterior

Main arteries, veins, and branches around the shoulder

subclavian artery: main artery from the chest leading down through the arm that branches into internal thoracic, vertebral, thyrocervical, transcervical, superior intercostal, and suprascapular.

axillary artery: a continuum of the subclavian artery in the axillary area that branches into highest thoracic, lateral thoracic, anterior humeral circumflex, posterior humeral circumflex, thoracoacromial, and subscapularis.

brachial artery: a continuum of the axillary artery and main artery of the arm. The branches are listed in the Arm and forearm section.

subclavian and axillary vein: the continuous vessel running alongside the subclavian and axillary arteries. The branches are not consistent and are rarely described in orthopaedic procedures.

cephalic vein: large vein between the deltoid and pectoralis muscles.

Nerves

brachial plexus: a large complex of nerves from the lower cervical and upper thoracic (C-5 to T-2) spinal segments. This nerve plexus includes:
superior, medial, and inferior *trunk*
anterior and posterior *division*
medial, lateral, and posterior *cord*
lower and upper subscapular nerve
musculocutaneous nerve
radial nerve
ulnar nerve
dorsal scapular nerve
axillary nerve
medial nerve
scapular nerve
long thoracic nerve

Ligaments around the shoulder region

At the sternoclavicular joint, the sternoclavicular ligament
At the acromioclavicular joint, acromioclavicular ligament, coracoacromial ligament, and coracoclavicular ligament (the conoid and trapezoid ligament)
At the glenohumeral joint, glenoid labrum and coracohumeral ligament

shoulder girdle: a general term for the soft tissue around the glenohumeral joint.

conjoined tendon: the common origin of two tendons from the coracoid process of the scapula leading to the arm and forearm. In surgery it is detached temporarily to gain access to the shoulder joint.

Surgical procedures for the shoulder
Eponyms

The following list of eponyms for surgical procedures is arranged according to the area of injury or deformity. In most instances the arthroplasties can be referred to as capsulorrhaphies of the shoulder.

Arthroplasties for acromioclavicular separations

Bosworth
Dewar and Barrington
Mumford-Gurd
Neviaser

Arthroplasties for anterior shoulder dislocations

Bankart	Magnuson-Stack
Bristow	Nicola
Cubbins	Putti-Platt
du Toit and Roux	Speed
Eden-Hybbinette	Trillat

Arthroplasties for posterior shoulder dislocations

McLaughlin
Scott
Wilson and McKeever

For high-riding scapulae (Sprengel deformity)

Chang and Farahvar
Green
Inclan-Ober
Robinson
Schrock
Woodward

Arthrodeses for shoulder stabilization

Brittain	Steindler
Gill	Watson-Jones
Putti	

Muscle transfers for paralysis of scapula

Chaves	His-Haas
Chaves-Rapp	Whitman
DeWar and Harris	Saha
Dickson	Vastamäki
Henry	

Posterior bone block elbow

Boyd
Putti
Putti-Scaglietti

Alphabetic listing

acromionectomy: excision of all or part of the acromion, usually in cases of rotator cuff injuries.

acromioplasty: repair or partial removal of the acromion.

Bankart procedure: capsular repair in the glenoid for chronic anterior dislocation of the shoulder.

Bateman procedure: for paralysis of the deltoid; a trapezius muscle transfer to the greater tuberosity.

Bosworth procedure: screw fixation of the clavicle to the coracoid for acromioclavicular separations.

Boyd and Sisk procedure: for stabilization of recurrent posterior shoulder dislocation; transfer of long head of biceps to posterior glenoid.

Braun procedure: for partial ankylosis of the shoulder, open tenotomy of the subscapularis. Also, for painful shoulder in stroke patients; section of subscapularis and pectoralis major tendons.

brisement: a closed manipulation of a stiff shoulder.

Bristow procedure: coracoid process transfer for chronic anterior dislocation of the shoulder.

Brittain procedure: extraarticular fusion of the shoulder.

Brooks and Saddon procedure: for paralysis of biceps; transfer of pectoralis major tendon to biceps.

Bunnell procedure: for paralysis of elbow flexion; transfer of triceps anterior to radial tuberosity. Also, for paralysis biceps transfer of sternocleidomastoid to long head of biceps.

Chaves-Rapp procedure: for long thoracic nerve palsy; transfer of the pectoralis major to inferior scapula.

clavicectomy: excision of all or part of the clavicle.

clavicotomy: surgical division of the collarbone.

Copeland and Howard procedure: for shoulder paralytic instability; fusion of scapula to ribs using tibial cortical grafts.

costectomy: excision of part or all of a rib for purposes of either a bone graft or approach to thorax.

costotransversectomy: excision of the transverse process of a vertebra and the neighboring rib for approach to the spine or cord.

Cubbins procedure: passage of the coracohumeral ligament through the humeral head for an old anterior dislocation of the shoulder.

Das Gupta procedure: technique of excision of scapula.

Debeyre procedure: for repair of rotator cuff tear, superior approach to supraspinatus in order to advance tendon.

Dewar and Barrington procedure: transfer of the coracoid tip to the clavicle for acromioclavicular separations.

du Toit and Roux procedure: a stapling procedure of the anterior shoulder capsule for chronic anterior dislocation of the shoulder.

Eden-Hybbinette procedure: a bone block to the anterior glenoid for chronic anterior dislocation of the shoulder.

Eden-Lange procedure: for spinal accessory nerve palsy; transfer of levator scapulae, rhomboid major, and rhomboid minor.

Eyler procedure: for paralysis of elbow flexor; transfer of flexor wad of five proximally on humerus facilitated with tendon fascia lata graft.

Fairbanks and Sever procedure: for internal rotation and adduction contraction of shoulder, resection of tendinous portion of pectoralis major

and minor, coracobrachialis, and short and long head of the biceps.

Gill procedure: intraarticular and extraarticular fusion of the shoulder.

Green procedure: soft tissue release and repair for high-riding scapulae.

Harmon procedure: for partial paralysis of deltoid; transfer of posterior origin to anterior part.

His-Haas procedure: for long thoracic nerve palsy; transfer teres major from humerus to chest wall.

Hovanian procedure: for paralysis of biceps; transfer latissimus dorsi to radial tuberosity. Also, for triceps weakness; a transfer of latissimus dorsi to triceps muscle.

Inclan-Ober procedure: soft tissue release and repair for high-riding scapulae.

Janecki and Nelson procedure: for scapular malignancy, radical resection that includes a portion of the clavicle, proximal humerus, and entire scapula.

L'Episcopo Zachary procedure: for internal rotation and adduction contracture of the shoulder; resection of anterior capsule and tendon of pectoralis major with transfer of triceps and latissimus dorsi tendon.

Magnuson-Stack procedure: stapling of the subscapularis for chronic anterior dislocation of the shoulder.

Marcove, Lewis, Horos procedure: for scapular malignancy, radical resection that includes a portion of the clavicle, proximal humerus, and entire scapula.

McKeever procedure: for open fixation of clavicle fracture, using a threaded wire.

McLaughlin procedure: for rotator cuff injury of shoulder, a technique of repair; a transfer of the subscapularis into a hatchet head deformity of the humerus for old posterior dislocation of the shoulder.

B.H. Moore procedure: for muscle imbalance in shoulder caused by stroke; posterior transfer of part of deltoid muscle.

J.R. Moore procedure: for posterior dislocation of humeral head in stroke; multiple anterior tendon and anterior capsule resection with bone graft to glenoid.

Mumford-Gurd procedure: resection of the distal clavicle for a chronic acromioclavicular separation.

Neviaser procedure: a transfer of the coracoacromial ligament to the clavicle for acromioclavicular separation.

Nicola procedure: transfer of the long head of the biceps tendon through humeral head for chronic anterior shoulder dislocation.

Ober and Barr procedure: for weakness of triceps; transfer of brachioradialis.

Phelps: for tumor, technique of partial resection of the scapula.

Putti-Platt procedure: subscapularis muscle and capsular repair for chronic anterior dislocation of the shoulder.

Putti procedure: fusion of the shoulder by two different methods.

Saha procedure: for paralysis of deltoid; transfer of trapezius and distal acromion to humerus below greater tuberosity. Also, for paralysis of subscapularis; transfer of two superior digitations of serratus anterior or transfer of pectoralis minor. Also, for paralysis of supraspinatus; a transfer of levator scapulae or sternocleidomastoid. Also, for paralysis of infraspinatus or subscapularis; a transfer of latissimus dorsi or teres major.

scapulectomy: excision of all or part of the scapula.

Schrock procedure: soft tissue release and repair for high-riding scapulae.

Scott procedure: wedge bone block procedure for chronic posterior dislocation of the shoulder.

Speed procedure: ligamentous repair for sternoclavicular joint separations; also for chronic dislocation elbow, reduction and stabilization, using a folded expansion of triceps muscle.

Spira procedure: for paralysis biceps, transfer of pectoralis minor.

Steindler procedure: intraarticular fusion of the shoulder.

Tikhoff-Linberg procedure: for scapular malignancy, radical resection that includes a portion of the clavicle, proximal humerus, and entire scapula.

Trillat procedure: for anterior shoulder dislocation, osteotomy of coracoid with attachment to glenoid to act as bone block.

Weaver and Dunn procedure: for acromioclavicular separation, transfer of coracoacromial ligament to distal clavicle.

Whitman procedure: for long thoracic nerve palsy, stabilization of scapula with fascial strips attached to spinous processes.

Wilson and McKeever procedure: K-wire (Kirschner wire) fixation after open reduction of an old posterior shoulder dislocation.

Watson-Jones procedure: shoulder fusion using a piece of acromion.

Woodward procedure: soft tissue release and repair for high-riding scapulae.

Zeir procedure: for long thoracic nerve palsy; pectoralis minor transferred to scapula using a tensor fascia lata graft.

THE ARM AND FOREARM

Specifically, the arm is the portion of the upper limb between the shoulder and the elbow, and the forearm is between the elbow and the wrist. Most surgical procedures on the arm and forearm are of a general type, that is, nerve and vessel repairs and fracture fixations. Most tendon transfers are considered in Chapter 9.

Anatomy of the arm and forearm
(Fig. 8-8)
Humerus

The humerus, the arm bone, extends from the shoulder to the elbow.

spiral groove: groove in the bone for the radial nerve.

medial and lateral epicondyles: large prominences on either side of the elbow.

capitellum: provides articulation with the radial head.

trochlea: provides articulation with the ulna.

olecranon fossa: thin portion of the bone with an opening above the elbow joint.

epitrochlea: medial epicondyle.

Radius

The radius is the bone on the thumb side of the forearm.

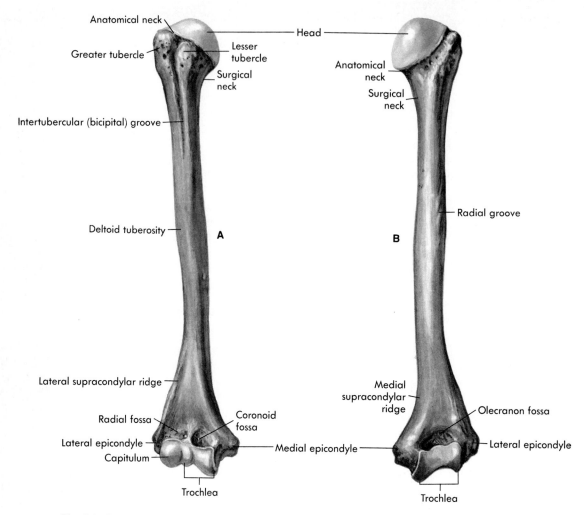

Anatomical neck

Greater tubercle

Lesser tubercle

Head

Surgical neck

Anatomical neck

Surgical neck

Intertubercular (bicipital) groove

Radial groove

Deltoid tuberosity

A

B

Lateral supracondylar ridge

Medial supracondylar ridge

Olecranon fossa

Radial fossa

Coronoid fossa

Lateral epicondyle

Capitulum

Medial epicondyle

Lateral epicondyle

Trochlea

Trochlea

Fig. 8-8. Right humerus. **A,** Anterior view. **B,** Posterior view. (From Seeley RR, Stephens TD, and Tate P: Anatomy and physiology, St Louis, 1989, Times Mirror/Mosby College Publishing.)

radial head: the articular portion of the radius to the elbow.

biceps tuberosity: point of insertion of biceps tendon.

styloid process: the distalmost portion of radius.

Lister tubercle: a prominence on the distal dorsum of the radius.

Ulna (Fig. 8-9)

The ulna is the bone of the forearm on the little finger side of the wrist, prominent at the elbow.

olecranon: prominent ulnar portion at the elbow.

coronoid process: anterior part of the ulna at the elbow joint at the brachialis insertion.

styloid process: the distalmost portion of the ulna, prominent on turning the wrist downward.

Muscles of the arm

rotator cuff: see under Shoulder anatomy.

biceps muscle: a two-belly muscle that flexes the elbow; extends from the scapula to the radius.

triceps muscle: a three-belly muscle that extends

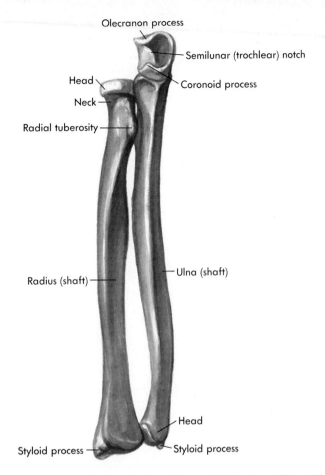

Fig. 8-9. Ulna and radius of the right forearm. (From Seeley RR, Stephens TD, and Tate P: Anatomy and physiology, St Louis, 1989, Times Mirror/Mosby College Publishing.)

the elbow; its origin is at the scapula, down the arm to the ulna.

brachialis muscle: flexes the elbow from the arm to the ulna.

coracobrachialis muscle: pulls the arm in and up; extends from the scapula to the arm.

Muscles of the forearm

Many muscles of the forearm that affect hand function are discussed in Chapter 9. Others that relate to forearm function are the following.

extensor wad of three: muscles that extend the wrist and flex the elbow.

brachioradialis muscle: located on the lateral side of the forearm; helps flex the elbow.

extensor carpi radialis longus: long muscle that extends the wrist.

extensor carpi radialis brevis: short muscle that extends the wrist.

flexor wad of five: muscles that flex the wrist and fingers and pronate the forearm—flexor carpi ulnaris, palmaris longus, flexor digitorum superficialis, pronator teres, and flexor carpi radialis; see Chapter 9.

supinator muscle: located at the proximal forearm; brings the palm up in supination.

pronator quadratus: flat muscle at the distal forearm that turns the palm down in pronation.

anconeus: small muscle on the ulnar side of the elbow.

Blood vessels (Fig. 8-10)

basilic vein: branches upward and laterally from ulnar side of forearm to front of elbow, winding around ulnar border of forearm to join the brachial vein which becomes the axillary vein.

brachial artery: main artery of the arm that divides at the elbow into the radial and ulnar arteries.

brachial vein: branches off axillary.

cephalic vein: branches off from axillary artery and vein on radial side; runs upward and medially to front of elbow and winds around and enters the axillary vein.

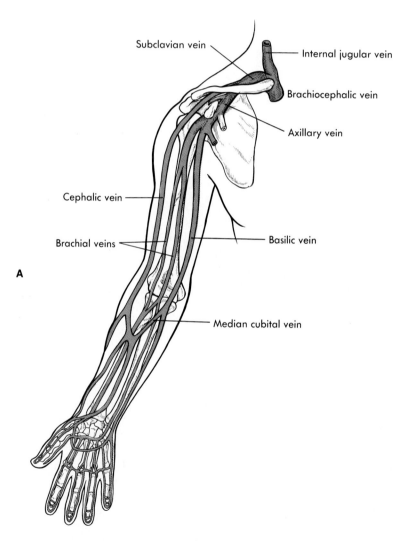

Subclavian vein — Internal jugular vein

Brachiocephalic vein

Axillary vein

Cephalic vein

Basilic vein

Brachial veins

A

Median cubital vein

Fig. 8-10. Blood vessels of the upper limb. **A,** Veins of the upper limb—the subclavian vein and its tributaries. The major veins draining the superficial structures of the limb are the cephalic and basilic veins. The brachial veins drain the deep structures.

median cephalic vein: near elbow area (where blood is drawn).

median basilic vein: near elbow area.

profundus: deep anterior brachial artery of the arm.

radial artery: one that travels deep into the muscle on the thumb side of the forearm.

radial vein: branches off from cephalic vein.

ulnar artery: one that travels deep into the muscle on the little finger side of the anterior forearm.

Other blood vessels, not defined, are (1) elbow—ulnar collateral, anterior and posterior ulnar recurrent, anterior and posterior radial recurrent, and (2) forearm—anterior and posterior interosseous.

axillary nerve: of the shoulder, supplying the deltoid and teres minor.

musculocutaneous nerve: of the arm, supplying the flexors of the elbow and sensation in the lateral forearm.

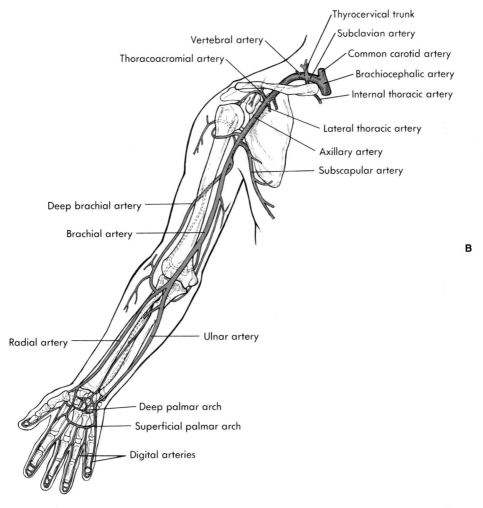

Fig. 8-10, cont'd. Blood vessels of the upper limb. **B,** Arteries of the upper limb—the brachiocephalic, subclavian, axillary, and brachial arteries and their branches. (From Seeley RR, Stephens TD, and Tate P: Anatomy and physiology, St Louis, 1989, Times Mirror/Mosby College Publishing.)

radial nerve: in the back of the arm and lateral forearm, supplying elbow, wrist, and finger extensor function and most of the posterior sensation of the arm, forearm, and hand.

median nerve: supplies motor function to the wrist and finger flexors, some thumb intrinsics, and sensation for the palm, thumb, index and long fingers, and radial side of the ring finger.

ulnar nerve: supplies the ulnar side of the forearm flexors, hand intrinsic muscles, and sensation in the little finger and the little finger side of the ring finger.

cutaneous nerve of the arm brachial cutaneous nerve): posterior, medial, and lateral.

cutaneous nerve of the forearm antebrachial cutaneous nerve): posterior, medial, and lateral.

Other undefined nerves are posterior interosseous (deep radial), anterior interosseous, and superficial radialis.

Ligaments

ulnar and radial collateral ligament: on the medial and lateral side of the elbow.

orbicular ligament: surrounding the radial head and holding it to the ulna at the elbow.

oblique ligament: a part of the radial collateral ligament of the elbow.

interosseous membrane: thick, fibrous tissue between most of the length of the radius and ulna.

laceratus fibrosus: expansion of fibers of the biceps tendon at the elbow; becomes an important structure in some injuries.

Surgery of the arm and forearm

Amspacher and Messenbaugh procedure: for malunion of humeral fracture; a distal rotation osteotomy.

arthrodeses of the elbow: two procedures are Staples and Steindler arthrodeses.

Bosworth procedure: resection of a portion of the radial head ligament and muscle attachment for tennis elbow.

Boyd and Anderson procedure: for biceps distal tendon rupture; a method of reattachment.

Boyd and McLeod procedure: for tennis elbow; excision of a part of the orbicular ligament.

Campbell procedure: for arthritic radial capitellar joint; resection of capitellum and radial head with imbrication of capsule over bone.

Campbell and Akbarnia procedure: for tumor of distal radius; resection of distal radius with replacement using tribial bone graft.

Ellis procedure: for reduction of intraarticular volarly displaced wrist fracture; a technique of screw plate fixation.

Fowles procedure: for chronic posterior dislocation of elbow; a posterolateral approach with detachment of all tight structures and possible V-Y plasty of triceps.

French procedure: for malunion ulna; distal ulnar osteotomy with screw and wire fixation.

Froimson and OH (keyhole) procedure: for chronic tendonitis of long head of biceps; a keyhole is fashioned in the bicipital groove and then used to insert a knotted portion of biceps tendon.

Gill procedure: for nonunion of ulna; a massive sliding graft technique.

Hassman, Brunn, and Neer procedure: for recurrent elbow dislocation; plastic repair of lateral capsuloligamentous structures.

Hitchcock procedure: for rupture of the long head of biceps, a method of reattachment.

Hohmann procedure: for tennis elbow.

Kapel procedure: triceps and biceps tendon formed into ligaments for a chronic dislocated elbow.

Liebolt procedure: for subluxing distal radial/ulnar joint; using tendon graft.

MacAusland procedure: arthroplasty of the elbow for a recurrent dislocation.

Milch procedure: for radial shortening; an ulnar shortening by step cut resection of distal shaft of ulna. Also, for pronation deformity; an osteotomy of distal ulna with fixation in supinated position; also humeral osteotomy for cubitus valgus deformity.

Nirschl procedure: for chronic lateral epicondylitis; excision of hypercapsular tendon segment of extensor carpi radialus brevis and decortication of anterolateral condyle.

Osborne and Cotterill procedure: capsular reefing for a chronic dislocated elbow.

Reichenheim-King procedure: transplantation of the biceps tendon into the coronoid process for a chronic dislocated elbow.

Speed and Boyd procedure: for irreducible Monteggia fracture; reconstruction of orbicular ligament and plating of ulnar fracture.

Spittler procedure: for forearm amputations; a biceps muscle cineplasty.

Steindler flexorplasty: transfer of the flexor wad of five muscles in the elbow to a higher level for loss of voluntary elbow flexion; Eyler flexorplasty is a variation of this procedure.

Stewart procedure: for radial navicular arthritis; excision of radial styloid.

Wilson procedure: for wrist contracture; excision of carpal bones.

THE SPINE

The spine is one of the most intricate parts of the human body. Lying in close contact with the spine are the three main neural components, specifically, the central and autonomic nervous systems and the peripheral nerves. There are 31 pairs of spinal nerves along the length of the cord. The *central nervous system* component occupying the spinal canal is the spinal cord. This structure gives rise to many nerve roots, which, after exit from the spine, become the *peripheral nerves*. The *autonomic nervous system* is composed of small nerve branches arising from the central nervous system and supplying *ganglia*, which are clusters of cells near but outside the bony limits of the vertebrae. The *sympathetic* and *parasympathetic nervous systems* are subdivisions of the autonomic nervous system, which is concerned with autonomic control of visceral organs and peripheral vascular control. The peripheral nerves contain the sensory fibers, voluntary muscle fibers, and fibers of the autonomic nervous system. The sensory nerves, which conduct most of the various sensations that one experiences, are in a *dermatome distribution*. The voluntary muscle supply is through a *myotome* distribution. Most peripheral nerves contain a mixture of sensory and motor fibers. The physician must know the anatomy of the spinal cord and its peripheral branches like a road map, with its many interchanges and destinations. With this knowledge, the physician will be able to detect any deficit on a sensory and motor examination.

Protecting the cord and spinal nerves are the meninges, membranes that invest the cord and composed of the dura mater, pia mater, and arachnoid; along with a hollow flexible skeleton made up of bony segments known as vertebrae. These are separated by intervertebral disks to permit motion. A complex arrangement of ligaments provides stability and further protection for the spinal cord. A second complex feature is seen in the muscles that both support and move the back.

The nerves from and to the spinal cord exit from and enter between the vertebrae through openings called foramina. Each individual vertebra making up the spinal column depends on the others to function normally, because should one part of the spine change in character (as in a fracture) or space allowed (as in a disk herniation), it affects the other parts as well. Although conservative or nonsurgical management is the preferred treatment for most spinal disorders, surgical intervention may sometimes be indicated.

The orthopaedist sees patients with nerve dysfunctions associated with disk herniation or other disk disorders that create impingement on nerves. The treatment may be preventative or rehabilitative in nonsurgical management, or operative if conservative measures fail.

General anatomy of the spine

The 33 vertebrae composing the spinal segments are divided into five regions, with the segments numbered from top to bottom. They are the cervical, thoracic, lumbar, sacral, and coccygeal regions of the spine.

It is very important to understand the designation of vertebrae, intervertebral disks, and nerves when making reference in writing. The proper description is as follows:

Vertebrae	Intervertebral disks	Dermatomes and nerve roots
C-1, L-5	C2-3, L4-5	C1, L4
T-4, S-2	T3-4, S1-2	T3, S2

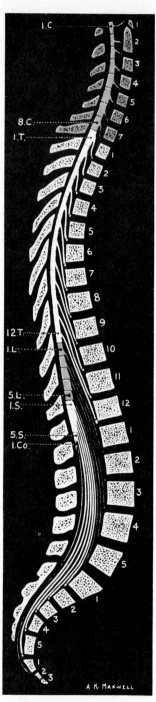

Fig. 8-11. Diagram showing the relation of the segments of the spinal cord and nerves to the segments of the vertebral column. (From Hamilton WJ, editor: Textbook of human anatomy, ed 2, London, England, 1976, The Macmillan Press, Ltd.)

These specific designations may be abbreviated without first being written out in tables and clinical or technical data, but it should be clear as to what part of the spinal anatomy is being referred.

cervical spine: seven spinal segments (C-1 to C-7) between the base of the skull (occiput) and the thoracic spine. The cervical spine differs from the rest of the vertebrae in two major aspects: (1) in each vertebra there is a lateral mass of bone containing a large artery (vertebral artery), and (2) there are jointlike margins called the *joints of Luschka* at the posterolateral aspects of the vertebral bodies.

thoracic (dorsal) spine: 12 spinal segments (T-1 to T-12) incorporating the 12 ribs of the thorax. Other than a slight increase in size from top to bottom, they are fairly uniform in appearance.

lumbar spine: five mobile segments of the lower back (L-1 to L-5). These are the largest of the vertebral segments and provide most of the bending and turning ability of the back, in addition to bearing most of the weight of the body.

sacral spine (sacrum): the five fused segments of

the lower spine that connect to the pelvis and have four foramina on each side.

coccygeal spine (coccyx): remaining three or four, somewhat fixed, fused segments at the end of the spine (tailbone) that articulate with sacrum above.

Except for the coccyx, sacrum, and the first cervical spine, there are anatomic parts that are common to all 33 spinal segments. Moving from anterior to posterior (front to back), the main vertebral parts are the following.

vertebral body (Fig. 8-12): from a lateral view it is the main rectangular portion; from an overhead view, oval.

pedicle: the first portion of the posterior spine arising from the vertebral body.

pars interarticularis: the posterior continuation of the spinal arch from the pedicle; the facets are located just above and below the pars interarticularis.

facets: mostly vertical platelike projections from the midpart of the spinal arch.

foramen: an opening allowing for the egress of

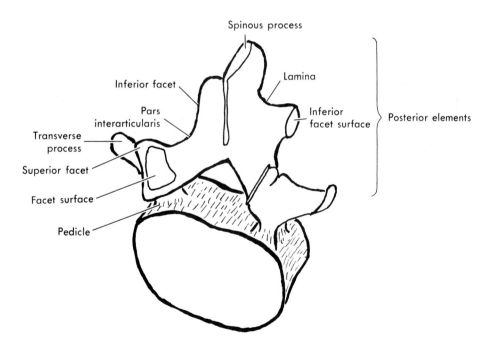

Fig. 8-12. Vertebral body and posterior elements.

spinal nerve roots from between two vertebrae.

lamina: a part of the spinal ring that covers the spinal cord or nerves posteriorly.

spinal process: the most posterior extension of the spine arising from the laminae.

transverse process: bony process arising from midportion of the spinal ring just posterior to the pars interarticularis.

Cervical spine anatomy
Bones and landmarks

atlas: the first cervical vertebra (C-1), lying directly under the skull, by which the head articulates with the neck. The main connection to the vertebra below is a pivot around the odontoid process that extends upward from the body of the second cervical vertebra. The atlas is held onto the odontoid by the anterior arch anteriorly and by the transverse ligament posteriorly.

axis: the second cervical vertebra (C-2), about which the first cervical vertebra rotates, allowing head movement. It bears the *odontoid process,* the projecting part of the second cervical vertebra, which allows the first cervical vertebra (atlas) to rotate.

carotid tubercle: prominence of the transverse process of C-6 felt on the lateral side of neck.

cricoid ring: cartilage ring above trachea and below the thyroid cartilage, the first cricoid ring is at the level of C-6.

hyoid bone: small, vertically oriented bones lateral to trachea, located at the level of C-3.

joints of Luschka (uncovertebral joints): structures peculiar to the cervical spine, in which jointlike structures are formed by the apposition of posterolateral portions of adjacent vertebral bodies.

lateral mass: the lateral expansion of the spinal ring in the cervical spine, where there is a specific place through which the vertebral artery travels.

occiput: the base of the skull.

thyroid cartilage: widening expanse of cartilage above the trachea, the top marks the level of C-4, the bottom C-5.

Muscles

strap muscles: a general term applied to the ribbonlike muscles in the anterior neck; they include omohyoid, sternohyoid, sternothyroid, and thyrohyoid.

longissimus colli: long muscle immediately anterior to the cervical spine.

platysma: thin outer muscle of the anterior lower face and the neck.

sternocleidomastoid: large externally visible muscle of the anterior neck, enabling head to turn to either side.

posterior neck muscles: splenius, spinalis, and semispinalis.

scalenus: the deep lateral muscles of the anterior neck, including anterior scalene m. (scalenus anticus), middle scalene m. (scalenus medius), and posterior scalene m. (scalenus posticus).

Arteries and veins

vertebral artery: large artery that travels in the lateral masses of the cervical spine and eventually supplies the lower brain stem.

carotid artery: main artery to the head that divides into external and internal carotid arteries.

other arteries and veins: transcervical, facial, superior thyroid, and inferior thyroid.

jugular vein: large obvious vein in the neck.

Nerves

cervical plexus: plexus of nerves that supply the neck muscles with branches named by muscles supplied, a portion of which is called the ansa cervicalis.

occipital nerve: nerve from the back of the neck that supplies motor function and sensation to the forehead; two parts—greater and lesser.

spinal accessory nerve (eleventh cranial): the nerve from the brain stem that supplies the sternocleidomastoid muscles.

phrenic nerve: nerve arising from the three branches in the neck (C-3 to C-5); supplies the diaphragm.

vagus nerve (tenth cranial): the long nerve in the anterior neck traveling with the carotid artery;

responsible for many organ functions in the chest and abdomen.

other nerves: transcervical, supraclavicular, posterior rami, facial, greater auricular, and hypoglossal (twelfth cranial).

Other structures

nuchal ligament: large midline posterior ligament in the neck from the base of the skull to the seventh cervical vertebra.

interspinous ligament: ligament between each of the spinal processes.

esophagus: portion of the gut between the mouth and stomach encountered in anterior neck fusion.

trachea: the windpipe.

thyroid gland: near the "Adam's apple"; responsible for secretion of hormone that is involved in regulation of the rate of the metabolism.

triangles: for surgical approaches and other considerations, the anterior half of the neck is divided into triangles—anterior, digastric, posterior, submental, and carotid.

Thoracic spine anatomy

thorax: the chest or rib cage; also refers to the space containing the lungs and heart. There are 12 vertebral segments and ribs; the lower two are called floating ribs.

costo-: combining form denoting relation to ribs.

costovertebral angle: juncture of tissue inferior and lateral to the twelfth rib and vertebral body.

costovertebral joint: junction of the rib with the thoracic spine.

costochondral junction: junction of the rib into cartilage in the anterior chest. NOTE: Most of the ribs have attachment to the cartilage rather than a direct junction with the breast bone.

sternum: the breast bone; further divided into three segments.
  manubrium: upper portion, proximal end.
  sternum: main portion.
  xiphoid: the daggerlike tip of sternum, distal end.

diaphragm: the muscle between the abdomen and thorax; main muscle of normal breathing.

intercostals: the muscles between the ribs.

other thoracic spine and chest muscles: pectoralis, semispinalis, rotators, latissimus dorsi, and spinalis.

Lumbar and lower spine anatomy
Bones

lumbar spine: the five movable spinal segments of the lower back and largest of the spinal segments.

sacral spine (sacrum): the five segments fused together as a solid bone and below the last lumbar segment position.

coccyx: the three, and sometimes four, segments of bone just below the sacrum; referred to as the tailbone; the end of the spinal column.

ilium: the largest of the three bones of the pelvis; this bony portion starts at the sacrum and goes anteriorly to the hip joint.

sacral gutter: the natural concavity produced by area between the spinous processes of the sacrum and the sacroiliac joint.

sacroiliac joint: the junction between the sacrum and the ilium; resembles a large ear.

sacral ala: lateral portions of the sacral bone.

Disk and spinal canal

interspinal or intervertebral disk: the structure that normally occupies the space between two moving vertebrae. It is more prominent in the cervical and lumbar spines. It is much like a radial tire. The centermost portion of the disk (nucleus pulposus) is normally composed of a clear, gelatinous material that varies in consistency from a firm jelly material to a very thick and less pliable substance. This core is then surrounded by numerous layers of fibrous (fibrocartilaginous) material called the *anulus fibrosus*. That structure goes to the normal margins of the vertebral body. There is a thick ligament, approximately 2 mm, that comprises the anterior part of the vertebral body, called the *anterior longitudinal ligament,* and on the spinal canal side posteriorly is the *posterior longitudinal ligament.*

spinal canal: the space between the vertebral body anteriorly and the lamina and spinal process posteriorly. The spinal cord and nerve roots extend to the level of the second lumbar segment in adults and the second sacral segment in infants. Below this level are numerous nerve roots from the spinal cord. The lower portion of the nerve sheaths of the spinal canal resembles a horse's tail and is referred to as such (*cauda equina* is the Latin derivation). The cord is attached to its coverings at the second sacral level by a single filament called the *filum terminale*. The sac, including from the brain to the second sacral level, is called the *meninges*. The thick, outer portion of that sac is called the *dura* or *dura mater*. The more flimsy inner coverings are the *arachnoid* (Latin for spiderlike) and are the weblike membrane coverings. The dura and nerve roots extend out to the foramina to the level of the second sacral segment. This saclike covering is called the *nerve sleeve*. Any space within the dura from the first cervical to the second sacral level is considered the *theca*.

spinal cord: specifically, the orthopaedist does not deal with the spinal cord—that is for the neurosurgeon. However, some affections of these parts may cause musculoskeletal problems.

   long tracts: the nerve fibers that connect the spinal cord with the brain; main spinal nerve pathways.

   pyramidal tract: carries the voluntary muscle messages from the brain.

   dorsal column: the main, normal sensory tract to the brain.

   spinal thalamic tract: the main tract of pain to the brain.

   dorsal lateral column: the main tract of position and tone to the brain.

   gray matter (anterior and posterior horns): the nerve cell bodies to muscle and sensory outflow and input, respectively.

ligamentum flavum: a yellowish ligament that runs between the laminae; it is important as a surgical structure in that a portion is usually removed during an exploration of the spinal canal.

Muscles

iliopsoas muscle: large muscle starting at L-1 and becoming wider as it picks up segments from the lower lumbar spine; combines with the iliacus muscle before attaching to the lesser trochanter of the hip.

quadratus lumborum: a muscle lateral to the iliopsoas muscle of the spine running from the lower ribs to the ilium.

posterior spinal muscle segments: upper and lower posterior serratus m., spinalis m., semispinalis m., and rotators.

abdominal muscles: important for back support and abdominal muscle tone; these muscles are rectus abdominis, external oblique, internal oblique, and transversus.

artery of Adamkiwwicz: relatively large feeder of the lumbar spinal cord, usually at T_9 to T_{11} level; not the only blood supply to the cord at that level.

Surgery of the spine

The two major types of back surgery as applied to orthopaedics are the removal of disk fragments or protrusions and the fusion of two or more vertebral segments. The definitions of disk surgery are given to present some important distinctions between procedures on the cervical spine versus the lumbar spine and to clarify the misuse of terms related to spinal surgical procedures.

Before certain procedures on the spine, such as a herniated disk, conservative measures are initially taken in the form of nonoperative management using traction, weights, and bed rest. When these measures do not help, a nonsurgical procedure called a *myelogram* may be done by the attending physician or radiologist. This is often done in conjunction with and preceding the decision for surgery. The patient is placed on a tilting table and, after introduction of a needle into the subarachnoid space (in lower lumbar spine), cerebrospinal fluid is withdrawn for analysis and then one of several types of radiopaque contrast materials is injected. This material infiltrates up and down the spinal canal outlining the nerve root, nerve sleeves, dural sac, and at higher levels, the spinal cord. Multiple x-ray views can be obtained at any given level to best outline the offending structure. Both *lumbar* and *cervical myelographies* can be studied with the lumbar punctures. A *cisternal myelogram* is one in which contrast material is injected into one of the upper spaces in the neck, but it is rarely necessary. Tumors or other disorders of the thoracic area are generally picked up in the lumbar myelogram. Contrast material may be an oil-based material that must be withdrawn at the end of the procedure or a water-soluble material that is absorbed by the body and does not require withdrawal.

Those procedures specifically carried out by neurosurgeons are not listed except those that are a concurrent part of an orthopaedic procedure. The following spinal surgical procedures are performed by orthopaedic surgeons.

chemonucleolysis: intradiskal procedure for lumbar disk herniation and degenerated disk; under direct x-ray control, a chemical that denatures the protein or protein sugar complex in the disk space is injected. The injected disk tends to dissolve itself, and the remaining cartilage cells repopulate the disk and produce ground substance similar in composition to normal nucleus pulposus, or continued degeneration and scar formation takes place. This procedure is designed to speed up the process of relief of compression of the nerve root without surgery. The procedure carries the risk similar to standard diskectomy via laminectomy.

laminectomy: the most commonly used term for the approach to the disk or nerve roots. It is a procedure to remove the entire lamina on both sides of and including the spinous process. This procedure may be performed at more than one level to approach the spinal cord and nerves for conditions including tumors and herniated disks. The spinal canal is approached from both sides, and the term is often inappropriately used in reference to the following two lesser procedures.

hemilaminectomy: the excision of only the right or left lamina, the posterior bony covering of the nerves.

laminotomy (Fig. 8-13): formation of a hole in

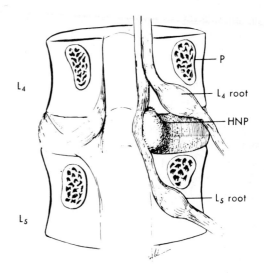

Fig. 8-13. Diagram of herniated nucleus pulposus *(HNP)* as seen from back with spinous processes and laminae removed from pedicles *(P)*. Note that disk protrusion between fourth and fifth lumbar vertebrae impinges on fifth lumbar nerve root. (From Brashear RH, and Raney BR: Shand's handbook of orthopaedic surgery, ed 9, St Louis, 1978, the CV Mosby Co.)

the lamina without disruption to the continuity of the entire lamina to approach the intervertebral disk. This is the most common approach to a herniated disk and is often mistakenly called a laminectomy.

laminoplasty: the lamina are hinged laterally and sutured to adjacent lateral muscles in an attempt to provide a larger epidural space.

diskectomy: the excision of intervertebral disk material that may be described as herniated, implying "bulging" or "ruptured" through the ligaments. If the central fragment of disk material has torn through a hole in the ligament, it is called an extruded fragment or extruded disk. The term *herniated nucleus pulposus* (HNP) is a catchall phrase for all of these conditions. In the neck a fresh (soft) disk excision is usually done through a posterior approach *(laminotomy)*. However, many cervical disk problems are more chronic and may be approached anteriorly to include a spinal fusion.

foraminotomy: a procedure carried out in conjunction with disk surgery. The foramina (openings for the individual nerves to pass from the spine) may become narrowed because of disk impingement, intervertebral collapse, and spondylolisthesis. In any event the surgical widening of the foramen is an attempt to relieve these pressures on the nerve roots.

decompression: in relation to the spine this procedure is carried out to relieve pressure on the spinal cord or nerve roots. The pressure may result from fracture fragments, disk fragments, tumors, or infections. The approach may be anterior, lateral, or posterior.

decompression laminectomy: a posterior approach decompression done by removing the lamina and spinous process.

spinal fusion: a procedure for fusing two or more spinal segments with or without removal of an intervertebral disk. The indications are commonly nerve root irritation in the cervical and lumbar spines, scoliosis in the thoracic and lumbar spines, and spinal instability or arthritis at any level. The excision of an intervertebral disk does not necessarily lead to symptomatic chronic degenerative arthritis or instability and is not in itself an indication for spinal fusion. However, it is often the case that disk surgery and spinal fusions are done concurrently for a variety of reasons. Fusions are sometimes done to provide stability when mechanics have been disturbed by old fractures or by infection (tuberculosis, mycoses, and so on). The lumbosacral region is the most common area for back fusions.

anterior spinal fusion: usually done for osteoarthritis associated with nerve root irritation in the cervical spine. A bone graft is taken from the iliac crest and inserted anteriorly. Some variations of this procedure include the Robinson, Cloward, and dowel procedures. The Kellogg-Speed lumbar spinal fusion is an anterior approach for spondylolisthesis, rarely used. The Dwyer procedure is another anterior approach to the spine for scoliosis. It is a fusion with fixation by a string of staples and wires.

Robinson and Riley: an extensive anterior approach for fusion of C-1 to C-3 or lower.

Whitecloud and Larocca: extensive anterior approach to cervical spine for fusion using a fibular bone graft.

posterior spinal fusion: a fusion of the cervical, thoracic, or lumbar regions primarily fusing the lamina and sometimes the facet joints, using iliac or other bone graft.

Callahan: individual wire fixation of a strut bone graft to involved facets.

posterolateral fusion: a fusion of both the lamina and transverse process, using the iliac bone for graft, usually in the lower lumbar and first sacral segments.

posterolateral interbody fusion (PLIF): lumbar spine fusion that includes a posterolateral fusion and an interbody fusion accomplished through the posterior approach.

Harrington rod fusion: an instrumentation fusion using a straight, stiff rod for distraction or compression; associated with a posterior spinal fusion in the thoracic or thoracolumbar spine for scoliosis or trauma.

Hibbs spinal fusion: a lumbar spinal fusion that includes fusing the spinous process, lamina, and facet for stabilization.

posterior cervical spinal fusion: spinal fusion done from the back, using the lamina and sometimes facets and spinous processes of the neck.

Robinson and Southwick: a posterior fusion with or without bone graft material.

Roger fusion: posterior cervical fusion using iliac cortical and cancellous grafts.

posterior lumbar spinal fusion: spinal fusion done from the back using the lamina and sometimes the facets and spinous processes of the lower back.

Albee: fusion of the spine using grafts across the spinous processes in spondylolisthesis.

Bosworth: a fusion using an H-shaped bone graft in spondylolisthesis.

Gill: removal of the posterior spinal arch in spondylolisthesis.

Gill, Manning, and White: a procedure sometimes combined with a posterolateral spinal fusion.

Miscellaneous procedures on the spine

coccygectomy: excision of the coccyx (tailbone).

coccygotomy: incision into the coccyx.

commissural myelorrhaphy: a longitudinal division of the spinal cord to sever crossing sensory fibers and produce localized analgesia.

cordotomy: incision into the nerve fiber tract within the spinal cord for relief of pain; usually a neurosurgical procedure.

corpectomy: for metastatic bone disease, excision of vertebral body with interposition of prosthesis or bone graft.

eggshell procedure: evacuation of vertebral body with or without bone graft replacement.

facetectomy: excision of an articular facet of a vertebra.

Getty procedure: for decompression of lumbar spinal stenosis; excision of lamina and portion of facet.

Hodgson procedure: anterior approach to C_1 and C_2 area for drainage of tuberculous abscess.

Leeds procedure: for scoliosis, segmental wiring of a kyphotically contoured square-ended Harrington rod.

myelotomy: a procedure for severing tracts in the spinal cord for localized analgesia.

rachicentesis: lumbar puncture for examination of the spinal fluid; rachiocentesis.

rachiotomy: incision into a vertebral canal for exploration.

rachitomy: surgical or anatomic opening of the vertebral canal.

radiculectomy: excision of a rootlet or resection of spinal nerve roots.

rhizotomy: division of the roots of the spinal nerves.

spondylosyndesis: surgical immobilization or ankylosis by fusion of the vertebral bodies with a short bone graft in cases of tuberculosis of the spine. Also called spondylodesis, Albee procedure.

spondylotomy: incision into a vertebra or vertebral column. Also called rachiotomy.

Overton: a dowel graft that is applied across facet joints.

Localio procedure: for sacral tumor; a method of partial excision of the sacrum.

Luque instrumentation: for scoliosis spine fusion; a method of fixation.

MacCarthy procedure: for sacral tumor; a method of excision of the sacrum.

Zielke instrumentation: for scoliosis spine fusions; a method of fixation.

THE PELVIS AND HIPS
The pelvis

The pelvis is a large basinlike structure that supports the lower abdominal viscera, contains the birth canal, and acts as a weight-bearing bridge between the spine and the lower extremities. It is often referred to as the *pelvic girdle*. It is composed of a bilateral set of three bones that are completely fused and are on either side of the sacrum. The largest and uppermost bone is the ilium, the lowermost and strongest is the ischium, and the anteriormost is the pubis. In the outer center of these fused bones is the hip socket, called the acetabulum, the "true" anatomic hip and socket for the ball-and-socket joint.

Most hip surgical procedures involve structures immediately neighboring the acetabulum. The anatomic structures involving the pelvis that are occasionally encountered in hip procedures are listed first, followed by anatomic structures directly related to hip procedures.

Anatomy of the pelvis
Bones

pelvic girdle: a general term that denotes the entire bilateral bony pelvis; the ring that the pelvis makes with its articulation to the sacrum (sacroiliac joint) is called the pelvic ring.

sacroiliac: joint space between the sacrum and the two ilia, junction of the pelvis to the spine.

innominate bone: composed of three fused bony subunits, called the ilium, pubis, and ischium, that are attached to the sacrum and coccyx to form the pelvis.

ilium: wide platelike bone that forms the top of the pelvis just below the waistline; generally referred to as "the hips."

iliac crest: the outer, uppermost margins of the ilium; the four iliac spines are sharp points of strong muscular attachments: anterosuperior, anteroinferior, posterosuperior, and posteroinferior iliac spines.

greater sciatic notch: the large notch on the posterior surface of the ilium below the posteroinferior iliac spine where the sciatic nerve exits.

gluteal lines: refers to the three curved lines across the outer surface of the ilium, anteriorly, posteriorly, and inferiorly.

iliopectineal line: a ridge inside the pelvis that denotes the entrance into the birth canal, with a concave inner surface called the *iliac fossa*.

ala of the ilium: the outer flair of the ilium; resembles a wing.

pubis (pubic bone): the anterior increased shape of bone of the pelvis, which meets its counterpart from the other side at a point called the *symphysis pubis*.

symphysis pubis: the hard portion of bone between the two pubic bones and just above the genital area.

superior pubic ramus: top portion of the pubic bone.

inferior pubic ramus: lower portion of the pubic bone.

ischium: a U-shaped bone of the lower part of the pelvis, which forms a ring.

ischial tuberosity: the prominent, hard portion of bone at the base of the ischium, felt when sitting erect.

ischial spine: prominence of bone of strong ligamentous attachment above the tuberosity; main significance is in obstetrics.

obturator foramen: formed in adult life when the ischium and pubis become a solid bony continuum, producing a hole or ring that is the largest foramen in the body.

Muscles

Most of the pelvic muscles affect the hip or abdominal motion and are described in this section. However, those muscles of the lower abdominal wall surrounding the bladder, uterus, and rectum are sometimes encountered in orthopaedic procedures; they are the levator ani, pubococcygeal, transverse urethral, and cremaster (in scrotum).

sphincter ani: muscle that controls defecation; loss of control of this muscle is a serious sign of herniated disk disease.

Ligaments

Poupart inguinal ligament: anterior ligament at the groin fold from the anterosuperior iliac spine to the pubic tubercle.

sacrotuberous ligament: ligament from the sacrum to the ischial tuberosity; small sacrosciatic.

sacrospinous ligament: from iliac spine to sacrum.

anterior sacroiliac ligament: large ligament between the sacrum and the ilium.

Blood vessels

Most large blood vessels within the pelvis are not encountered in orthopaedic practice. The aorta divides into the common iliac arteries at about the level of the fourth lumbar vertebra. Branches within the pelvis include the hypogastric, superior and inferior gluteal, iliac (which becomes the femoral at the inguinal ligament), and pudendal.

Miscellaneous terms

peritoneum: inner membrane lining of the abdominal cavity.

inguinal: refers to the area of the groin. The precise line is from the anterosuperior iliac spine to the pubis; this is the line of the natural fold of skin in the groin. Terms relating to the area include inguinal nerve, hypogastric nerve, ilioinguinal nerve, and inguinal canal.

Nerves

lumbar plexus: arises from the second through fourth lumbar vertebrae, with two major nerves.
  femoral nerve: arises from L-2, L-3, and L-4 and supplies most of the knee extensors.
  obturator nerve: arises from L-2, L-3, and L-4 and supplies many of the thigh adductors.

sciatic plexus: the major plexus of nerves arising in the pelvic area to include nerves from L-4 and L-5 and nerves of the first three sacral levels.

Major injuries or disorders of this plexus are rare, but it is important to understand that this plexus forms the sciatic nerve, which eventually becomes the tibial and common peroneal nerves. Most "sciatica" is actually a nerve root irritation in the spinal column.

sciatic nerve: the large nerve developed by the sacral plexus supplying the hip rotators, knee flexors, and entire leg and foot muscles, as well as most of the sensation.

pudendal nerve: arising from just below the sacral plexus, traveling along the ischium (Alcock canal), and supplying the lower pelvic muscles that do not affect hip motion but affect sexual function.

cluneal nerve: inferolateral, inferomedial, and superior sensory nerves of the buttocks and thighs.

The hip

The average person refers to the prominent part of the pelvis that flares out just below the waistline (iliac crest) as the "hip." However, the hip portion of the pelvis is the lesser part of the entire pelvic mass; it is 5 inches below the iliac crest and is called the acetabulum, or "true" hip. The three bones of the pelvis merge to form the cup-shaped depression of the hip joint, which holds the femoral head in place. The proximal femur (thigh bone) and its components are described here as the major elements of the hip function and not as part of the lower extremities.

Anatomy of the hip
Bones

acetabulum: cup-shaped depression in the mid-outer pelvis known as the hip; this is the socket of the ball-and-socket joint of the hip.

superior dome: the weight-bearing portion of the acetabulum.

fovea centralis: central depression in the center of the acetabulum and origin of the ligamentum teres.

triradiate cartilage: structure present only during growth; the meeting point of the ischium, ilium, and pubis.

posterior lip: posterior part of the acetabulum, which sometimes breaks off in a dislocation of the hip.

femur: as related to the hip, is considered the upper, proximal 4-inch segment of bone.

femoral head: the ball and topmost part of the ball-and-socket joint of the hip; in a growing child may be referred to as the *capital epiphysis.*

femoral neck: the area below the femoral head where the bone narrows into a tubelike structure about 2 inches long.

greater and lesser trochanters: part of the femur just distal to the neck where the bone widens into two large prominences, the lower, smaller, and medial of which is the lesser trochanter; the greater trochanter is the larger, lateral prominence. In thin persons the greater trochanter can be felt at about the level of the palm of the hands when the arms are resting by the sides. It is often used as a landmark in physical and x-ray examinations.

intertrochanteric: refers to any region between the two trochanters; a large number of fractures of the hip occur in this region.

subtrochanteric: refers to the widened part of the shaft just below the lesser trochanter.

Muscles

gluteus maximus muscle: the large buttock muscle that helps to extend the hip.

gluteus medius and minimus muscles: the deeper significant muscles that abduct the hip and prevent a waddling gait.

iliopsoas muscle: a combination of the iliacus and psoas muscles arising from the anterior back and inserting into the lesser trochanter. These large hip flexors are often involved in hip reconstructive procedures.

rectus femoris muscle: anterior thigh muscle of the quadriceps group; attaches across the hip joint.

sartorius muscle: the muscle stretching from the anterolateral pelvis (anterosuperior iliac spine) to the medial tibia, crossing two joints; it enables the person to assume a cross-legged position.

adductors: a group of five muscles that pulls the thigh inward (adduction); these include the adductor magnus, adductor longus, adductor brevis, pectineus, and gracilis muscles.

external and internal rotators: a group of muscles originating at the pelvis around the hip, helping to control internal and external rotation; these muscles are the internal and external obturator gemelli (superior and inferior gemellus), quadratus femoris, and piriformis.

tensor fascia lata muscle: the most lateral hip abductor muscle.

Ligament

ligamentum teres: the round ligament between the middle of the femoral head and the center of the acetabulum (fovea centralis).

Arteries

femoral artery: the major artery from the point of exit from the pelvis to the point of exit behind the knee. Near the hip it gives off a branch called the deep femoral (profundus) artery and from this, one branch supplies the femoral head, the artery that arises from the lateral side of the deep femoral artery and supplies the lateral and anterior femoral neck. This is the major blood supplier to the femoral head in late childhood and adult life. A branch of the femoral artery is the medial circumflex artery, which arises from the deep femoral artery and supplies the posterior femoral head in early childhood.

superior gluteal artery: a large artery from the internal iliac artery within the pelvis supplying the gluteus maximus and lesser muscles outside the pelvis.

inferior gluteal artery: large artery from the internal iliac artery within the pelvis; supplies the gluteus medius and minimus.

obturator artery: a branch from within the pelvis that supplies some of the adductor muscles after exiting through the obturator foramen.

Nerves

All three nerves supplying the thigh and leg also supply the hip. As a result many patients with hip problems complain of thigh, calf, and even foot pain. The large nerves passing near the hip are the following.

femoral nerve: supplies sensation to the anterior thigh, medial leg, and the muscle for knee extension.

obturator nerve: supplies sensation to the medial side of the thigh and the muscles for pulling the thigh inward (adducting).

sciatic nerve: supplies sensation to the posterior thigh and hip extensors; the more distal branches (common peroneal and posterior tibial) are discussed under Thigh arteries and veins.

Surgery of the pelvis and hips

Most of the surgery performed on the hip is directed toward making the hip a mobile, painless, weight-bearing joint. Surgical procedures designed to remodel the hip or replace the parts involved are described in this section. Surgical procedures to fuse the hip or to change the direction of alignment of the femur or pelvis are defined in the following sections.

Hip arthroplasty

A hip arthroplasty is a procedure designed to directly change the contour of or to replace the hip joint (acetabulum) and/or femoral head. This term is so general that it includes most procedures for congenital dysplasia of the hips and all procedures that involve prosthetic replacement. For example, the term *total hip arthroplasty* is used often to denote the total joint replacement procedure. Nonprosthetic procedures are listed first.

shelf procedure: a bending of the outer acetabulum (hip joint) so it more completely covers the femoral head. This is commonly done for congenital dysplastic hips, where the acetabulum is not well rounded and allows the femoral head to displace. It is then necessary, in many instances, to reduce the hip and then perform a shelf procedure, using a bone graft to maintain a new position of the lateral acetabulum. Some types of operative shelf procedures are Albee, Bosworth, Ghormley, Gill (type I, II, III), Chiari, Frank Dickson, Lowman, Wiberg, Steel, Colonna, and Hay-Groves.

capsular arthroplasty: many procedures for a dislocation of the hip involve soft tissue manipulation only and include curetting of the acetabulum and muscle transfers but do not involve bony osteotomies such as are seen in the shelf procedures. One of these procedures is the Colonna capsular arthroplasty.

cup arthroplasty: surgical remodeling of the femoral head and the acetabular socket with the insertion of a metal cup. This procedure is usually reserved for younger persons with severe deforming diseases of the hip after trauma; mold arthroplasty.

femoral head prosthesis: insertion into the femoral shaft of a metallic or synthetic component that resembles the femoral head. In present usage it replaces the femoral head in an older person who has a normal acetabulum but a recent fracture of the hip.

total hip arthroplasty (low friction arthroplasty): a joint replacement involving an internal prosthesis by removing the diseased joint and replacing the acetabular component with either metal or plastic materials and a metal prosthesis of the femoral segment. This type of procedure is usually reserved for older individuals who are suffering from osteoarthritis, avascular necrosis, or other degenerative diseases of the hip. See Internal prostheses for a description of the many types used.

Closed hip reduction procedures for congenital dysplasia of the hip (CDH)

These are manipulations in an infant or child to reduce a dislocated hip. The method of reduction, followed by the casted position after reduction, varies.

Crego: use of skeletal traction until a closed manipulation with minimal force becomes possible.

Lorenz: both a method of reduction and the frogleg position cast applied following the reduction.

Ridlon: method of reducing a congenital dislocated hip and then using a Lorenz cast.

Lange: positioning the hip in abduction, internal rotation, and extension after a closed reduction.

Wingfield frame: used in a gradual method of closed reduction.

Open hip reduction

An open hip reduction is a procedure that, when listed by itself, implies the need to reduce a hip under direct surgical vision but with minimal reconstruction of the capsule. Some open techniques include Calandriello, Ferguson, Howorth, Scaglietti, and Somerville.

Iliopsoas transfers

This strong hip flexor is sometimes transferred to act as a hip abductor in conditions of muscle imbalance and hip dislocation. Two such procedures are the Mustard and the Sharrard.

Osteotomies

The osteotomies of the hip are listed here for reference, but some are defined more fully in this chapter under Osteotomy.

Amstutz and Wilson	MacEwen and Shands
Blount	McCarroll
Blundell Jones	McMurray
Borden, Spencer, and	Müller
Herndon	Osgood
Brackett	Pauwels
Chiari	PauwelsY
derotation	Pemberton
dial	Platou
Dimon	Salter (innominate)
Gant	Sarmiento
Ghormley	Schanz
Hass	Schede
Irwin	Southwick
Langenskiöld	Steel-triradiate
Lloyd-Roberts	Sutherland-Greenfield
Lorenz	Whitman

Arthrodeses

The arthrodeses are listed for reference but some are defined more fully under General surgery of joints.

Abbott	Badgley
Abbott-Fisher-Lucas	Blair
Albee	Brittain

Chandler	Kickaldy and Willis
Davis	Schneider
Gant	Stamm
Ghormley	Trumble
Henderson	Watson-Jones
Hibbs	John C. Wilson

Other pelvic and hip procedures

acetabuloplasty: any surgical remodeling of the cup side of the hip joint.

Bleck procedure: for excessive hip internal rotation when walking; a recession of the iliacus and psoas tendon to anterior capsule of hip.

Campbell procedure: for abdominal and hip flexion contracture; excision of a part of the anterior ilium after a soft tissue release.

Chandler procedure: for hip adduction gait; intrapelvic obturator neurectomy.

Couch, DeRosa, and Throop procedure: for hip adduction gait; transfer of the adductor tendon to ischial tuberosity.

coxotomy: surgical opening of the hip joint.

Dimon and Hughston procedure: for comminuted intertrochanteric hip fracture; a method of reduction with valgus placement and use of a high angle nail.

Dunn procedure: for displaced slipped capital femoral epiphysis, removal of "hump" and fusion of epiphysis.

Girdlestone resection: excision of the femoral head and neck for a fractured intertrochanteric hip joint and other diseases.

Graber-Duvernay procedure: boring holes leading to the center of the femoral head for the purpose of promoting circulation.

hebosteotomy: incision into the pubis; hebotomy.

Heyman-Herndon procedure: for displaced slipped capital femoral epiphysis, a shortening of the femoral neck with correction of deformity.

ischiectomy: surgical excision and removal of a part of the ischium.

ischiohebotomy: surgical division of the ischiopubic ramus and ascending ramus of the pubis.

ischiopubiotomy: incision into the ischial pubic junction.

Karakousis and Vezeridis procedure: for malignancy of pelvis; resection of hemipelvis and head of femur preserving neurovascular structures.

Legg procedure: for paralysis of gluteus maximus; posterior portion of tensor fascia lata muscle is transferred to a more posterior position.

McCarty procedure: for chordoma of sacrum; resection of a portion of sacrum.

Menson and Scheck procedure: for osteoarthritis of the hip; release of the pericapsular muscles. Also called "hanging hip" procedure.

Ober-Barr procedure: for paralysis of gluteus maximus; a fascia lata graft still attached to fascia lata and flap transferred to erector spinae m.

pubiotomy: surgical incision and division in the pubic bone.

Radley, Liebig, and Brown procedure: for malignancy of ischium; resection of tuberosity and lower portion of pubis.

Sarmiento procedure: for intertrochanteric fracture of the hip; use of osteotomy cut in the distal fragment to achieve valgus nail plate fixation.

Selig procedure: for hip adducted gait; intrapelvic obturator neurectomy.

Soutter procedure: for abdominal and hip flexion contracture; release of the soft tissues about the iliac crest.

Staheli procedure: for congenital hip dysplasia; shelf procedure using iliac crest bone graft for buttress.

Stener and Gunterberg procedure: for chordoma of sacrum; resecting portion of sacrum.

Sutherland procedure: for internal rotation deformity of the hip; transfer of semitendinosus and semimembranosus to lateral posterior septa of thigh.

Thomas, Thompson, and Straub procedure: for gluteus medius paralysis; transfer of external abdominal oblique to the tensor fascia lata.

Veleanu, Rosianu, and Ionescu procedure: for hip adduction gait; combination of adductor tenotomy and obturator neurectomy.

THE LOWER LIMBS
Anatomy of the lower limbs
Bones

femur (Fig. 8-14): thigh bone; largest bone in the body.

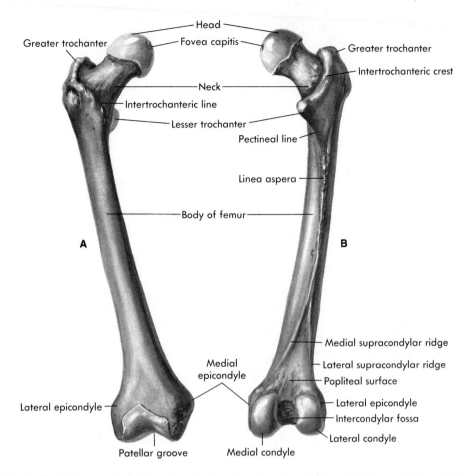

Head
Greater trochanter — Fovea capitis —
— Greater trochanter
— Intertrochanteric crest
Neck
Intertrochanteric line
Lesser trochanter
Pectineal line
Linea aspera
Body of femur
A
B
Medial supracondylar ridge
Lateral supracondylar ridge
Medial epicondyle
Popliteal surface
Lateral epicondyle
Lateral epicondyle
Intercondylar fossa
Lateral condyle
Patellar groove
Medial condyle

Fig. 8-14. Right femur. **A,** Anterior view. **B,** Posterior view. (From Seeley RR, Stephens TD, and Tate P: Anatomy and physiology, St Louis, 1989, Times Mirror/Mosby College Publishing.)

linea aspera: a line of prominent bone in the posterior proximal and middle femur for insertion of the gluteus maximus.

femoral condyles: the two prominences at the distal end of the femur, called the medial and lateral femoral condyles. The space between the condyles, called the *intercondylar notch,* contains the cruciate ligaments within the knee.

adductor tubercle (adductor tuberosity): the knobby prominence of the medial femoral condyle, which is easily felt by pressing on the medial side of the knee 5 cm above the joint.

patella (Fig. 8-15): the kneecap, a round to ovoid bone within the quadriceps (knee extensor) tendon. It has a posterior cartilaginous surface for articulation with the femoral condyles known as the *medial* and *lateral facets.*

tibia (Fig. 8-16): the large leg bone on the medial side between the knee and ankle.

trochlea: the groove that holds the patella in line on the distal femoral joint surface.

fibula (Fig. 8-16): the smaller bone on the lateral side between the knee and ankle.

tibial plateau: the surface that articulates with the femur; may be subdivided into the medial and lateral plateaus.

anterior and posterior tibial spines: little prominences of bone inside the knee joint; attachment for the anterior and posterior cruciate ligaments.

anterior tibial tubercle: the large knob just below

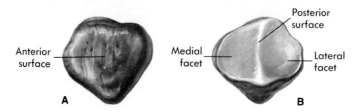

Fig. 8-15. Right patella. **A,** Anterior view. **B,** Posterior view. (From Seeley RR, Stephens TD, and Tate P: Anatomy and physiology, St Louis, 1989, Times Mirror/Mosby College Publishing.)

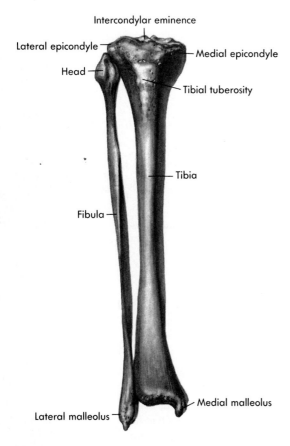

Fig. 8-16. Right tibia and fibula, anterior view. (From Seeley RR, Stephens TD, and Tate P: Anatomy and physiology, St Louis, 1989, Times Mirror/Mosby College Publishing.)

the anterior knee joint; the point of insertion for the quadriceps (knee extensors) muscles.

Chaput tubercle: the anterior tubercle of the distal tibia at the ankle joint. Also called *tubercle of Tillaux-Chaput*.

fibular facet (proximal tibiofibular facet): the flat portion of bone on the lateral side of the proximal tibia for articulation with the fibula.

fibular neck: narrow part of the fibula just below the proximal enlargement of the bone.

Gerdy tubercle: prominence of bone superior and lateral to the anterior tibial tuberosity; used as reference point in some knee surgery.

medial malleolus: the large prominence on the inner side of the ankle and part of the tibia.

posterior malleolus: a structure that cannot be seen or felt but is the posterior joint aspect of the tibia. It may fracture by itself or, more commonly, in association with other ankle fractures.

lateral malleolus: the distal end of the fibula, which is the outer prominence of the ankle.

Muscles

adductor muscle: the medial muscle of the thigh responsible for pulling the thigh toward the midline.

quadriceps muscle: the four divisions of muscles that are the bulk of the anterior thigh that become a tendon, that surrounds the patella and ends on the tuberosity of the tibia. They function in extending the knee and, in the case of the rectus femoris, help to flex the hip. The quadriceps femoris group of muscles includes the vastus lateralis, vastus medialis, vastus intermedius, and rectus femoris.

hamstring muscle: three posterior thigh muscles, originating mostly at the pelvis and posterior femur, that help flex the knee. They are given this common name because when they reach the knee joint they are mostly tendinous. The three hamstring muscles are:

biceps femoris: outer hamstring.

semitendinosus: inner hamstring.

semimembranosus: inner hamstring.

popliteus muscle: a muscle in the posterior superior tibia that has its tendon insertion into the posterior femur. It is important in lateral injuries of the knee in that the structure may be involved or encountered on arthrographic examination or as a part of surgical procedure.

pes anserinus: the distal tendon portion of the gracilis, sartorius, and semitendinosis muscles, which at their attachment on the proximal medial tibial side are similar to a goose's foot in appearance.

Muscle compartments

Muscles act in groups to bring about movements, primarily as agonists, antagonists, synergists, and prime movers. There are many muscle groups and compartments throughout the body. The most commonly referred to muscle groups are in the leg, because swelling within the compartments leads to irreversible muscle change and loss of motor function. Therefore the four compartments of the leg are defined here and the function and names given of the muscle groups of the lower extremity.

anterior compartment: contains the muscles responsible for dorsiflexion of the ankle and the large and lesser toes; included are the tibialis anterior, extensor hallucis longus, extensor digitorum longus, and peroneus tertius.

lateral compartment: contains the muscles that evert or plantar flex the ankle; they are the peroneus longus and the peroneus brevis.

deep compartments: contain the flexors of the toes and ankle and are known as the tibialis posterior, flexor digitorum longus, and flexor hallucis longus.

posterior compartments: contain the triceps surae muscles, which make up the bulk of the calf; included are the following:

gastrocnemius: the most posterior muscle of the calf, leading to the Achilles tendon, that flexes both the ankle and knee.

soleus: the larger deep ankle flexor of the calf leading to the Achilles tendon.

plantaris: the smaller ankle flexor that leads to the Achilles tendon over the medial side.

gastrocsoleus muscle: refers to the combination of the two largest muscles contributing to the Achilles tendon.

Achilles tendon: the heel cord that is the extension from the triceps surae group of muscles.

Ligaments

The knee is an encapsulated joint that has several layers of fascial tissue. The deeper layer is referred to as the *joint capsule,* but numerous ligaments and tendons make up this capsule (Fig. 8-17).

medial collateral ligament: strong fibrous ligament on the medial side of the knee connecting the femur with the tibia. There is a *superficial* and a *deep ligament* in most knees. The posterior oblique ligament is composed of fibers that arise from the medial collateral ligament and attach more posteriorly in the joint.

lateral collateral ligament: strong fibrous ligament of the lateral knee joint with fibers from the femur to the tibia and fibula. This ligament is sometimes called the tibial collateral, but caution should be taken to distinguish this from the ankle ligaments.

anterior and posterior cruciate ligaments: the two deep ligaments within the knee that are crossed.

ligaments of Henry and Wrisberg: small ligaments of attachment for the meniscus in the posterior knee.

proximal tibiofibular ligament: ligament between the fibular neck and tibia.

tibiofibular ligament: when used without distinction as to distal or proximal, refers to the ligaments just above the ankle; these ligaments are divided into the anterior, middle, and posterior tibiofibular ligaments.

ligamentum mucosa: not a true ligament but the thin, filmy membrane that sometimes divides the knee joint.

Arteries and veins (Fig. 8-18)

femoral artery and vein: large artery and vein of the thigh that originate in the groin area; they penetrate posteriorly through fascia above the

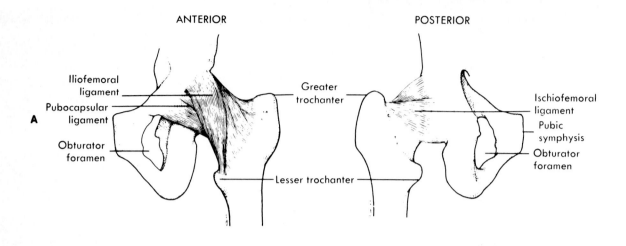

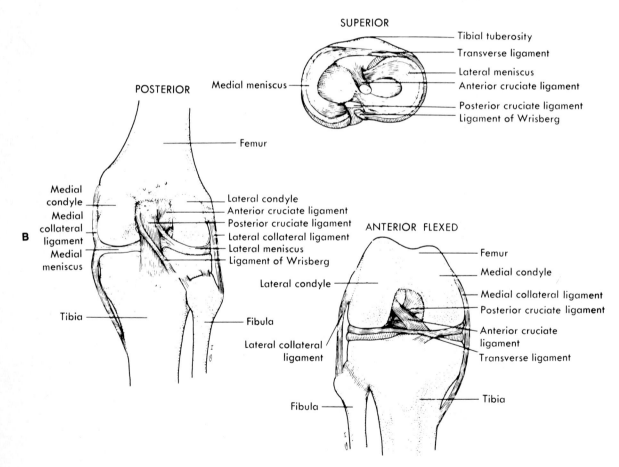

Fig. 8-17. Major joints in terms of disease and surgical sites. **A,** Hip. **B,** Knee. (From Hilt NE, and Cogburn SB: Manual of orthopedics, St Louis, 1980, The CV Mosby Co.)

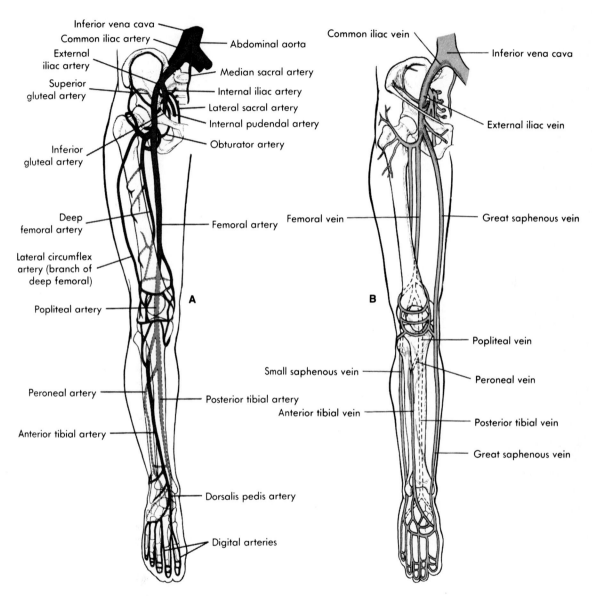

Fig. 8-18. Blood vessels of the pelvis and lower limb. **A,** Arteries of the pelvis and lower limb—the internal and external iliac arteries and their branches. The internal iliac artery supplies the pelvis and hip, and the external iliac artery supplies the lower limb through the femoral artery. **B,** Veins of the pelvis and lower limb—the right common iliac vein and its tributaries. (From Seeley RR, Stephens TD, and Tate P: Anatomy and physiology, St Louis, 1989, Times Mirror/Mosby College Publishing.)

knee (Hunter canal) and become the popliteal artery and vein.

deep femoral artery: the largest branch of the femoral artery in the upper thigh that travels closely to the femur and gives off numerous circumferential branches around that bone; the branches are referred to as the *perforating arteries*.

highest genicular artery: large branch from the femoral artery supplying the muscles and joints on the medial aspect of the knee. Branches above the knee may be referred to as medial and lateral superior genicular, medial and lateral inferior genicular, anterior and posterior tibial recurrent, and fibular arteries.

saphenous vein: large vein of the subcutaneous tissue in the medial thigh; continuous to the medial side of the ankle.

popliteal artery and vein: continuation of the femoral artery and vein as they emerge behind the knee, dividing distally to that joint and giving off the anterior tibial artery and posterior tibial artery.

anterior tibial artery: main artery of the anterior leg supplying the extensors and peroneal muscles.

posterior tibial artery: large artery of the posterior leg supplying most of the muscles of the calf and deep spaces; a major branch is the peroneal artery.

peroneal artery: travels along the posterior fibula supplying deep calf muscles and collateral circulation of the leg.

other arteries of the leg near the ankle: perforating, anterior and posterior medial malleolar, and anterior and posterior lateral malleolar arteries.

Other structures

medial and lateral menisci: referred to as the semilunar cartilages, which are fibrocartilaginous structures interfacing the medial and lateral rim of the femorotibial joint; serve to help distribute the weight load on the two cartilaginous surfaces by changing shape and position during motion.

infrapatellar fat pad (retropatellar fat pad): a distinct mass of fat behind the patellar tendon extending into the anterior joint of the knee. Also called *Hoffa fat*.

suprapatellar pouch: the extension of the anterior knee joint to about 12 cm above the joint line.

prepatellar bursa: a bursa in the fat in front of the kneecap.

interosseous membrane: a very strong fibrous membrane between the fibula and tibia, extending throughout most of the length of the bones.

plica: a fold, pleat, band, or shelf of synovial tissue; minor structures but may be large enough to produce symptoms and demand surgical attention. Specific locations include the transverse suprapatellar, medial suprapatellar, mediopatellar (also called medial patellar shelf), and infrapatellar plica (also called ligamentum mucosa, which does not produce symptoms).

Nerves of the lower limbs

deep peroneal nerve: nerve that supplies voluntary function of the toe and ankle extension; the sensory branch is between the first and second toes.

saphenous nerve: nerve branch from the femoral nerve; supplies only sensation to the medial leg.

sural nerve: large sensory nerve of the calf deriving branches from both the peroneal and posterior tibial nerves.

sciatic nerve: nerve of the posterior thigh, supplying muscles of the posterior thigh and dividing into the common peroneal and posterior tibial nerves.

posterior tibial nerve: nerve of the posterior leg that supplies the outer and deep calf muscles and eventually the muscles of the foot and sensation on the sole of the foot.

common peroneal nerve: a brief segment of nerve that divides into the superficial and deep peroneal nerve just distal to the fibular head.

superficial peroneal nerve: nerve that supplies the voluntary muscle function which turns the ankle out; also supplies sensation on the dorsum of the foot.

Surgery of the lower limbs
The thigh

Caldwell and Durham procedure: for quadriceps rupture, a transfer of the biceps femorus tendon to quadriceps tendon.

D'Aubigne procedure: for tumor of femoral condyle or tibial plateau, use of attached patella to act as graft for joint surface.

Enneking procedure: for malignancy of distal femur or proximal tibia, resection of affected bone and use of graft taken from healthy bone and fixation with rod and patellar screws.

Lewis and Chekofsky procedure: for malignant tumor of proximal femur, resection of proximal femur.

Wagner procedure: for correction of leg length discrepancy (LLD); a method of shortening the femoral or tibial diaphysis; or shortening the metaphysis of the femur or tibia; or lengthening the femur or tibia.

White procedure: for leg length discrepancy; a method of shortening the femur.

The knee

Knee injuries account for a large percentage of the surgical procedures of the lower limbs because many muscles arising in the thigh and leg affect that joint. Often more than one procedure is indicated at the same time. Over the years some of the combinations of procedures have acquired eponymic designations. To give a general purview of surgery of the knee, the single procedures and their modifications are listed first, and the combined procedures are listed last.

Knee surgery for internal derangement

Campbell procedure: use of fascial strip from quadriceps tendon to replace anterior cruciate ligament.

Cho procedure: for anterior cruciate deficiency, intraarticular use of semitendinosis tendon.

Clancy: for anterior cruciate deficient knee, use of midpatellar tendon with attached patellar and tibial bone.

Ellison procedure: extraarticular repair to replace anterior cruciate function, rerouting iliotibial band under the lateral collateral ligament.

Ericksson procedure: for anterior cruciate instability; midportion of patellar tendon and portion of bone redirected through tibia and into posterior lateral femoral condyle.

five-in-one repair: five procedures for severe ligamentous injuries to the knee; includes a medial meniscectomy, medial collateral ligament repair, vastus medialis advancement, semitendinosus advancement, and a pes anserinus transfer. Also called *Nicholas procedure.*

Fox-Blazina procedure: extraarticular repair to replace anterior cruciate function by rerouting the iliotibial band under the lateral collateral ligament and placing it distal to original attachment.

Hey-Groves procedure: a reconstruction of the anterior cruciate ligament using tensor fasciae latae graft.

Hughston and Degenhardt: for posterior cruciate deficient knee, use of medial head of gastrocnemius.

Hughston and Jacobson: for posterolateral instability, advancement of bony attachment of fibular collateral ligament and popliteus tendon to a superior and anterior direction.

Jones procedure: repair of the anterior cruciate ligament using a portion of the patella and patellar ligament. A *Lam modification* of this procedure is also used.

ligamentous advancement: implies a soft tissue procedure only. The ligament is detached and then pulled up or down and reattached to bone. This is done for the medial and lateral collateral ligaments.

Lindeman procedure: for anterior cruciate ligament rupture; gracilis tendon transfer as a replacement.

Loose procedure: for anterior cruciate instability with pivot shift; portion of iliotibial band is redirected through lateral femoral condyle and around lateral joint.

MacIntosh procedure: using infrapatellar and quadriceps tendon for transfer over posterior lateral femoral condyle for anterior cruciate ligament replacement. Also, iliotibial band used in reconstruction to provide anterior cruciate stability.

Marshall procedure: for anterior cruciate ligament laxity; portion of patellar tendon and fascia is directed through notch and over lateral femoral condyle.

Mauck procedure: detachment of a segment of the tibia containing the medial collateral ligament and replacement of that block of bone in a position that tightens the ligament.

meniscectomy: excision of the medial or lateral meniscus. There are other menisci in the body, but meniscectomies are usually done on the knee. A *partial meniscectomy* is the removal of the torn portion only or a definite attempt to leave meniscal margins of an even width.

Muller procedure: for posterolateral instability; reinforcement with iliotibial band graft.

over-the-top procedure: for anterior cruciate deficiency; any procedure that places the transferred ligament over the lateral femoral condyle rather than through the condyle.

Paddu procedure: for anterior cruciate deficient knee; intraarticular use of gracilis and semitendinosis tendons.

Paulos procedure: for anterior cruciate deficient knee; use of medial patellar tendon and retinaculum through tibial grove.

reverse Mauck procedure: detachment of a segment of the femur containing the medial collateral ligament and insertion of this block of bone into a position that tightens the ligament.

Slocum procedure: a pes anserinus transfer (pes transfer). This is commonly done in association with other procedures and involves a change in the direction of pull of tendons inserting just below the medial knee joint; designed to help replace dynamic stability in ligamentous laxity.

triad knee repair (O'Donoghue procedure): a repair involving the anterior cruciate ligament, medial collateral ligament, and a medial meniscectomy.

vastus medialis advancement: a procedure done rarely by itself but more commonly in association with procedures for ligamentous laxity of the knee and/or chronic subluxing patella. It is

a tightening of the vastus medialis muscle.

Zarins and Rowe: for anterior cruciate deficient knee; simultaneous "over the top" use of semitendinosis and iliotibial band with posteromedial and posterolateral capsular reefing.

Knee surgery for chronic subluxation of the patella

Campbell procedure: fascial tissue transfer and vastus medialis reefing.

Emslie-Trillat procedure: medial displacement of anterior tibial tuberosity on a bone pedicle for subluxing patella.

Hauser procedure: inferomedial displacement of a block of bone with the infrapatellar tendon attached.

Hughston procedure: lateral release with quadricepsplasty and patellar tendon transfer as needed.

Maquet procedure: anterior tibial tuberosity displacement on bone pedicle for patella alta.

Roux-Goldthwait procedure: medial displacement of the lateral portion of the infrapatellar tendon.

Sargent procedure: lateral release and advancement of vastus medialis over patella with attachment to exposed, bleeding patellar surface.

Silfverskiöld procedure: for knee flexion contracture (in cerebral palsy); transection of medial and lateral head of gastrocnemius muscle and motor branch to medial gastrocnemius.

Southwick slide procedure: medial displacement of bony attachment of the patellar tendon, replacing the lateral defect with bone from the medial side.

Stanisavljevic procedure: for congenital dislocating patella; massive patellar tendon and quadriceps refashioning.

West and Soto-Hall procedure: patellectomy and medial advancement of the quadriceps mechanism for patellar osteoarthritis.

Patellar surgery

Cave and Rowe procedure: for osteoarthritis of the patella; partial patellectomy with fold of infrapatellar fat sewn onto the posterior patella.

Codivilla procedure: for neglected quadriceps tendon rupture, direct repair and advancement of fold from superior quadriceps mechanism.

Magnuson procedure: for unstable fracture of the patella; arthroplasty of the knee (fascia) in an attempt to remodel, and use of encircling metal wire.

Martin procedure: for patellar fracture; fixation with a wire loop.

McLaughlin procedure: for quadriceps or patellar tendon rupture, a reinforcing encircling wire is attached to patella or tibia respectively.

Miyakawa procedure: patellectomy with fabrication of a fold taken from the thick tissue well superior to the patella and reinforcing the patellar area to provide better mechanical force.

patellar or **femoral condylar shaving (skiving):** a direct removal of diseased cartilage from the patella and femoral cartilage, usually done in combination with treatment of other chronic knee injury problems.

patellectomy: removal of the kneecap.

patellectomy (partial): this procedure has two different meanings: (1) the total removal of cartilage from the patella, and (2) a removal of a portion of the bone following a fracture.

Scudari procedure: for fresh quadriceps rupture, repair with reinforcing flap from superior quadriceps mechanism.

Total knee arthroplasty

Total knee arthroplasty is the replacement of both sides of the knee joint by metal or plastic components. See under Internal prostheses in this chapter for various types of prostheses.

Quadricepsplasty

Any repair or reapproximation of the quadriceps mechanism is called a quadricepsplasty.

Tendon transfers

Surgical releases for muscle imbalance or knee contractures are referred to as tendon transfers.

Baker procedure: patellar tendon advancement; semitendinosis transfer for knock-kneed gait caused by internal rotation deformity of the hip.

Bickel and Moe procedure: translocation of the peroneus tendon.

Caldwell and Durham procedure: for quadriceps paralysis; transfer of biceps femorus to quadriceps mechanism.

Chandler procedure: patellar tendon advancement.

Ecker, Lotke, and Glazer procedure: for neglected infrapatellar tendon rupture; transfer of gracilis and semitendinosis for reinforcement.

Eggers procedure: transfer of the biceps femoris tendon associated with capsular releases and soleus neurectomy.

Galleazzi procedure: for chronic subluxation of the patella; transfer of the semitendinosus.

Hughston procedure: for chronic subluxation of the patella; patellar tendon transfer fixed by staple and redirection of vastus medialis.

Kelikian procedure: for old patellar tendon rupture; transfer of the gracilis tendon.

Sutherland procedure: for internal rotation deformity in hip affected by cerebral palsy; lateral transfer of medial hamstring.

Tachdjian procedure: for hamstring tightness in cerebral palsy; plastic lengthening of hamstring sheaths and tendons.

Genu recurvatum procedures

Brett and Campbell: tibial osteotomies.

Heyman procedure: reinforcement of posterior capsule using multiple tendon transfers; soft tissue release and transfers.

Perry procedure: posterior capsular repair with multiple tendon transfers.

Knee arthrodeses

Brittain
Charnley
Key
Lucas and Murray
Putti

Ankle arthrodeses

Blair
Campbell
Charnley

Chuinard and Petersen
Horwitz and Adams
sliding

Tibial osteotomies

Campbell
Cotton
Coventry
Ferguson-Thompson-King
Brett
Pott
Lucas and Cottrell

Lower limb (below knee) surgery

Anderson procedure: for unequal leg lengths; tibial lengthening using an external skeletal fixator.

Anderson and Hutchins procedure: for unstable tibial fractures; a method of skeletal pins and casting for fixation.

Bosworth procedure: for anterior tibial epiphysitis; insertion of bone pegs into the tibial tubercle.

Brett procedure: for malunited proximal tibial fractures with knee recurvatum; bone graft applied to opened anterior tibial plateau hinged posteriorly.

Brown procedure: for congenital absence of tibia; transfer fibula to femoral intercondylar notch.

Carroll procedure: bone graft replacement of the distal end of the fibula for tumors.

d'Aubigne procedure: for tumors; a method of excision of femoral condyle or tibial plateau.

Fahey and O'Brien procedure: for excision of tumor; technique of excision of a portion of the shaft of a bone.

Forbes procedure: for nonunion tibial fracture; iliac bone graft to tibia.

Gruca procedure: for congenital absence of the fibula; construction of an ankle mortise by splitting of the fibula.

Langenskiold procedure: for partial absence of fibula; fusion of distal tibia and fibula.

Malawer procedure: for malignancy of proximal fibula; resection of proximal fibula.

Wagner procedure: for leg-length disparity; shortening of proximal tibia or distal femur.

Wilson and Jacobs procedure: for comminuted tibial plateau fractures; replacement technique for the lateral side using iliac crest graft.

Ankle and foot

Baker procedure: for Achilles tendon tightness; relaxation of proximal tendon with a rectangular sliding slot incision.

Bosworth procedure: for repair of old rupture of Achilles tendon; fashioning direct tendon graft from median raphe (central portion of tendon).

Bugg and Boyd procedure: for repair of old Achilles tendon rupture; use of fascia lata graft.

Chrisman and Snook procedure: repair of lateral collateral ligament of ankle using peroneus brevis tendon. Also called modified Elmslie procedure.

DuVries procedure: for chronic instability of deltoid ligament of ankle; cross-shaped imbrication of deltoid ligament.

Ellis Jones procedure: for subluxing peroneal tendon; reconstruction of retinaculum using portion of Achilles tendon.

Evans procedure: for lateral collateral ligament instability of ankle; use of peroneus brevis tendon.

Hauser procedure: for Achilles tendon tightness; partial incision at two levels with passive stretching and casting.

Hoffer procedure: for spastic inversion of foot; transfer of anterior tibial tendon to cuboid.

Jones procedure: an ankle repair of the fibular collateral ligament using the peroneus brevis muscle.

Kaufer procedure: for spastic inversion of foot; transfer of posterior tibial tendon to peroneus brevis.

Lindholm procedure: for repair of ruptured Achilles tendon; fashioning of fascial flaps from superior tendon.

Lynn procedure: for repair of Achilles tendon rupture; use of fanned out portion of plantaris tendon to cover direct repair.

Ma and Griffith procedure: for Achilles tendon rupture; percutaneous technique of suture repair.

Majestro, Ruda, and Frost: for spastic posterior

tibial tendon; intramuscular lengthening.

McReynolds procedure: for comminuted calcaneus fracture; open reduction and fixation with staple, using a medial approach.

Pierrot and Murphy procedure: for dorsiflexion of the ankle weakness; transfer of Achilles tendon anteriorly on calcaneus.

Staples-Black-Brostrom procedure: for acute, severe ankle sprain; method of repair of lateral collateral ligaments.

Strayer procedure: for tight heel cord; gastrocnemius lengthening leaving soleus intact.

Tohen procedure: for spastic equinovarus deformity of foot; transfer of conjoined extensor hallucis longus and anterior tibial tendon to second or fifth metatarsal.

Valpius and Compere procedure: for Achilles tendon tightness; proximal inverted V-shaped lengthening.

Warner and Farber procedure: for trimalleolar fractures with large posterior fragment; detachment of the fibula from tibia to get screw fixation of posterior fragment.

White slide procedure: for Achilles tendon tightening in spastic hemiplegia, anterior fibers of the Achilles tendon are cut distally, and medial fibers are cut proximally. The foot is then dorsiflexed, producing the slide.

SKIN GRAFTS

Skin grafts are of three major categories: split-thickness skin graft (STSG), full-thickness skin graft (FTSG), and pedicle and rotational flaps.

Split-thickness skin graft

A split-thickness skin graft is 0.015 inch, or 0.4 mm thick. Taking a graft this way leaves behind viable skin from the donor site and living cells in the graft. However, both donor site and the graft will appear different from normal surrounding skin. Names associated with skin grafts are Blair-Brown, Douglas (mesh), Dragstedt, and Ollier-Thiersch.

Full-thickness skin graft

A full-thickness skin graft is a procedure that, throughout the entire surface of the graft, includes all the epidermis and therefore all the smooth skin coverage. This leaves behind a *donor site* that will need some form of closure or a split-thickness skin graft; for example, if a small necrosed area on a finger needs full skin coverage, a small ellipse of skin could be removed from the forearm; this is called a *pinch graft,* and the wound edges are closed.

Names associated with full-thickness skin grafts are Braun, Davis, Esser (Stent), Krause-Wolfe, Reverdin, and Wolfe.

Pedicle grafts and rotational flaps

A pedicle graft is a layer of fat, dermis, and epidermis, raised from a portion of the body having a sufficient blood supply to keep it alive. Pedicles are often used to cover large tissue defects, areas of exposed tendons, or areas where there will be considerable wear on the skin. The intended purpose of a pedicle is to eventually transfer this loose piece of skin and fat to cover another portion of the body. A flap is another name for pedicle, although the term connotes a local use in some cases; for example, a *rotational flap* is a rearrangement of the skin and fat in one area to cover a local defect.

A *delayed flap* is used for stimulation of the blood supply. An incision in the skin and fat with reapproximation of the wound margins into their original position is carried out. In a second or third procedure the flap is raised on a pedicle that is still attached, but now the distal part of that flap can be laid on another portion of the body. For example, a U-shaped incision is made in the leg and closed; 3 weeks later that skin is raised through the same incision and the flap that develops is laid down on an open area of the opposite leg. This is called a *cross-leg pedicle graft.*

Other terms referring to pedicle grafts and flaps are bilobed, compound, compound lined, double pedicle, Verdan, jump, marsupial, tumbler, Tait, and island pedicle.

SURGICAL BLOCKS

The term *local anesthesia* is sometimes used to indicate a regional anesthesia. In precise parlance local anesthesia indicates the injection of anesthetic agents at the site of the procedure. Regional anesthesia is infiltration of anatomic structure(s) proximal to the location of the procedure. Those used for orthopaedics are the following:

axillary block: injection of anesthetic agent into the nerves immediately around axillary artery, approached from the axilla; used for elbow, forearm, and hand procedures.

epidural block: infiltration of anesthetic agent into spinal canal but outside of the dura; can be used for so-called continuous drip anesthesia, where a catheter is left in place during procedure so that if more anesthesia is required it can be administered without repositioning the patient.

intravenous block: application of double tourniquet and the infiltration of anesthetic agents directly into vein to produce anesthesia in the limb below the tourniquet. Also called *Bier block*.

scalene block: injection of anesthetic agent into brachial plexus at the point of scalene muscles; used for shoulder and other upper limb procedures.

spinal block: infiltration of anesthetic agent into the spinal canal within the dura in the lumbar region. The proper positioning of patient during anesthetic infiltration is important in ensuring correct and sufficient anesthesia for procedures on the pelvis and lowers limbs.

SURGICAL APPROACHES

A surgical approach implies the type of incision made by the surgeon to do a particular procedure. Many surgical approaches have been described by various surgeons whose names are applied to those approaches. However, those approaches are not all original and have been modified and improved over the years. Anatomically, the direction of the incision may be modified by another surgeon, whose name then becomes attached to that incision, although in fact it is oriented to the same area of the bone of joint. In many instances an experienced surgeon may decide to plan an individualized approach in a given situation.

This prior consideration to surgical intervention may be described by the anatomic location and direction of the incision, for example, anterolateral or posterolateral approaches. More frequently the anatomic terms are favored in describing where an incision is to be made, even though the eponyms are also used for a particular anatomic area described.

Approaches are listed by anatomic location, eponyms, and common uses for the incision. Those interested in the technique of an incision will use other references. At the end of this section is a list of common incision shapes.

Shoulder

anterior axillary approach: usually used for repair of anterior shoulder dislocations; Roberts.

anteromedial approach: used for repair of shoulder and acromioclavicular joint injuries; Cubbins, Callahan, and Scuderi, Roberts, Thompson and Henry, saber-cut.

deltoid splitting approach: used to approach the rotator cuff and subacromial bursa.

transacromial approach: used to approach the rotator cuff and bursa; Codman, Darrach-McLaughlin, saber-cut.

posterior approach: used for repair of a posterior dislocation of the shoulder and lateral scapula. Abbott and Lucas, Bennett, Harmon, Kocher, McWhorter, Rowe, Yee.

Humerus

anterolateral approach: an approach to the bone and radial nerve; Thompson and Henry.

anteromedial approach: an approach to the median and ulnar nerves.

posterior approach: an approach used to visualize the humerus, triceps, and radial nerve; Henry.

Elbow

posterolateral approach: for elbow dislocations, radial head and distal humeral fractures, and arthroplasties; Kocher.

anterolateral approach: for exploration of the radial nerve; Henry.

medial approach: for exploration of the ulnar nerve and medial epicondyle; Campbell, Molesworth and Campbell.

anterior and anteromedial approach: for exploration of the median nerve, brachial artery, and other soft tissues; often associated with fractures.

posterior: for fractures of the distal humerus; Bryan and Morrey.

Forearm

posterior approach: in the proximal forearm used for fixation of proximal ulnar fractures and an approach to radial fractures; Thompson approach.

posterolateral approach: approach used for radial head fractures, some ulnar fractures, and exploration of the deep radial nerve; Boyd.

anterior approach: used for visualization of most of the forearm muscles that flex the fingers and for internal fixation of fractures of the radius; Henry approach.

posterolateral (distal) approach: used for some distal forearm fractures, tendon transfers, and excision of the distal ulna; Gordon.

Wrist

dorsal approach: on the back side of the wrist this approach is used for tendon transfers, fusions, and ganglionectomies.

volar approach: approach from the palmar aspect of the wrist, used for carpal tunnel releases, tendon explorations, and some bony procedures.

medial approach: an approach to the ulnar side of the wrist used for some tendon transfers and for the Darrach procedure; Smith-Petersen.

lateral approach: used on the radial side of the wrist for tendon transfers, radial styloidectomy, and visualization of the navicular bone.

Hand

Surgical approaches are too numerous and complicated to describe here. Refer to Edmonson AS and Crenshaw AH, editors: Campbell's operative orthopaedics, ed. 7, vol. I, St Louis, 1987, The CV Mosby Co., pp. 119–129.

Spine

posterior approach: used for laminectomies and spinal fusions at any level; Hibbs, Wagoner.

anterior approach: when used to approach the cervical, cervicodorsal, dorsal, and lumbar spines, it is designed to provide sufficient surface for multiple segmental spinal fusions; Hodgson, Roaf.

anterior approach: for specific cervical spinal explorations and fusions; Southwick and Robinson, Bailey and Badgley, Whitesides and Kelly, Henry (to the vertebral artery).

dorsolateral approach: an approach to the dorsal spine by costotransversectomy, usually done for fractures and other affections of the spinal cord.

anterolateral approach: an approach to the dorsal spine by rib resection to explore the spine anteriorly and in some cases to do spinal fusions and decompressions of the spinal cord.

Pelvis

Avila approach: anterior approach along the iliac crest to reach the anterior sacroiliac crest.

Radley, Liebig, and Brown approach: to the ischium.

Hips

anterolateral approach: for open reduction and internal fixation of the femoral neck, prosthetic replacement, and some congenital dysplasia surgery; Smith-Petersen, Van Gorder, Wilson, Cave, Callahan, Fahey.

lateral approach: for internal fixation of hip fractures and prosthetic replacement; Callahan, Charnley-Müller, Fahey, Harris, Hay, McLaughlan, Murphy, Ollier, Watson-Jones.

Senegas (modified Ollier): for acetabular fractures; an extensive exposure of the involving detachment of the greater trochanter.

posterior approach: for prosthetic replacement and repair of some pelvic fractures; Abbot, Gibson, Guleke-Stookey, McFarland and Osborne, Moore, Osborne.

medial approach: for congenital dysplastic hip surgery and other iliopsoas tendon approaches; Ludloff, Young.

Femur

anterolateral approach: used for rod or plate fixation fractures; Thompson.

lateral approach: used for fracture fixation; Eycleshymer and Schoemaker.

posterior approach: used for some muscle surgery and fixation of fractures; Bosworth.

posterolateral approach: used for muscle procedures, fracture fixation, and nerve explorations; Eycleshymer and Shoemaker, Henry.

Knee

All approaches to the knee are for ligamentous and bony reconstruction, meniscectomies, and vascular explorations. The posterior approaches are more specifically devoted to neurovascular surgery but may also be used in ligamentous and bony reconstructive procedures.

anterior approach: Coonse and Adams, Bosworth, Putti, Jones and Brackett, Insall.

anterolateral approach: Kocher, Henderson.

anteromedial approach: Abbott and Carpenter, Langenbeck.

medial approach: Aufranc, Cave, Henry, Bosworth.

lateral approach: Bruser lateral, Aufranc, Henry, Hoppenfield, de Boer, Pogruna, and Brown.

posterolateral approach: Henderson.

posterior approach: Abbott, Osgood, Brackett and Osgood, Putti and Abbott.

posteromedial approach: Banks and Laufman, Henderson.

transverse approach: Cave, Charnley, Cozen, Sir Henry Platt, McConnell.

Leg

posterolateral approach: for peroneal nerve and muscle surgery and for some bone grafts; Harmon, Henry, Huntington.

posterior approach: approach to the superomedial region of the tibia and gastrocnemius muscle; Banks and Laufman.

posteromedial approach: for neurovascular exploration and internal fixation of fractures; Phemister.

anterior approach: for internal fixation of fractures; this is an exploration of the anterior deep spaces.

Ankle

anterior approach: for tendon repairs, transfers, and some ankle fusions; Kocher, Ollier.

lateral and posterolateral approach: used for repair of fractures, ligamentous injuries, and some tendon transfers; Kocher, Gatellier and Chastang.

medial and posteromedial approach: used for ankle fractures, tendon transfers, and correction of clubfeet; Broomhead, Colonna and Ralston, Koenig and Schaefer, Garceau.

Surgical incisions described by appearance

J shaped	curvilinear
L curved	double
S-flap	linear
T shaped	longitudinal
T-tube	saber-cut
U shaped	split
Y incision	transverse
Z-plasty	

REPLANTATION-MICROSURGERY

Microsurgery, the use of a binocular microscope to perform surgery, is a relatively new area for the skilled orthopaedic surgeon. It has been used extensively within other specialties but only recently adapted to a variety of orthopaedic conditions. Microtechniques are applied to nerve repair, vascular repair, replantation, free tissue transfers, and spinal surgery.

The integration of this technique provides the surgeon with a three-dimensional telescopic view of the operating field at magnifications of structures 2½ to 25 times the size. Nylon sutures of high tensile strength, finer than human hair, are used to reattach small blood vessels and nerves. Keeping vessels open and carefully avoiding constriction are the goals of this procedure. Use of the technique requires extreme patience and perseverance on the part of the microsurgical team.

Replantation of traumatically severed extremities has become a common practice in orthopaedic surgery, a breathrough in musculoskeletal trauma management. The reintegration of tissues by way of microsurgical techniques has successfully restored functional use and eliminated the need for amputation in many cases. Hand and knee surgery have benefited greatly from microsurgery.

Replantation is truly a team effort, involving many hours of work with no room for compromise. The surgeon must spend many hours practicing and developing the skill and then use extreme patience and good judgment during application. The team approach is used to allow replacements during the long procedures.

Although other tissues heal in a short time, healing of blood vessels and nerves may take from 1 to 2 years. Other technologic developments, such as the *laser scalpel,* are also being used in surgical procedures.

AMPUTATIONS

The least desirable procedure for any surgeon is an amputation of a part; however, sometimes it becomes necessary. An *amputation* is the removal of a part through bone, and a *disarticulation* is the removal of a part through a joint space. Both of these terms are interpreted by most as the same procedure, but there is a distinction.

Most amputations take place in the lower limbs and may be indicated by traumatic injury, burns, infection, loss of blood supply, or malignancy. Amputation may also be indicated when a nonfunctioning limb could be replaced by a functional prosthetic device or when a congenital defect could be improved cosmetically or functionally by the removal of a part.

The level of amputation is often based on preservation of as much of the residual limb as would heal well with the vascular and peripheral circulation intact. The most common levels fall into the following categories: above elbow (AE), above knee (AK), below elbow (BE), and below knee (BK).

In the present nomenclature the description for limb absences can be reversed, that is, a leg, complete, is a complete leg amputation; if there is a partial amputation, it can be stated as to the level, for example, partial arm (upper one third). Any amputation through an epiphysis or closer to a joint is considered a complete amputation; an amputation of the distal third to the distal growth plate (growth plate scar in an adult) is considered a complete leg amputation (Tables 3 and 4).

Following such a procedure the patient is fitted right away with an artificial limb for the remaining stump. The aftertreatment of the stump is most important in the adjustment and rehabilitation of the amputee, as are the psychologic aspects.

Before and after a prosthesis (artificial limb) is

Table 3. Amputation levels, upper limb

New terms (with abbreviations)	Current terms	Eponyms
Shoulder (Sh), complete	Forequarter	Littlewood
Arm (Arm), complete	Shoulder disarticulation	Larrey, Dupuytren, Lisfranc
Arm (Arm), partial (upper ⅓)	Short (upper-third) AE	
Arm (Arm), partial (middle ⅓	Medium (mid-third) AE	
Arm (Arm) partial (lower ⅓)	Long (lower-third) AE	
Forearm (Fo), complete	Elbow disarticulation	
Forearm (Fo), partial (upper ⅓)	Short (upper-third) BE	
Forearm (Fo), partial (middle ⅓)	Medium (mid-third) BE	
Forearm (Fo), partial (lower ⅓)	Long (lower-third) BE	
Carpal (Ca), complete	Wrist disarticulation	
Carpal (Ca), partial	WD, with some carpals still present	
Metacarpal (MC), complete		
Metacarpal (MC), partial	Partial hand amputations, usually	
Phalangeal (Ph), complete	without precise differentiation	Kutler
Phalangeal (Ph), partial		

Note: An amputation at the MCP joints of the ring and little fingers would be designated as Ph, 4,5, complete; an amputation of the same two fingers at the PIP joints would be Ph, 4, 5, partial.

From Kay HW: A nomenclature for limb prosthetics, Orthot Prosthet J 28(4):37-47, 1974.

Table 4. Amputation levels, lower limbs

New terms (with abbreviations)	Current terms	Eponyms
Pelvic (Pel), complete	Hemicorporectomy	
Hip (Hip), complete	Hemipelvectomy	King and Steelquist, Jaboulay, Gordon-Taylor, Sorondo-Ferré
Thigh (Th), complete	Hip disarticulation	Béclard, Boyd, Pack
Thigh (Th), partial (upper ⅓)	Short (upper-third) AK	Alouette
Thigh (Th), partial (middle ⅓)	Medium (mid-third) AK	
Thigh (Th), partial (lower ⅓)	Long (lower-third) AK	Kirk
Leg (Leg), complete	Knee disarticulation	Gritti-Stokes, Morestin, Callander, Pollock,
Leg (Leg), partial (upper ⅓)	Short (upper-third) BK	Carden, Batch, Spittler and McFaddin
Leg (Leg), partial (middle ⅓)	Medium (mid-third) BK	
Leg (Leg), partial (lower ⅓)	Long (lower-third) BK	Carne
Tarsal (Ta), complete	Ankle disarticulation	Syme, Pirogoff, Guyon, Hancock, MacKenzie
Tarsal (Ta), partial		Chopart, Le Fort, Malgaigne, Vladimiroff-Mikulicz, Tripier
Metatarsal (MT), complete	Known collectively as partial foot amputations	Lisfranc, Hey
Metatarsal (MT), partial		
Phalangeal (Ph), complete		
Phalangeal (Ph), partial		

From Kay HW: A nomenclature for limb prosthetics, Orthot Prosthet J 28(4):37-47, 1974.

prescribed for an amputee, the physical medicine and rehabilitation team is an important link in teaching the patient prosthetic training. Prostheses have come a long way in appearance, fit, and functional use, and often it is not evident that a person is using a prosthesis. Chapter 7 discusses the many types of prostheses available. The following list of general terms applies to amputations.

General Terms

open amputation: any amputation in which the wound is left open for drainage, as opposed to a closed amputation.

closed amputation: any amputation in which the wound is closed at the time of initial or secondary surgery.

cineplastic (kineplastic) amputation: amputation that includes a skin flap built into a muscle (the biceps being the most common); a portion of the prosthetic mechanism is activated by the muscle.

fish mouth amputation: one in which the skin flaps extend distally to the bone amputation level, giving the appearance of a fish mouth.

guillotine (chop) amputation: amputation making a straight cut through the limb.

disarticulation: any amputation in which the limb is severed through a joint.

circular amputation: one in which a perfect circular incision is made.

stump revision: any surgery designed to revise the shape or scar of an amputation stump.

Syme amputation: The term is used to describe a special method of incision and closure for amputations at other locations, but describes a below-ankle amputation (removal of foot).

ASSOCIATED SURGICAL TERMS

ablate: to completely excise or amputate; the surgical destruction and removal of a part is referred to as ablative surgery, for example, the excision of a large tumorous mass and the surrounding soft tissue.

advancement: surgical or traumatic detachment of muscle, tendon, or ligamentous structure followed by reattachment at a more advanced point.

anastomosis: restoration of continuity of any vessel or organ; usually refers to the suturing of a tubular structure such as a blood vessel creating the passage between two distinct parts, such as end-to-end anastomosis.

anesthesia: loss of sensation or loss of consciousness as a direct result of the administration of a systemic drug agent. The term also describes the local or systemic loss of sensation caused by trauma or other injury.

approximate: to bring together or into apposition; this term is commonly used to refer to suturing of tissues or the repositioning of fractures.

aseptic: free from bacteria; aseptic technique is any technique designed to prevent contamination by bacteria.

aspiration: withdrawal of fluid from any open or closed space.

autopsy: a postmortem and pathologic examination of the body by dissection; necropsy.

biopsy: the excision of a section of living tissue for microscopic examination and diagnosis. This may be performed on any tissue; for example, a bone marrow biopsy is performed by closed method (use of a needle or trochar); the terms *needle biopsy* and *closed biopsy* are often used. In the same sense an *open biopsy* is one in which the tissue is examined before excision, and all or a sample of that tissue is sent for microscopic inspection.

The purpose of a biopsy is to determine the etiology and test for systemic, neoplastic, or reactive conditions. A biopsy is not made on normal anatomic tissue or where there is trauma or inflammation.

brisement (brēz-maw): the forcible breaking up of joint capsule, usually for conditions of partial fibrous ankylosis such as frozen shoulders.

callotasis: for limb length disparity, a transverse section of the bone of the short limb is stabilized with an external skeletal fixator and then the limb is gradually lengthened over a period of weeks.

catheterization: insertion of a tube into a cavity or blood vessel for drainage.

cauterization: the use of an electric current to stop local bleeding. This term also denotes the use of caustic materials such as silver nitrate to reduce local tissue granulation, as seen in open wounds.

cautery: an instrument designed to stop bleeding by destroying tissue through heat, electricity, or corrosive chemicals.

curettage: procedure in which a sharp, scraping instrument is used to remove abnormal tissue, growths, or obtain diagnostic specimens.

curette: a sharp, scraping, spoon-shaped instrument used in currettage.

debridement (debrēēd-maw): cleansing a wound of devitalized, contaminated, or foreign material.

decompression: surgical relief of pressure to any structure.

dehiscence: a separation or splitting of the edges of a surgical wound, where the expectation was for the wound to remain closed.

delayed primary closure (secondary closure): the closure of an open wound by intention after the initial surgery or injury; this is often done when the risk of infection is very high.

dismemberment: amputation of a limb.

dissection: separation of tissue for any reason. *Sharp dissection* is the use of a sharp instrument to facilitate dissection. *Blunt dissection* refers to the separation of tissues along natural lines of cleavage by the use of the fingers or other blunt instruments.

drainage: removal of fluid from a cavity. This term is often used to refer to material arising from open surgical wounds. *Dependent drainage* is an active effort to position a patient so that gravity will carry fluid away from the wound via catheterization.

ebonation: stripping of one tissue from another. In orthopaedics this refers to a surgical or pathologic removal of hard, bony loose cartilage from the surface of bone.

electrocautery: surgical instrument used to control bleeding of a surgical wound. The use of this instrument is called *electrocauterization.*

enucleate: to remove whole and clean in its entirety an organ, tumor, or cyst by shelling out.

evacuate: to empty a cavity.

excise: to cut out.

exploration: the examination by direct surgical visualization; surgery done for the express purpose of examining tissue is called exploratory surgery.

extirpation: the removal in its entirety of diseased tissue, a structure or mass; excision.

extraction: process of removal by pulling out.

extubation: the removal of a tube; used to refer to the tube inserted into the windpipe during anesthesia.

fixation: as applied to orthopaedics, implies the use of internal or external fixation, which is the use of metallic devices inserted into or through bone to hold a fracture in a set position and alignment while it heals.

fulguration: the use of high frequency electrocautery to destroy tissue during surgical procedures.

fusion: the uniting of two bony segments, whether a fracture or a vertebral joint.

granulation: the proliferation of numerous small blood vessels at a wound site to give the general appearance of a raw, red tissue. This is a normal healing process in that this rich vascular bed can modulate into normal tissue or act as a base for skin grafts or primary closure. Granuloma is a pathologic reaction to a foreign body or organism and should not be confused with granulation.

imbrication: the overlapping of tissue structures in closure of a wound and in repair of defects to improve the tightness of a structure.

implant: any substance inserted into the tissue for an indefinite period; this includes all internal prostheses, internal fixation devices, and other materials not absorbed by the body.

incision and drainage (I&D): surgical incision into a cavity, usually for purpose of removing purulent (infected) material; most common example is the lancing of an abscess.

infiltration: usually refers to local injection of anesthetic solutions or fluids into soft tissue permeation; may be a result of failure of intravenous fluids to go into the vein correctly.

infusion: introduction of any solution such as saline into a blood vessel or cavity.

injection: introduction of material, nutrients or medicine, into tissues of the body by the use of a syringe and needle.

in situ: in orthopaedics, the fixation of a fracture in the position that it presents at the time of injury, usually a nondisplaced fracture; also used to describe a lesion that is highly localized.

in toto: in total; removal of an organ, cyst, or tumor in its entirety.

intubation: insertion of a tube into the trachea for entrance of air during surgical procedure; for example, endotracheal entubation.

in vitro: living organism in artificial environment (glass test tube) as used in the laboratory.

in vivo: living organism within the human body as in a malignancy.

irrigation: washing out of a wound or cavity with a solution. *Closed suction irrigation* is a specific system by which irrigating tubes are surgically implanted in a wound and used continuously after the time of surgery.

laser (*l*ight *a*mplification by *s*timulated *e*mission of *r*adiation): a device used in surgical procedures consisting of a resonant optical cavity in which a substance is stimulated to emit light radiation; and a mirror which reflects the rays back and forth so molecules will emit more radiation. Finely directed laser light sources can be used to cut tissue, coagulate vessels, or cause the adhesion of one tissue surface to another.

lavage: the copious washing out or irrigation of a wound or cavity.

ligation: tying off; used particularly in reference to the tying of blood vessels at a surgical wound.

ligatures: sutures used to tie off blood vessels.

manipulation: the planned and carefully managed manual movement of a joint or fracture to produce increased joint motion or better position and alignment of the fracture. This term is sometimes used to denote a precise sequence of movements of a joint to determine the presence of disease or to reduce a dislocation.

marsupialization: incision into a cystic lesion with incorporation of the walls of the cyst to the exterior edges of the skin to produce constant drainage.

morcellation: breaking up of tissue for easier removal, or to leave in place but in a refashioned shape such as bone graft material.

palliative: surgical procedure or use of medications to treat the symptoms without curing the disease process; used relative to the treatment of terminal conditions seen in cancer.

paracentesis: needle puncture into a cavity to aspirate fluid; usually done in the abdominal and thoracic cavities.

per primam: the healing of a surgical or traumatic wound by first intention, after closure. This means that the closure of the wound is successful and that there is no reopening of the wound due to failure of healing.

-pexy (suffix): fixation by solid tissue attachment. In orthopaedics the most common term using this root is *scapulopexy,* a procedure whereby the scapula is fixed directly to the ribs.

phantom pain: the sensation of pain following amputation that seems to be in the part that has been removed. Eventually the patient is able to localize the pain to the stump and loses the sense of the presence of the amputated part.

primary closure: the closure of the wound edges at the time of trauma or surgery.

prosthesis: this term has a very broad meaning and includes all artificial limbs as well as materials implanted in the body to replace the structure, function, or appearance of that missing structure.

reefing: a folding in or overlapping of soft tissue by surgical suture designed to make that structure tighter.

reflect: in the surgical sense means to fold back tissue such as a muscle belly to expose deeper structures.

release: incision into any soft tissue to produce relaxation of that tissue, for example, tendon release.

resection: partial excision of soft tissue or segment of bone; also the removal of a portion of diseased nerve tissue, called a nerve resection.

retraction: a pulling back of tissue, whether done mechanically at the time of surgery or by scar formation after surgery; for example, a scar that is indented inward toward the body is considered a retracted scar.

revision: any surgical reconstruction of soft or hard tissue. A revision may be done at the time of

initial trauma if damaged tissue is removed and normal structures are repositioned to compensate for that destruction. The term is more commonly used to describe a later surgical effort to reposition various tissues.

rongeur: to cut into bone with a sharp biting instrument called a rongeur, usually to remove bone that is diseased or obstructing visualization of deeper structures.

saucerization: creation of a saucerlike depression in bone in an effort to remove diseased bone. This is most commonly done for bone infections, and the wound is usually left open for drainage.

secondary closure: closure of a wound that had been left open after previous trauma or surgery. This is also called *delayed primary closure* and is done often when there is a high risk of infection.

sepsis: the presence of bacterial infection in blood or tissue from any source. This term is often used to describe the systemic condition resulting from an infection, for example, septicemia.

septic: contaminated with bacteria. A septic wound, otherwise known as a *dirty* wound, is one in which there is an existing infection with purulent material.

-stasis (suffix): to control flow or progression, for example, hemostasis.

stasis: condition arising from a static circumstance. For example, a stasis ulcer is one that is created in a patient kept in the same position for any length of time where blood or fluids stagnate.

subcutaneous: the fatty and fibrous tissues beneath the thick layers of skin.

subcuticular: the thick layer of skin below the epidermal layers. A subcuticular suture is used to close the skin by a continuous suture that pulls the deep layer of skin together, with the suture exiting at each end of the wound only.

sulcus: any normal groove or depression in bone or soft tissue.

suspension: usually refers to a soft tissue procedure designed to help hold some anatomic structure in a more functional position; tenodesis.

suture: any threadlike, pliable material that is used to close soft tissue; catgut, nylon.

tamponade: method to control bleeding by direct pressure.

-tome (suffix): meaning any instrument that cuts.

tourniquet: any instrument used to compress blood vessels to slow or stop circulation. If light pressure is applied by tourniquet, there will be congestion in the venous system. This is often used to help draw blood for laboratory testing. More secure tourniquet pressure, designed to stop all blood flow to a part, is used to prevent bleeding.

toxic: poisonous. This term is often used to describe the systemic condition of a patient with infection.

transect: to cut across the long axis of a tissue. For example, a tendon transection is often done to release the pull of that tendon at its point of insertion.

transfusion: term commonly used to describe the intravenous infusion of whole blood or blood components; however, any solution may be transfused.

transposition: the repositioning of an intact and attached tissue segment from one place to another. This term is often used in describing soft tissue and bone graft procedures.

-tripsy (suffix): surgical crushing, for example, an osteotripsy is a procedure done in the foot to relieve a corn or callus caused by prominence of bone under the skin.

vest-over-pants closure: closure of fascia, particularly near joints, where one layer is closed on top of another to produce tightening or pull on the joint capsule.

viable: alive or capable of living; used to describe healthy tissue that appears to be intact.

9

The hand

Where is there available a precision instrument that can either gently pick up eggs or lift 200 pounds; detect the weight of only four grains of sand, temperature differences of 1 degree, and the distance between two points less than 0.1 inch apart; be remote controlled, self-powered, and transportable to any part of the world? This priceless tool is available at no cost to almost all humankind—the hand.

A description of the intricate anatomy of the hand cannot be completely simplified. The sequence of definitions given here will help to define the basics of hand control and function. Some diseases or surgery are briefly annotated in Chapter 8 but more fully defined in the second part of this chapter.

ANATOMY OF THE HAND
Muscles

There are large muscles in the forearm that insert into the bones of the hand by means of their tendons (Figs. 9-1 and 9-2). These *extrinsic muscles* cause the hand and fingers to flex and extend (close and open). The *intrinsic muscles* are small and originate within the hand. These control positioning and to a large extent functional coordination of the fingers. In normal hand function all these groups work together in intricate unison.

extrinsic wrist flexors: flexor carpi ulnaris, palmaris longus, flexor carpi radialis; insert on the metacarpals, carpal bones, and ligaments; they cause strong wrist flexion.

extrinsic wrist extensors: extensor carpi radialis longus, extensor carpi radialis brevis, extensor carpi ulnaris; insert on the metacarpals.

extrinsic finger flexors: flexor digitorum profundus, flexor digitorum sublimus or superficialis, flexor pollicis longus (thumb); insert on either the distal or the middle phalanges of the digits and cause powerful finger or thumb flexion.

extrinsic finger extensors and thumb abductor: extensor digiti quinti proprius, extensor digitorum communis, extensor indicis proprius, extensor pollicis longus, extensor pollicis brevis, abductor pollicis longus; insert on the bones and extensor hoods of the fingers and thumb and cause extension of the digits.

thenar muscles: opponens pollicis, abductor pollicis brevis, flexor pollicis brevis deep and superficial head, the deep head sometimes called first palmer interosseous: (intrinsic muscles of the thumb); arise from the carpal bones and ligaments at the base of the palm and insert on the proximal phalanx or on the thumb metacarpal. They function to bring the thumb out and away from the palm and to oppose it to the other fingers. One intrinsic muscle arises from the metacarpals and crosses deep in the palm to the thumb. This adductor pollicis muscle pulls the thumb forcefully back in toward the palm (adduction).

hypothenar muscles: opponens digiti quinti or minimi, flexor digiti quinti, abductor digiti quinti; a less important group of intrinsic muscles that arise from the carpal bones and insert on the little finger, metacarpal, and proximal phalanx.

other intrinsic muscles: lumbricals, dorsal interossei, volar interossei; arise from the metacar-

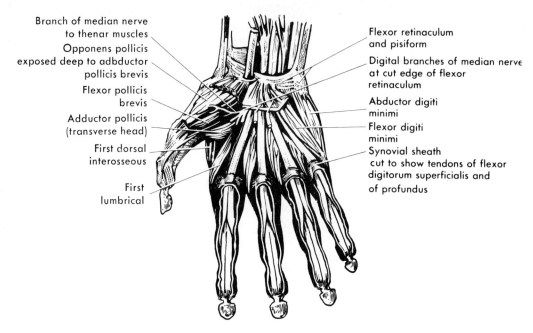

Fig. 9-1. Muscles of the anterior aspect of the human hand; the palmar aponeurosis has been removed. (From DiDio LJA: Synopsis of anatomy, St Louis, 1970, The CV Mosby Co.)

pals or from the flexor tendons and insert into the finger dorsal (extensor) mechanism and base of the proximal finger bone. They are responsible for spreading and bringing together the fingers and for firm coordination of motion at each finger joint.

other muscles in the forearm: brachioradialis, pronator teres, supinator, anconeus, and pronator quadratus; these do not extend to the hand but affect the position of the hand by actions such as rotation of the forearm (pronation and supination).

Ligaments

There are numerous ligaments named for the bones to which the ligaments are attached.

carpal tunnel: tunnel in wrist created by the volar carpal ligament. This space contains the flexor tendons to the fingers and thumb as well as the median nerve.

collateral ligament: any ligament running along the sides of a joint adding lateral stability; named for a specific bone or joint.

deep transverse metacarpal ligament: specific distal ligaments between the second, third, fourth, and fifth metacarpophalangeal volar plates.

digital retinaculum: the covering fascia of the finger flexors.

extensor and flexor retinaculum: the heavy fascial tissue that covers the outer layer of the forearm and wrist and prevents the tendons from bowstringing away from the wrist.

extensor retinaculum: broad band of superficial fascia over the dorsum of the wrist; helps to restrain the extensor tendons.

extensor tendon compartments: the 6 fascial compartments on the dorsum of the distal radius for the wrist extensors. Numbering from radial to ulnar are the following:

abductor pollicis longus and extensor pollicis brevis

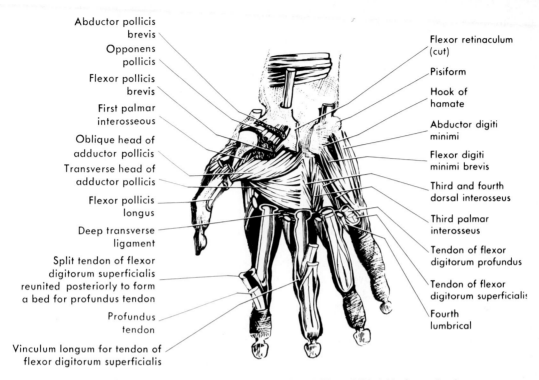

Abductor pollicis brevis
Opponens pollicis
Flexor pollicis brevis
First palmar interosseous
Oblique head of adductor pollicis
Transverse head of adductor pollicis
Flexor pollicis longus
Deep transverse ligament
Split tendon of flexor digitorum superficialis reunited posteriorly to form a bed for profundus tendon
Profundus tendon
Vinculum longum for tendon of flexor digitorum superficialis

Flexor retinaculum (cut)
Pisiform
Hook of hamate
Abductor digiti minimi
Flexor digiti minimi brevis
Third and fourth dorsal interosseus
Third palmar interosseus
Tendon of flexor digitorum profundus
Tendon of flexor digitorum superficialis
Fourth lumbrical

Fig. 9-2. Muscles of the anterior aspect of the human hand. (From DiDio LJA: Synopsis of anatomy, St Louis, 1970, The CV Mosby Co.)

extensor carpi radialis brevis and longus

extensor pollics longus

extensor digitorum communis and extensor indicis proprius

extensor digiti quinti

extensor carpi ulnaris

palmar fascia: complex interwoven fascia in the palm of the hand. It is part of the expansion of the palmaris longus. and protects the delicate structures in the hand.

superficial transverse intermetacarpal ligaments: the expansion of the palmar fascia in the region of the distal metacarpals.

volar carpal ligament: the ligament that spans the arch of the carpal bones and covers and binds down the nine long flexor tendons of the thumb and fingers and also covers the median nerve. Also called *transverse ligament, transverse carpal ligament*.

web ligament: expansion of the palmar fascia between the base of the fingers.

Nerves

lateral cutaneous nerve: (of forearm) sometimes provides sensation to the lateral side of the thumb metacarpal area.

median nerve: the nerve that crosses under the small volar carpal ligament, supplies all the small muscles of the thumb except the adductor and the deep head of the flexor pollicis brevis, and provides sensation for most of the palm and volar thumb, long and index fingers, and thumb side of the ring finger.

radial nerve, superficial branch: this nerve supplies sensation only; sensory distribution is over the dorsum of the thumb, index finger, long finger, and radial side of the ring finger.

ulnar nerve: the nerve crossing the wrist through

the Guyon canal and supplying the adductor pollicis, deep head of the flexor pollicis brevis, and all small muscles of the hand, except the thumb and first two lumbricals. The sensation supplied is to the little finger and the little finger side of the ring finger.

Fingers

cutaneous ligaments: ligaments that restrain the skin during finger motion. These include the Cleland and Grayson ligaments.

cuticle: the skin edge immediately covering the base of the fingernail.

dorsal digital artery and nerve: the branches of artery and nerve in the dorsum of the finger.

dorsal (extensor) hood: the fanlike expansion of the extensor communis tendon over the dorsum and sides of the *metacarpo*phalangeal (MCP) joints. This complex structure brings together intrinsic and extrinsic tendons to control interphalangeal (IP) joint extension and MP joint flexion or extension.

  lateral bands: the portions of the intrinsic muscle tendons that run laterally across the proximal phalanx to the dorsum of the distal interphalangeal (DIP) and proximal interphalangeal (PIP) joints.

  dorsal expansion: the fibers spreading laterally at the base of the dorsal hood.

  central slip (tendon): the portion of the extensor tendon that inserts into the middle phalanx.

germinal matrix: the cells located at the base of the nail that generate the tissues that eventually form the nail.

Grayson ligaments: fibrous tissue bands of the finger extending from the volar DIP and PIP joint area to the lateral skin.

hyponychia: the tissue immediately under the distal portion of the nail.

nail plate: the hard portion of the dorsum of the finger and thumb. This rigid outer covering extends approximately 8 mm under the nail fold and arises from the nail bed.

nail bed: tissue immediately under the nail.

nail fold: a fold of skin supporting the nail at its most proximal portion (base).

paronychium: the skin on either side of the nail.

proper volar digital nerve and artery: the nerves and arteries after they have divided in the palm and travel along the two volar sides of the finger.

pulleys: thickened portions of flexor tendon sheaths that hold the tendons in place. Depending on the orientation of the fibers of the pulley, they are labeled as annular or cruciate. The most proximal pulley is located on the distal metacarpal and is labeled annular 1 (A1), then annular 2 through 4. The cruciate pulleys are similarly labeled C1 through C3 (Fig. 9-3).

pulp: the tissue of the volar distal finger.

septa: fibrous tissue structures in the fingertips.

skin creases: indentations in the skin at the point of natural motion points of the finger. The digital skin creases are labeled proximal, middle, and distal.

subungual space: the potential space between the nail and nail bed, common site for a hematoma.

vinculae: blood vessel bridges to the flexor tendons having a *vinculum breve* and *longum.*

volar plate: a thick cartilaginous structure over the volar surface of each of the finger and thumb joints.

hypothenar eminence: prominence caused by intrinsic muscle mass on little finger side of the palm.

intermediate bursa: occasionally seen anatomically as the bursa containing the index finger flexor tendon sheath.

midpalmar space: a deep potential space on the little finger side of the palm.

palmar skin crease: the skin crease in the palm caused by natural folds in the skin. These are labeled as distal palmar (DPC), midpalmar, and thenar (the "life line").

thenar eminence: the prominence caused by intrinsic muscle mass on the thumb side of the palm.

thenar space: the potential space on the thumb side of the hand deep to the tendons and nerves.

ulnar bursa: the sac containing the tendon sheaths of the index, long, ring, and little fingers in the palm and extending to the end of the little finger.

Cleland ligaments: fibrous tissue bands on the lateral side of the fingers that stabilize the skin

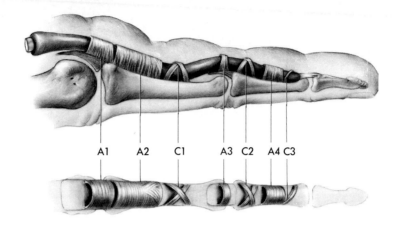

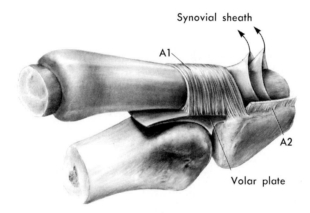

Fig. 9-3. This anatomic diagram of various parts of flexor sheath is helpful in understanding gliding of tendon. Maintenance of second annulus (A2) and fouth annulus (A4) is essential to retain appropriate angle of approach and prevent "bowstringing" of flexor tendons or tendon graft. (From Doyle JR and Blythe W: In American Academy of Orthopaedic Surgeons: Symposium on tendon surgery in the hand, St Louis, 1975, the CV Mosby Co.)

during finger movement, dorsal to Grason's ligament.

Landsmeer ligaments: fibrous tissue bands on the lateral side of the fingers that help to synchronize the motion of the two distal joints; also called oblique retinacular ligaments.

web space: skin web between the base of the fingers.

eponychium: thin skin covering base of the nails on the dorsal surface.

lunula: half-moon-shaped color change at the base of the nails.

unguis: the nail.

subungual: under the nail.

knuckle pad: the thick skin over the dorsum of the DIP and PIP joints of the finger.

snuffbox (anatomic snuffbox): the area of the lateral wrist, bounded by the extensor pollicis longus and abductor pollicis longus.

Palm

radial bursa: bursa containing the flexor pollicis longus tendon sheath located in the palm and thumb.

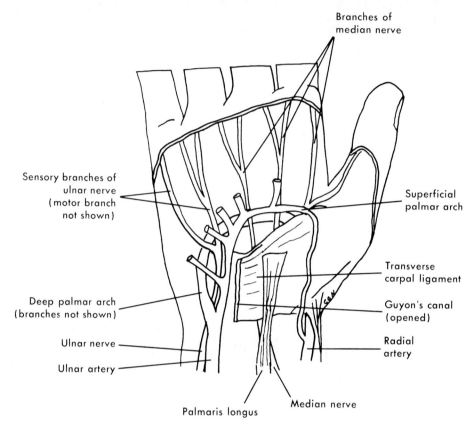

Branches of
median nerve

Sensory branches of
ulnar nerve
(motor branch
not shown)

Superficial
palmar arch

Transverse
carpal ligament

Deep palmar arch
(branches not shown)

Guyon's canal
(opened)

Ulnar nerve

Radial
artery

Ulnar artery

Palmaris longus

Median nerve

Fig. 9-4. Major arterial and nerve supply to the hand. Note the median nerve crossing under the carpal tunnel and the separate structure of the Guyon canal.

radial artery: major artery on the thumb side of the palm and wrist.

ulnar artery: artery on the little finger side of the palm and wrist.

superficial and deep palmar arterial arch: the superficial and deep connecting arcades of the radial and ulnar artery in the palm.

common digital arteries and nerves (Fig. 9-4): the main branch of the various nerves or arteries in the palm; these then divide into the proper digital arteries and nerves.

palmar fascia: thick outer fascia of the palm.

Guyon canal: space between the hamate and pisiform bones for ulnar artery and nerve, covered by ulnar side of volar carpal ligament. Floor is the pisohamate ligament.

Bones (Fig. 9-5)

phalanx: any given bone of the thumb of finger, namely, the *distal, proximal,* or *middle phalanx* of the fingers and the distal or proximal phalanx of the thumb. The *tuft* is the terminal bony expansion of the distal phalanx.

metacarpals: the five long bones of the palm, numbered one through five starting with the thumb.

carpus: the eight carpal bones of the wrist. The distal row leading from the thumb side is composed of the trapezium (or greater multangular), trapezoid (lesser multangular), capitate, and hamate. The proximal row leading from the thumb side is composed of the scaphoid (navicular bone), lunate (semilunar), triquetrum (triangular), and pisiform.

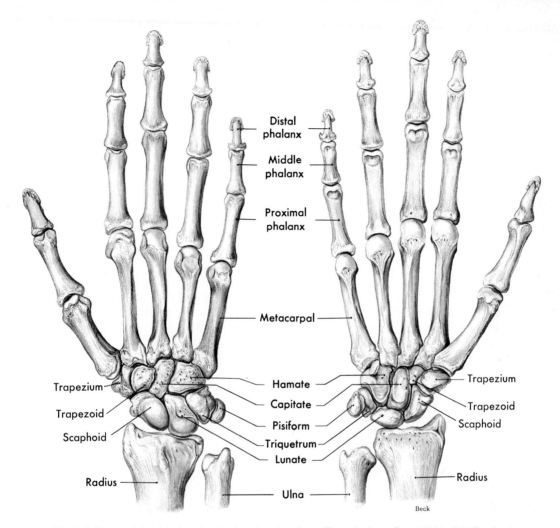

Distal phalanx

Middle phalanx

Proximal phalanx

Metacarpal

Trapezium

Trapezoid

Scaphoid

Radius

Hamate

Capitate

Pisiform

Triquetrum

Lunate

Ulna

Trapezium

Trapezoid

Scaphoid

Radius

Beck

Fig. 9-5. Bones of the right hand and wrist, dorsal surface. (From Anthony C and Kolthoff N: Textbook of anatomy and physiology, ed 9, St Louis, 1975, The CV Mosby Co.)

sesamoids: small bones in some of the tendons of the thumb.

ZONES

zone I: anatomic structures distal to the insertion of the sublimus tendon into the middle phalanx.

zone II: anatomic structures in the region from just proximal to the A1 pulley up to zone I. Also called *no man's land.*

zone III: anatomic structures in the region from carpal tunnel to zone II. This is the region of the arterial arch and the origin of the lumbricals.

zone IV: the carpal tunnel.

zone V: anatomic area of the wrist proximal to the carpal tunnel.

In Appendix A (Orthopaedic abbreviations) are listed many abbreviations frequently used because of the length of the Latin terms. Only a few of these abbreviations are recognized by the Joint Commission on Accreditation of Health Organizations (JCAHO). Therefore it is suggested that the full Latin name be spelled out at the outset and abbreviated when used again in context.

DISEASES OF THE HAND

Most of the diseases that affect the bones and joints of the hand are described in Chapter 2. The specific terminology for deformities caused by rheumatoid arthritis, nerve injuries, and congenital defects related to the hand is listed here. The terminology for diseases of the hand comprises many words not specific to other parts of the anatomy and is divided as follows: (1) arthritic deformities, (2) deformities from nerve injuries, (3) congenital deformities, (4) infections of the hand, and (5) other specific terms.

Arthritic deformities

attenuation (attrition) of tendons: erosion and eventual rupture of tendons by diseased synovium or bony spurs.

boutonnière deformity: A fixed deformity of the finger consisting of flexion of the proximal interphalangeal joint and extension of the distal interphalangeal joint. A result of rheumatoid destruction of the extensor tendon mechanism at the proximal interphalangeal joint and also secondary to trauma without arthritis.

intrinsic minus deformity: hyperextension of the metacarpophalangeal joint associated with flexion of the other joints of the fingers; may result from any interruption of intrinsic function.

intrinsic plus deformity: position of the hand in which the metacarpophalangeal joint is flexed and the proximal interphalangeal joints are extended. This is caused by intrinsic muscle tightness, is commonly seen in rheumatoid arthritis, and is associated with other deformities.

mallet finger: drop of the distal phalanx due to traumatic or arthritic damage to the extensor tendon over the distal interphalangeal (DIP) joint.

opera glass hand: a rare, very advanced stage of arthritis in which the joints are destroyed and the bones become thin, fragile, and shortened.

radial drift: the position toward which the metacarpals tend to drift in rheumatoid arthritis—the alignment of the hand deviates toward the thumb; may apply to the thumb but usually specified.

swan neck: the posture of the finger with hyperextension of the proximal interphalangeal joint and flexion of the distal interphalangeal joint, as seen in rheumatoid arthritis or traumatic rupture of the distal insertion of the extensor tendon, and may also be congenital because of laxity in the ligaments.

tophus: accumulation of any crystalline material in the soft tissue; seen commonly in gout.

ulnar drift: the position of the fingers in rheumatoid arthritis; the fingers point away from the thumb and are often associated with radial drift at the wrist.

Deformities caused by nerve injury

clawhand or intrinsic minus deformity: posture of hyperextension of the metacarpophalangeal joints and flexion of other finger joints resulting from loss of the intrinsics; seen in median and in ulnar nerve loss, in which the exact deformity takes various shapes depending on the level of nerve loss. Reference is often made to high median nerve loss and low median nerve loss. The low palsy involves only the intrinsic muscles of the hand, whereas the upper palsy eliminates flexion of the thumb, index, and long fingers. Also called *benediction posture*.

ulnar clawhand: claw position (hyperextension of the metacarpophalangeal joint) of the ring and little fingers and loss of abduction of the thumb. NOTE: In a *high ulnar nerve palsy* the deformity is less apparent because of the extrinsic (forearm) muscle involvement. In a low ulnar nerve palsy only the intrinsic muscles are involved.

wrist drop: loss of extensor control of the fingers and wrist caused by radial nerve palsy.

Congenital deformities

camptodactyly: bent finger; commonly referred to as a congenital flexion deformity of the proximal interphalangeal joint of the little finger.

clinodactyly: varus deformity of the PIP or DIP joint of the little finger.

clubhand (radial clubhand, talipomanus): position of the hand in strong flexion and radial deviation, caused by partial or complete absence of the radius and thumb.

Kirner deformity: spontaneous incurving of the terminal phalanx of the fifth digit.

lobster-claw deformity: absence of the central rays (metacarpals and fingers), resulting in a lobster-claw appearance.

macrodactyly: overgrowth in size and diameter in one or more digits.

Madelung deformity: congenital or traumatic shortening of radius due to relative overgrowth of the distal ulna. Wrist is flexed and ulnarly deviated.

Poland syndrome: absence of the pectoral head of the pectoralis major muscles associated with deformities in thumb ray or fingers.

polydactyly: excess number of fingers; tends to be hereditary.

supernumerary digits: extra nubbins of fingers or thumb, usually possessing no function.

symphalangism (multiple): congenital fusion of multiple PIP joints.

symphalangism (true): congenital fusion of a single PIP joint.

syndactyly: fusion of two or more fingers in which there may be involvement of soft tissue only (simple) or that may include a fusion of bone or cartilage (complex).

Streeter dysplasia: condition involving congenital tight circular bands of skin, congenital amputations, and syndactyly (fused fingers).

Classification of upper limb anomalies

The International Federation of Societies for Surgery of the Hand (IFSSH) has adopted a classification system for limb anomalies that affect hand function. An example is given for each.

Group I: failure of formation of parts (transverse arrest, phocomelia longitudinal arrest, radial clubhands)

Group II: failure of differentiation of parts (syndactyly)

Group III: duplication of parts (duplicate thumb)

Group IV: overgrowth (macrodactyly)

Group V: undergrowth (bradydactyly)

Group VI: congenital constriction band syndrome (congenital constriction band syndrome)

Group VII: generalized skeletal abnormalities (dwarfism, Klippel-Feil syndrome).

Infections of the hand

The hand has many structures that are vulnerable to infections. When edema and swelling place pressure on muscles, tendons, vessels, and nerves, function is disrupted and compartmental ischemia could result. Adhesions or fibrosis following infection may reduce hand function temporarily or permanently. Terms related to infections are the following.

collar button abscess: abscess around the metacarpal head areas.

deep space infection (palmar space infection): refers to infection of the thenar or midpalmar spaces.

eponychia: infection at the base of the nail.

felon: bacterial infection of the nail pulp.

herpetic Whitlow (aseptic felon): pulp infection with herpes simplex virus, common in children and dental hygienists.

horseshoe abscess: infection spread from the thumb to the little finger or vise versa, traveling by way of bursal spaces.

Melanie infection: a synergistic infection by two organisms; leads to gangrene.

paronychia: bacterial infection of the skin folds at the sides of the nail.

subungual abscess: infection between the nail and the nail bed.

tenosynovitis: bacterial infection of the tendon sheath or bursa.

Other specific terms

Bouchard node: thick nodular swelling due to bone spurs in the proximal interphalangeal joints, not necessarily associated with systemic arthritis.

carpal bossing: prominence seen particularly at the dorsal index metacarpal-carpal joint; may be painful but usually causes no symptoms.

carpal tunnel syndrome: decreased sensation,

pain in palm and forearm, and, occasionally, weakness in thumb movements due to compression of the median nerve at the transverse carpal ligament.

de Quervain syndrome: an inflammation in the abductor pollics tendon sheath at the wrist.

Dupuytren contracture (palmar fibromatosis): inflammatory process of the palmar facia, occasionally extending into the fingers, in which severe contractures and nodular proliferation (skin dimples) may result. There are three phases; proliferative (nodular), involutional, and resolved. In the resolved state the remaining constricting tissue is referred to as bands.

flexor origin syndrome (reverse tennis elbow): tendonitits of pronator teres and wrist and finger flexor muscle origin on medial epicondyle of elbow.

ganglion: a clear, viscid, fluid-filled sac found near the wrist joints or fingers, arising from capsuloligamentous structures; rarely associated with other diseases; most commonly found on dorsum of wrist.

glomus tumor: small vascular lesion that is usually very painful and associated with hypersensitivity to pressure or temperature; usually in fingertip.

Heberden node: a thick nodular swelling due to bone spurs in the distal interphalangeal joints; not necessarily associated with systematic arthritis.

inclusion cyst: a noninfectious process following healed laceration or puncture wound; germinal matrix of dermal growth, causing mass comprised of desquamated dermal cells.

Keinbock disease (lunatomalacia): spontaneous loss of blood supply and collapse of lunate, usually seen in young adults.

mucous cyst: a misnomer; this is a ganglion of the distal interphalangeal joint, which makes a cyst under the skin in the eponychial area.

Prieser disease: spontaneous loss of blood supply and collapse of scaphoid, usually seen in young adults.

stenosing tenosynovitis: a bulbous swelling of the tendon, causing the tendon to catch as it passes through the pulley (the thick fibrous tunnel that holds the tendon in place); sometimes caused by rheumatoid arthritis. Also called *trigger fingers, snapping tendons.*

trapeziometacarpal arthritis: an arthritis at the base of the thumb; often occurs in the absence of systemic disease or previous trauma. Most common in women.

trigger finger: tumescence of flexor tendon associated with a thick stenosing sheath; usually located in the distal palm. Causes the finger to catch as it extends.

SURGERY OF THE HAND

Surgical procedures of the hand are described more on an anatomic basis than by eponyms. All terms, including eponyms, are listed according to the goals of the surgical procedure.

Arthrodeses of the fingers

Moberg arthrodesis: finger joint fusion using a small squared bone peg.

Potenza arthrodesis: finger joint fusion using bone peg taken from the adjacent phalanx or metacarpal.

Arthrodeses of the wrist

Abbott arthrodesis: using only cortical bone grafts. Also called Abbott-Saunders-Bost arthrodesis.

Brockman-Nissen arthrodesis: intraarticular wrist fusion.

Carroll arthrodesis: rabbit ear-shaped bone graft fusion.

Gill-Stein arthrodesis: extraarticular fusion using the dorsal distal radius as the graft. Also called radiocarpal arthrodesis.

Haddad-Riordan arthrodesis: intraarticular fusion using iliac crest bone graft.

Liebolt arthrodesis: fusion using chips of bone graft.

Nalebuff arthrodesis: fusion that includes use of a Steinmann pin.

Seddon arthrodesis: intraarticular fusion involving resection of the distal ulna.

Smith-Petersen arthrodesis: fusion that includes resection of the distal ulna.

Wickstrom arthrodesis: fusion of the wrist using bone graft inserted into both the radius and carpus.

Arthroplasty

Arthroplasty is reconstruction of joints to restore motion and stability. Joint destruction is commonly found in rheumatoid arthritis, and arthroplasties of various joints are frequently done by hand surgeons.

metacarpophalangeal joint arthroplasty: Vainio, Tupper, Fowler, or Swanson (implant) arthroplasty.

carpometacarpal joint arthroplasty: for the thumb. Also called Eaton-Littler arthroplasty.

proximal interphalangeal joint arthroplasty: Carroll and Taber, or Curtis arthroplasty.

wrist arthroplasty: Darrach procedure or volar shelf arthroplasty (Albright and Chase).

implant arthroplasty: a prosthetic replacement of joints by metallic or silicone-rubber parts, usually for arthritic conditions or traumatic ankylosis. Swanson silicone-rubber arthroplasty is a popular choice. Some other prosthetic devices for the hand and wrist are *AMC total wrist (Volz), Steffe, Swanson.*

Grafts (nerve, bone, skin)

The general grafts of nerve, bone, and skin used in forearm and hand injuries are listed here with the grafts and other procedures for fingertip amputations. Procedures involving tendons and tendon grafts are often interrelated and are listed in the next section.

nerve cable graft: a multi-strand free nerve graft (taken from elsewhere in the body); usually done in the forearm to bridge a large gap in one of the three main nerves.

Gillies and Millard technique: metacarpal lengthening and transfer of local flap.

Hauser transplant: metacarpal head transplant.

Russe graft: a bone graft procedure to a scaphoid nonunion; used to stimulate union of a nonunited fracture.

distal finger amputation revision: procedure performed following traumatic amputation involving the distal phalanx (fingertip) by the following techniques.

fingertip flaps: to preserve sensation.

Kutler: lateral double V-Y advancement.

Atosoy: volar single V-Y advancement.

Wolfe-graft: (free skin [pinch] graft): a section of full-thickness skin placed on the open area.

cross-finger flap: a section of skin with its blood supply intact from a neighboring finger used to cover open area.

thenar flap: one raised from the thumb side of the base of the palm.

pedicle flap: a procedure that will permit an island of skin and subcutaneous tissue to be transferred from one place to another on its own vascular supply, using multiple operative stages.

pedicle grafts: a term used for pedicle flaps but also includes *pedicle bone grafts. Island pedicle grafts and neurovascular pedicle grafts* are pedicle, skin, or subcutaneous tissue containing blood and nerve supply, thus providing sensation for the skin graft.

TENDON SURGERY OF THE HAND

Broadly speaking, there are two types of tendon procedures: (1) restoration of tendon function by direct repair of a tendon, its advancement, or its transfer and (2) freeing of tendon from scar tissue, restrictive bands, or abnormal lining tissues. Because of these basic categories, tendon grafts and advancement procedures are listed here contextually and not in alphabetic order.

tendon advancement: done when the damage segment of a tendon is so near its insertion that a direct tendon-to-bone rather than tendon-to-tendon repair is necessary. One such technique is the *Wagner* advancement of the profundus tendon.

tenodesis: the fixation of a tendon onto two bony locations to keep a joint from flexing or extending beyond a selected range. This procedure lends itself to prevention of hyperextension of the metacarpophalangeal joints in ulnar claw deformity. Two commonly done are the Fowler and Riordan procedures.

tenorrhaphy: the repair of a lacerated tendon, either immediate or delayed.

tendolysis: often called tenolysis; a tendon release. It describes two different types of procedures: (1) one in which the tendon is freed from scar tissue or entrapment so that it may move properly, and (2) tenosynovectomy, whereby all or part of the sheath of a functioning tendon is excised.

Tendon repair

Numerous techniques and types of suture are used in repairing tendons. The specific technique is directed at gaining maximal strength with minimal scarring.

Becker: Multiple cross-stitching technique for approximation of fresh tendon edges.

Bunnell: a double figure 8 suture technique used in approximation of fresh tendon edges.

Kessler: loop system of tendon repair of fresh tendon edges.

Kleinert: modification of Bunnell technique, burying suture knot at tendon edge.

Tsuge: multiple cross-stitching technique for tendon reapproximation.

Verdan: multiple cross-stitching technique for tendon reapproximation.

Tendon grafts and transfers

A tendon transfer is the relocation of a tendon from one place to another. The tendon retains attachment to its muscle. By contrast, free tendon graft requires complete excision of a tendon and its repositioning in a new location. Tendon transfers may be static or dynamic.

static tendon transfer: transfer of a free tendon graft that is attached to two or more bony locations such that the active movement of one joint will cause the passive movement of some other joint. For example, a tendon appropriately inserted proximal to the wrist and in the fingers will cause flexion of the fingers if the wrist is extended.

dynamic tendon transfer: one that brings about motion by direct action of muscle contraction.

Tendon transfers are commonly required to replace or assist voluntary muscle function that is lost because of nerve injury, nerve disease, or direct and indirect sequelae of trauma to the muscle. Substantial numbers of transfers are used in central nervous system paralyses such as those caused by strokes and polio. Transfers are listed by categories that define function.

opponensplasty: for thumb opposition (pulling the thumb across the hand); Brand, Burkhalter, Groves, Goldner, Riordan, Phalen-Miller, Littler, Huber, and Fowler procedures.

thumb adduction: pulling the thumb to side of index finger; Boyes technique, Bunnell, Edgarton-Grand, and Royle-Thompson procedures.

thumb abduction: pulling thumb away from hand; Boyes technique.

finger extension: Boyes technique.

finger flexion: for flexion of the metacarpophalangeal joint (intrinsic transfer); Boyes, Fowler, Bunnell, Stiles-Bunnell, Riordan, and Pulver-Taft techniques, and Brand I and Brand II.

wrist extension: Boyes technique, using pronator teres to the extensor carpi radialis brevis muscle.

Tenosynovectomy

Tenosynovectomy refers to the excision of thickened tendon sheath and other tissue surrounding a tendon, commonly seen in infection, chemical irritation, and rheumatoid arthritis (synovectomy). It also refers to the following two procedures in hand surgery:

trigger finger release: a release of fibrous covering of tendon (pulley) at the base of the finger to prevent a tendon with nodular changes from snapping with motion of the finger. Also called snapping tendon release.

abductor pollicis longus release: a release of the fibrous canal surrounding the abductor pollicis longus at the wrist for symptoms of de Quervain syndrome (pain on abduction of the thumb). Also called de Quervain release.

Other tendon procedures

Boutonniere repair: a procedure designed to relieve the deformity of flexion at the proximal interphalangeal joints and hyperextension at the distal interphalangeal joints of the finger; Littler, Matev, and Fowler procedures.

Hunter rod: a long silicone tube implanted to allow the soft tissue to form a sheath around it. The rod is later removed, and a free tendon graft is inserted through the canal.

Kortzeborn procedure: this is a lengthening of the extensor tendons of the thumb and formation of a fascial attachment of the thumb to the ulnar side of the hand to relieve "ape hand" deformity.

swan-neck revision: surgery designed to eliminate a swan-neck deformity in the fingers by revision of tendons; Swanson revision, Littler modified tendon revision.

Other hand procedures

capsular release (capsulectomy): an incision of a joint capsule done to regain lost motion caused by contractures.

capsulodesis: in hand surgery the capsule, which may include the volar plate, may be tightened to help hold an affected joint in a position that can no longer be held voluntarily. This is done often for nerve injuries and is commonly called the Zancolli procedure (for clawhand deformity).

carpal tunnel release: a division of the strong ligamentous band (transverse carpal ligament) that covers the median nerve and flexor tendons of the finger and thumb. This is usually done to relieve pressure on the median nerve that may result from arthritis, trauma, or unknown causes. A *tenosynovectomy,* if necessary, may be done through the same incision.

carpectomy: the removal of the proximal row of carpal bones, usually indicated in some forms of arthritis or severe spastic contractures.

dermodesis: the removal of a segment of skin and then closure of the skin margins to shorten skin and restrict motion of a joint. It is frequently done in conjunction with a Zancolli capsulodesis for ulnar clawhand.

Dupuytren contracture release: named after a French surgeon, this surgical procedure is the excision of the contracted fibrotic bands of the palmar fascia. However, the skin is often adherent and recurrent deformity is a problem.

Specific techniques for resection of these bands are:

Luck procedure: percutaneous transection of fibrotic bands without removal of tissue.

McCash procedure: transverse skin incision with transection of bands and then passive stretch dressing applied, leaving the wounds open.

ganglionectomy: the excision of a ganglion, which usually occurs on the dorsum of the wrist or the base of the fingers.

K-wire fixation: in a Kirschner wire (K-wire) fixation small threaded or nonthreaded wires are used to transfix fractures or to produce traction with the use of an external appliance.

Krukenberg procedure: in the congenital absence of a hand the radius and ulna are surgically separated and covered with soft tissue so that the two bones will act as a claw.

mallet finger revision: designed to regain active extension of the distal interphalangeal joints of the finger.

Fowler release: technique used at the proximal interphalangeal joint for a mallet finger.

onychectomy: removal of a fingernail.

onychotomy: the method of cutting into a nail, usually to remove a mass under the nail.

Palmar fasciectomy, fasciotomy: the release, with or without resection of tissues, of shortened, thickened, and contracted fasciae in the palm or finger in flexion deformities resulting from Dupuytren contracture.

phalangectomy: the excision of a part or all of a phalanx because of trauma or arthritis. Rarely performed in the hand, more commonly done in the foot.

pollicization: any operation replacing a congenitally or traumatically missing thumb by reconstruction of the index, long, ring, or little finger such that it acts or functions as a thumb; Buck-Gramko, Riordan, Littler, Gillies, and Verdan procedures.

Ray amputation: a procedure to remove a metacarpal and all phalangeal segments of a finger distal to that metacarpal.

replantation: a microsurgical procedure that requires the reattachment of nerves, veins, and arteries to attempt restoration of function to a freshly severed part such as a finger.

revision polydactyly: polydactyly usually affects the thumb and little finger. Revision requires reattachment of specific tendons or ligaments; Marks and Bayne (thumb).

synovectomy: removal of synovium in joints. The procedure is done frequently for rheumatoid arthritis.

10

The foot

The foot is a fascinating anatomic structure that has a stable base capable of supporting large amounts of weight, and shift in any direction while structural support is still maintained. As weight is systematically shifted from the heel to the ball of the foot, forces increase to as much as 1¼ times the body weight, yet the bony arch still supports this weight. Responsible for this feat are the tarsals, metatarsals, and ligaments, which form a springy arch that gives supporting strength, aided by the dynamic balance of coordinated muscular counterforces. The two-way arch construction of the foot goes lengthwise from heel to toe and crosswise in the ball of the foot.

The orthopaedic surgeon treats many major problems related to the feet—congenital deformities (clubfeet), tendon lengthenings, fusions, and other complicated surgical procedures necessary for foot correction.

The feet are the most used parts of the locomotor system, and therefore subject to injury and abuse. The average person will walk an estimated 20,000 to 460,000 miles in a lifetime and for that reason will at some time seek the expertise of an orthopaedic surgeon or podiatrist. Injuries around the ankle joint receive the most attention and are discussed in Chapter 1.

Problems of the feet are so numerous that treatment and care has become a specialty in itself. The American Orthopaedic Foot Society has been directly responsible for establishing a subspecialty within the specialty of Orthopaedics devoted to the problems of the foot. This subspecialization has grown and is included in many residency programs. In larger institutions, the orthopaedist may work in association with the podiatrist in the care of patients with ankle- and foot-related problems.

Doctors of Podiatric Medicine (podiatrists) are specialists who are graduates of a 4-year doctoral level program and who devote their practice to the diagnosis and treatment of diseases and disorders in the human foot, offering instructions to patients in proper shoe fit and foot care. This may involve conservative management, surgery, biomechanics (prosthetic/orthotics corrections), or for patients with systemic diseases (diabetes) that affect the foot. The patient population consists of podopediatrics (children), podogeriatrics (elderly), podiatric sports medicine, and in general, anyone with foot disabilities.

This chapter discusses the anatomy, diseases, and surgery of the foot as seen by the orthopaedist and podiatrist. Specific terminology of podiatry is included with the general orthopaedic terminology of the foot.

ANATOMY OF THE FOOT
(Figs. 10-1—10-4)

The anatomy of the foot is listed in alphabetical order.

abductor hallucis: short muscle on medial side that pulls the great toe away from other toes and supports medial longitudinal arch.

Achilles tendon (heel cord): the long tendon of the calf composed of the gastrocnemius, soleus, and plantaris muscles and inserting into the calcaneus. Also known as the *triceps surae*.

adductor hallucis: short muscle that attaches to base of great toe, pulls it toward the second toe, and presents splaying of metatarsal bones.

anterior tibial tendon (tibialis anticus): long ten-

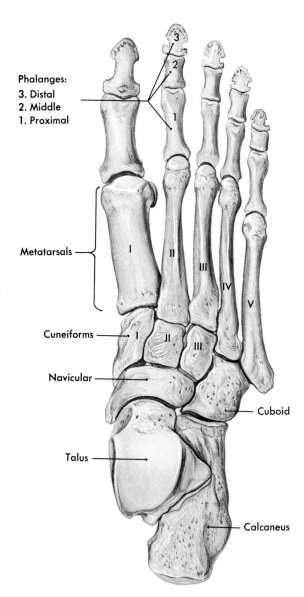

Phalanges:
3. Distal
2. Middle
1. Proximal

Metatarsals

Cuneiforms

Navicular

Talus

Cuboid

Calcaneus

Fig. 10-1. Bones of right foot viewed from above. Tarsal bones consist of cuneiforms, navicular, talus, cuboid, and calcaneus. (From Anthony C and Kolthoff N: Textbook of anatomy and physiology, ed 9, St Louis, 1975, The CV Mosby Co.)

don of anterior leg inserting into the medial cuneiform and first metatarsal; helps to dorsiflex the foot.

calcaneus: the heel bone; largest of the bones of the foot, joins with the talus and cuboid. The combining form is *calcaneo,* for example, calcaneotarsal ligament, calcaneofibular or fibulocalcaneal ligament.

cuboid: cube-shaped bone on the lateral side of the foot, just anterior to the calcaneus and articulating with the base of the fourth and fifth metatarsals.

cuneiforms: three wedge-shaped bones lying just proximal to the first three metatarsals and articulating with the navicular bone. These are called the first, second, and third cuneiforms or medial, lateral, and middle cuneiforms.

deltoid ligament: triangular ligament on the medial side of the ankle, running from the tibia to talus and calcaneous.

digital artery and nerves: terminal arteries and nerves that travel together on the sides of the toes.

dorsalis pedis artery: branch from the anterior tibial artery, going into the dorsum of the foot.

eponychium: the epidermal layer covering the nail root (cuticle).

extensor digitorum longus and brevis: long tendon from limb and short tendon from foot that pull the lesser toes up in dorsiflexion (extension) and stabilizes the lesser metatarsophalangeal joints. There is no brevis tendon to the fifth toe.

extensor hallucis longus and brevis: long tendon from limb and short tendon from foot that pulls the great toe up in dorsiflexion (extension) and stabilizes the first metatarsophalangeal joint.

fat pad: thick fibrous collection of fat on the plantar surface of the foot.

Feiss line: the line that travels from the medial malleolus to plantar aspect of the first metatarsophalangeal joint.

flexor digitorum longus and brevis: long tendinous insertion from the tibia and short muscle from the foot that insert into the distal and middle phalanges and plantarflex the toes and MP joints.

flexor hallucis longus and brevis: long tendon

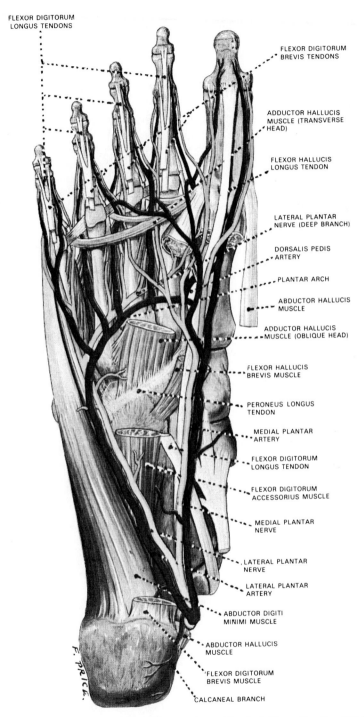

FLEXOR DIGITORUM
LONGUS TENDONS

FLEXOR DIGITORUM
BREVIS TENDONS

ADDUCTOR HALLUCIS
MUSCLE (TRANSVERSE
HEAD)

FLEXOR HALLUCIS
LONGUS TENDON

LATERAL PLANTAR
NERVE (DEEP BRANCH)

DORSALIS PEDIS
ARTERY

PLANTAR ARCH

ABDUCTOR HALLUCIS
MUSCLE

ADDUCTOR HALLUCIS
MUSCLE (OBLIQUE HEAD)

FLEXOR HALLUCIS
BREVIS MUSCLE

PERONEUS LONGUS
TENDON

MEDIAL PLANTAR
ARTERY

FLEXOR DIGITORUM
LONGUS TENDON

FLEXOR DIGITORUM
ACCESSORIUS MUSCLE

MEDIAL PLANTAR
NERVE

LATERAL PLANTAR
NERVE

LATERAL PLANTAR
ARTERY

ABDUCTOR DIGITI
MINIMI MUSCLE

ABDUCTOR HALLUCIS
MUSCLE

FLEXOR DIGITORUM
BREVIS MUSCLE

CALCANEAL BRANCH

F. PRICE.

Fig. 10-2. The arteries and nerves of the plantar surface of the foot. (From Hamilton WJ: Textbook of human anatomy, ed 2, St Louis, 1976, The CV Mosby Co.)

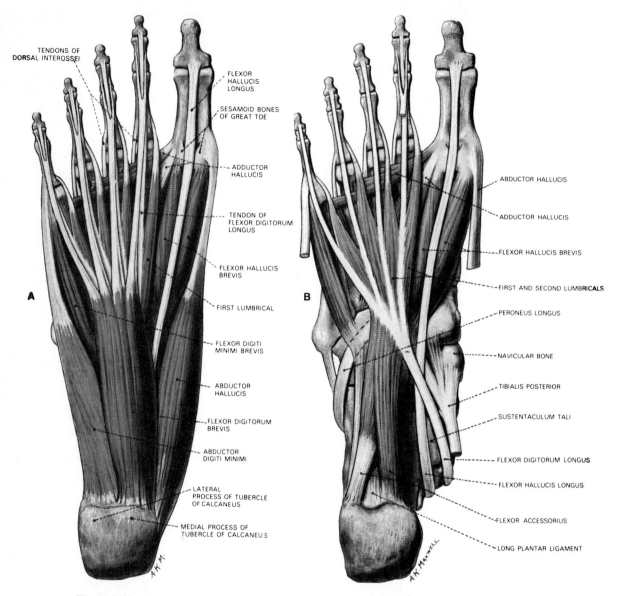

Fig. 10-3. Muscles of sole. **A,** First layer. **B,** Second layer. **C,** Third and fourth layers. (From Hamilton WJ: Textbook of Human Anatomy, ed 2, St Louis, 1976, The CV Mosby Co.)

from fibula and short muscle (flexor digitorum longus) from foot to great toe that acts as flexor of great toe in walking; supports medial longitudinal arch of foot and is important in equilibrium.

hallux: the great toe (*pl.* halluces).

hindfoot: calcaneal and talar portion of the foot (heel bone). Also called rear foot.

hyponychium: the free distal edge of the nail plate.

interossei muscles: group of small muscles be-

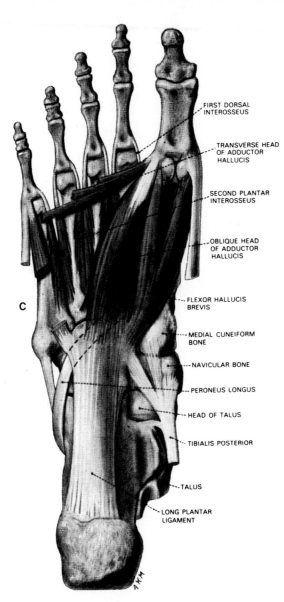

FIRST DORSAL INTEROSSEUS

TRANSVERSE HEAD OF ADDUCTOR HALLUCIS

SECOND PLANTAR INTEROSSEUS

OBLIQUE HEAD OF ADDUCTOR HALLUCIS

FLEXOR HALLUCIS BREVIS

MEDIAL CUNEIFORM BONE

NAVICULAR BONE

PERONEUS LONGUS

HEAD OF TALUS

TIBIALIS POSTERIOR

TALUS

LONG PLANTAR LIGAMENT

C

Fig. 10-3, cont'd. For legend, see opposite page.

tween the metatarsals that extends into the extensor hoods and flexors at the MTP joints.

intrinsic and extrinsic muscles: muscles that originate in the foot and maintain arches.

lateral collateral ligaments: three ligaments that give stability to the lateral aspect of the ankle joint; anterior talofibular ligament, calcaneo fibular ligament, and the posterior talofibular ligament.

lunula: half-moon-shaped (lighter) area at the proximal base of the nail next to the root.

malleolus: the prominence of bones on either side of the ankle. The medial and lateral malleoli come from the tibia and fibula, respectively. The posterior malleolus is deep to the Achilles tendon and is a part of the tibia.

metatarsals: the five long bones of the foot between the tarsals and the phalanges.

Meyer line: in a normal foot a line that passes through the big toe to midpoint of heel.

midtarsal joint: this joint is comprised of the navicular-talar and cuboid-calcaneus articulations and permits adduction-abduction and inversion-eversion motions of the forefoot.

nail bed: skin directly under the nail. Also called the *matrix.*

nail plate: hard portion of epidermis on dorsal side of hallux and phalanges from which the nails grow. Also called the *unguis.*

navicular: tarsal bone on medial side of foot that articulates proximally with head of talus and distally with three cuneiforms. Formerly called the *scaphoid.*

os trigonum: a small bone sometimes found just posterior to the talus and can be easily confused with a fracture of the posterior lateral tubercle of the talus. Also called *Bardeleben's bone.*

peroneal muscles (peroneus longus, brevis, and tertius): tendons arising from the muscles travel posterior to the lateral malleolus and insert into the dorsolateral and plantar aspects of the foot. After crossing the plantar aspect of the foot, the longus inserts into the base of the first metatarsal, the brevis inserts into the base of the fifth metatarsal, and the tertius into the dorsum of the foot about the cuboid.

phalanx: the toe; more specifically, the two distal bones of the great toe and three distal bones of the four small toes. The fifth toe is sometimes

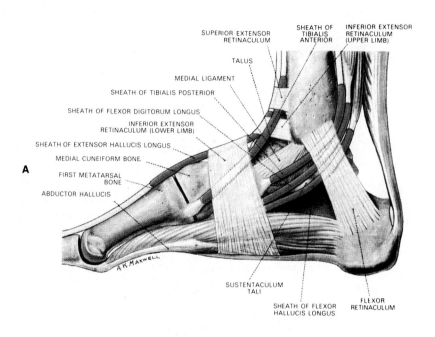

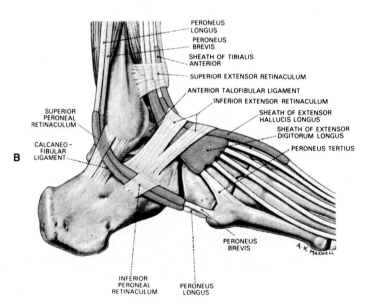

Fig. 10-4. A, Retinacula and synovial sheaths of ankle region, medial view. **B,** Retinacular and synovial sheaths of ankle region, lateral view. (From Hamilton WJ: Textbook of Human Anatomy, ed 2, St Louis, 1976, The CV Mosby Co.)

fused and has two phalanges only (*pl.* phalanges).

plantar fascia: dense fascia of the plantar aspect of foot arising from calcaneus and inserting into base of proximal phalanges. Also called *plantar aponeurosis.*

plantar nerve: terminal portion of posterior tibial nerve that divides into medial and lateral plantar nerves, giving off sensory branches to plantar side of foot and motor branches to intrinsic muscles of foot.

posterior tibial artery, nerve, and vein: travel through a fascial tunnel on the inner ankle (tarsal tunnel) and branch to supply the plantar aspect of the foot and toes.

posterior tibial tendon (tibialis posticus): long tendon from posterior leg passing along medial side of the foot, inserting diffusely into the plantar aspect of the midfoot.

quadratus plantaris: muscle of the plantar arch associated with the flexor digitorum longus.

ray: complex of the metatarsals and phalanges that, on anteroposterior x-ray view, appear as five rays.

sesamoid: two seed-shaped bones in the flexor hallucis brevis tendon located beneath the first metatarsal head, helping to plantarflex (flex) the great toe.

subtalar joint: this joint is comprised of the talarcalcaneus articulation and permits triplane movement of the rearfoot.

talus (astragalus): large bone beneath tibia that helps make up one third of the ankle joint, permitting the foot to go up or down. The talocalcaneal (subtalar joint) below the ankle joint allows the heel to turn in and out. The talonavicular ligaments (spring ligaments) originate from the talus.

tarsi: the seven proximal bones of the foot connecting the tibia and fibula to the five metatarsals. The combining form *tarso* is used often, for example, tarsometatarsal joints and ligaments (*sing.* tarsus).

web space: web of skin between and at the base of each toe.

DISEASES AND CONDITIONS OF THE FOOT

The pathologic and neuromusculoskeletal changes that take place in the foot can be the result of multiple entities. For one, there is stress and strain placed on the feet with overweight, overuse, improper shoe fit, and similar causes. The simple affectations of the foot can relate to dermal abrasions, blisters, ulcers, fissures, bunions, corns, calluses, fungi, and other infections. The more severe problems involve peripheral vascular (ischemia) diseases, metabolic disorders (diabetes, gout), musculoskeletal changes (deformities), and trauma (fractures, dislocations). All of these may cause or contribute to disability and inability to function. Diseases and conditions of the foot are listed alphabetically for reference. Other anatomic involvements are listed in Chapter 2.

accessory navicular: extra bone sometimes found on the medial side of the navicular bone. Also known as an *os navicularis.*

ainhum: condition where there is spontaneous lysis, usually of the fourth or fifth toe but sometimes other toes.

anonychia: absence of toenail(s).

athlete's foot (tinea pedis): fungus infection of skin on the plantar surface of the feet and between the toes and nails caused by one of the dermatophyte species (Trichophyton or Epidermophyton); disease consists of scaling, fissures, maceration, and eroded areas between the toes. Dermatomycosis pedis.

bunion: localized enlargement at the first metatarsal head area either because of malposition of the first metatarsal or because of overgrowth of bone at the first metatarsal head. This deformity may or may not affect the position of the great toe. If the great toe is affected, then one of the following designations would be appropriate:
hallux abductus with bunion
hallux adductus with bunion
hallux abductovalgus with bunion

bunion (dorsal): overgrowth of bone (exostosis) on the dorsal surface of the first metatarsal head or a dorsal malposition of the first metatarsal.

bunionette: similar to the bunion deformity but affecting the fifth metatarsal causing the metatarsal head to be prominent laterally; often referred to as a "tailor's bunion."

bursitis: inflammation of a fluid-filled sac that is normally present around a bony prominence to cushion it.

callosity: hard, thickened skin on the bottom of the foot like a clavus. Also called *tyloma, keratoma, callous (pl. callouses).*

clavus: any corn or hyperkeratotic tissue involving a toe; a reaction of skin to intermittent chronic pressure, producing extra layers of hard skin; caused by restrictive foot wear or by abnormal position or motion of the toes.

clavus (soft): soft skin thickening between the toes, usually between the fourth and fifth toes. Also called *heloma molle, soft corn, clavus mollum.*

claw toes: dorsiflexion of the metatarsophalangeal joints associated with hammertoe deformities and often with a clavus foot.

clubfoot: foot deformity resulting in the appearance of a golf club. The components include forefoot adduction with medial displacement of the talus, ankle equinus, and heel varus. The result is that the foot turns in with the heel pulled medially.

coalitions: a bridge between two bones; may be fibrous (syndesmosis), cartilage (synchondrosis), or bone (synostosis), for example, a calcaneonavicular bar which is a bridge between the calcaneus and navicular bones. Also called *tarsal bars.*

congenital bars: bridging of bone from one tarsal bone to another, with the most common being calcaneonavicular bars.

congenital rocker-bottom flatfoot: condition present at birth; abnormal equinus position of talus with valgus position of the heel, resulting in a foot that looks like a rocker and has a prominence below the medial ankle. Also called *congenital vertical talus, congenital convex pes valgus.*

dorsiflexed metatarsal: a metatarsal that is malpositioned so that its head is higher than the adjacent metatarsal heads, resulting in limitation of motion of the involved metatarsophalangeal joint.

dropfoot: paralysis of the dorsiflexor muscles of the foot causing toes to drag when walking. Also called *footdrop.*

Dupuytren contracture: a contracture of the plantar fascia of the foot; also, a flexion deformity of the toe caused by involvement of the plantar fascia.

equinus: abnormal position of flexion and used in combining form with other words to denote anatomic location; ankle equinus, forefoot equinus, metatarsus equinus.

exostosis: bony growth, protruding from the surface of bone.

foot cramps: an involuntary action involving a muscle-tendon reflex contraction, stretching the tendon, which sends nerve messages to spinal cord, which in turn stimulates the muscle even more, producing a painful cramp. This can be related to abnormal levels of minerals (calcium, potassium, magnesium), a decrease in blood supply to the muscle, a pinched nerve, holding the foot in pronation for a length of time, or a problem with the muscle itself.

forefoot equinus: plantarflexion of the forefoot on the rearfoot, producing a high arch foot with the apex of the deformity at the midtarsal joint.

forefoot valgus: an everted structural position of the forefoot that causes abnormal pronation of the foot.

forefoot varus: an inverted structural position of the forefoot that causes abnormal pronation of the foot.

ganglion: soft tissue mass filled with fluid usually coming from a joint or a tendon sheath.

gastrocnemius equinus: an abnormal tightness of the Achilles tendon that restricts dorsiflexion of the foot in the ankle joint. This can be congenital or acquired.

Haglund deformity: prominent posterosuperior aspect of the calcaneus. Also known as a *retrocalcaneal exostosis* or a "pump bump."

hallux abductus: great toe pointing toward second toe (transverse plane deformity).

hallux adductus: grcat toe pointing toward midline of body (transverse plane deformity).

hallux dolorosa: flatfoot condition resulting in pain of the great toe.

hallux extensus: fixed dorsiflexed position of the great toe.

hallux flexus: fixed flexion position of great toe.

hallux malleus: hammertoe deformity of the great toe; cock-up deformity of the distal interphalangeal joint.

hallux rigidus: painful, stiff metatarsophalangeal joint with limitation of motion and pain on dorsiflexion; caused by arthritic changes.

hallux valgus: great toe pointing toward second toe but rotated in frontal plane so that the nail plate is facing away from second toe.

hallux varus: great toe pointing toward midline of body but rotated in frontal plane so that the nail plate is facing second toe.

hammertoes: descriptive of a variety of deformities of the second to fifth toes; increased flexion of the distal toe, causing prominence of the bones of the dorsal aspect of the proximal interphalangeal joint.

hard corn: a particularly hard, thickened area of skin over the dorsum of the toe. Also called *heloma durum, clavus durum.*

heel spur: an overgrowth of bone at the plantar aspect of the calcaneus.

heloma durum: a hard, thickened area of skin over the dorsum of a toe. Also called *hard corn, clavus.*

ingrown nail: condition of the nail growing into the skin distally. Also called *unguis incarnatus, onychocryptosis.*

intractable plantar keratosis: well-defined callous tissue with a central core located beneath a metatarsal head and usually the result of abnormal pressure from the metatarsal.

macrodactyly: enlargement of a toe or toes.

mallet toes: flexion of the distal joint of the second to fifth toes, such that the toenails are pointing into the ground when walking.

metatarsal cuneiform exostosis: an overgrowth of bone usually involving the dorsal surface of the first metatarsal base and first cuneiform.

metatarsalgia: pain in the plantar aspect of the metatarsal area caused by a variety of disorders.

metatarsus abductus: turning out of the forefoot (metatarsals). Also called m. valgus.

metatarsus adductocavus: forefoot turned inward in association with a high arch, usually seen in clubfoot deformity that includes heel varus (talipes equinovarus).

metatarsus adductus: turning in of the forefoot (metatarsals). Also called m. varus.

metatarsus atavicus: abnormal shortness of the first metatarsal bone.

metatarsus latus: broad foot; widened forefoot.

metatarsus equinus: see equinus.

metatarsus primus varus: refers to wide splaying between first and second metatarsals and can be the cause of a bunion deformity.

Morton foot: short hypermobile first metatarsal. Also called *Morton syndrome.*

Morton neuroma: thickening of the plantar nerve just beyond the metatarsal head in the web spaces; most common between the third and fourth toes, followed by the second and third toes.

onychocryptosis: condition of nail growing into the skin distally. Also called *ingrown nail, unguis incarnatus.*

onychomycosis: fungus infection of the nail plate.

osteochondrosis: disruption of the blood supply to a growth center of a bone.
These have been given eponyms after the men who first reported them:
  Kohler disease: osteochondrosis of the navicular bone.
  Freiberg infraction: osteochondrosis of the metatarsal head.
  Sever disease: osteochondrosis of the calcaneus apophysis.

pachyonychia: thickening of toenails, commonly caused by a fungus or trauma. Also called *onychauxis.*

paronychia: an inflammation surrounding the nail plate.

peroneal spastic flatfoot: overall descriptive term

applied to many flatfeet, including congenital bony bars (bridges).

pes: generally speaking, the term *pes* (foot) is used as a prefix to denote an acquired affection of the foot, for example, pes planus, better known as *flatfoot*. The terms *pes* and *talipes* are generally interchangeable.

pes cavus: high arched foot.

pes planus: lowering of the longitudinal arch; flatfoot. There are two basic categories:

    flexible pes planus: flatfoot with general laxity in which the foot appears normal when not bearing weight but flattens with weight-bearing.

    rigid pes planus: nonflexible flatfoot that is present when not bearing weight and when bearing weight.

plantarflexed metatarsal: a metatarsal that is malpositioned so that its head is lower than the adjacent metatarsal heads, resulting in abnormal pressure, which may produce a plantar callus.

plantar wart: a virus affecting the plantar surface of the foot. Also called *verruca*.

polydactyly: congenital deformity, excess number of toes.

pronation: complex motion of the foot that produces *flattening* of the arch. This motion is normal during gait; however, excessive pronation can lead to pathologic changes of the foot.

rocker-bottom foot: deformity of the foot such that the arch is disrupted and looks like a rocker bottom. This may be a complication of clubfoot treatment or myelomeningocele.

stiff ray: immobility of all joints of any toe or toes.

supination: complex motion of the foot that produces an *increase* in the arch. This motion is normal during gait; however, excessive supination can lead to pathologic changes of the foot.

syndactyly: congenital fusion of two or more toes; may be bony or merely soft tissue.

talipes: generally speaking, the term *talipes*, meaning ankle and foot, is used as a prefix to denote an affection of the foot, for example, talipes equinovarus (clubfoot).

talipes calcaneocavus: high-arched foot with fixed dorsiflexion (pes c.).

talipes calcaneus: abnormally dorsiflexed hind-foot, with increased dorsiflexion of the calcaneus. Also called cavus foot (pes c.).

talipes calcanovalgus: abnormally dorsiflexed hindfoot with turning out of the heel (pes c.).

talipes calcanovarus: abnormally dorsiflexed hindfoot with turning in of the heel (pes c.).

talipes cavovalgus: high arch and turning out of the heel (pes c.).

talipes cavovarus: high arch associated with turning in of the foot (pes c.).

talipes equinovalgus: plantar flexion and turning out of the calcaneus (pes c.).

talipes equinovarus: turning of the heel inward with increased plantar flexion. More precisely, a clubfoot often having the components of talipes equinovarus with metatarsus adductus. This condition can result from disease, causing paralysis, or from unknown causes. Also called *clubfoot* (pes c.).

talipes planovalgus: depression of the longitudinal arch associated with heel valgus. Also called *pes planovalgus* (pes p.).

talipes planus: depression of the longitudinal arch; no specified heel valgus is implied by this term. Also called *pes planus, flatfoot.* A *flexible pes planus* is flatfoot with general laxity but no other specific disease process (pes p.).

SURGERY OF THE FOOT

A list of undefined procedures is given related to the foot. There are many types of procedures available for a single-condition, but not all are listed here; for example, of more than 50 operations for bunions, only a few are described. For easy reference, definitions of specific surgical terms are presented alphabetically.

Bunions

Akin
Austin
bunionectomy
chevron osteotomy
closing abductory wedge osteotomy (CAWO)
Hauser
Keller
Keller with prosthesis
Lapidus

Ludloff
Mayo
McBride
McKeever
Mitchell
opening abductory wedge osteotomy (OAWO)
Reverdin-Green
Silver
Stone
Wilson

Clubfeet (talipes equinovarus)

Barr and Record
Brockman
Dwyer
Garceau
Gelman
Heyman
McCauley
Phelps
Turco

Pes planus (flatfeet and related disorders)

Coleman
Grice
Grice and Green
Hammon
Hark
Harris and Beath
Herndon and Heyman
Hoke
Ingram
Kidner
Lowman
Miller
Osmond-Clarke
subtalar arthroereisis
Vulpius-Compere
White
Young

Achilles tendon lengthenings

Hauser
Vulpius-Compere
White
Z-plasty

Metatarsus varus

Fowler
Heyman
Lange
Peabody

Ingrown nails (onychocryptosis)

avulsion of nail plate
cotting
Frost
Heifetz
matrectomy
phenolization
Rose
Steindler
Suppan
Winograd
Zadik

Toe pathology

digital prosthesis
intermediate phalangectomy
osteotripsy
partial ostectomy
syndactylization
V-Y plasty
Z-plasty

Small toe deformities

Dickson-Diveley
DIP fusion
DuVries condylectomy
Gridlestone-Taylor
McElvenny
PIP fusion
Ruiz-Moro

Footdrop

Campbell
Gill

Surgical terms and definitions relating to the foot

Akin procedure: for bunion deformity, or deformed great toe; an osteotomy of the proximal phalanx of the great toe.

Austin procedure: for bunion deformity, and osteotomy in the form of a chevron made in the distal aspect of the first metatarsal; also referred to as a chevron procedure.

avulsion of nail plate: a nonpermanent removal of the nail plate, either partial or complete, without disrupting the matrix cells that produce the nail plate.

Barr procedure: for paralytic clubfoot; transfer of the posterior tibial tendon to the third cuneiform or metatarsal.

Barr-Record procedure: for clubfeet; subcutaneous plantar fasciotomy and tendon Achilles lengthening (TAL) done as separate procedures, with tibiotalar fusion.

Batchelor-Brown procedure: for flat feet; fusion of the subtalar joint using a fibular bone graft.

Berman and Gartland procedure: for metatarsus adductus; dome-shaped osteotomy of all five proximal metatarsals.

Brahms procedure: for mallet toe; transfer of flexor digitorum profundus to dorsum of proximal phalanx.

Brockman procedure: for clubfoot; a soft tissue release of the medial capsule of the foot as well as a release of the posterior tibial tendon.

bunionectomy: a general class of many different operations that are designed to correct bunion deformity.

Campbell procedure: for dropfoot or talipes equinus of certain origins; creates a posterior bone block to prevent plantar flexion.

chevron osteotomy: for bunion deformity; an osteotomy in the form of a chevron made in the distal first metatarsal.

Chopart amputation: of the forefoot through the talonavicular and calcaneocuboid joint.

closing abductory wedge osteotomy (CAWO): for bunion deformity; proximal metatarsal osteotomy with closure of wedge to bring first metatarsal closer to second metatarsal.

Cole procedure: for cavus foot deformity; an anterior tarsal wedge osteotomy with fusion.

Coleman procedure: for talipes valgus; soft tissue and tendon release associated with a subtalar fusion.

cotting: for ingrown nail; excision of a nail.

cylindrical osteotomy: to shorten long bones; a cylinder of bone is removed.

Dickson-Diveley procedure: for clawing of big toe; the distal interphalangeal joint is fused, and the extensor hallucis longus is transferred to the long flexor.

digital prosthesis: excision of interphalangeal joint with insertion of prosthetic device in that space.

DIP fusion: for mallet toes; removal of the distal interphalangeal joint and then fusion.

dorsal V osteotomy: for plantar callosity; an osteotomy at the neck of a lesser metatarsal to allow the metatarsal to assume a slightly higher position.

dorsal wedge osteotomy: for plantar callosity; an osteotomy at the base of a metatarsal to allow the metatarsal to move to a higher position.

Dunn-Brittain: for paralytic clubfeet; a method of triple arthrodesis excising most of the head of the talus.

Dunn-Brittain triple arthrodesis: removal of entire navicular bone.

DuVries plantar condylectomy: for plantar callosities; resection of plantar condyles from the lesser metatarsals.

Dwyer procedure: lateral closing wedge osteotomy of the calcaneus; associated with soft tissue release for clubfeet and other disorders.

Emslie-Cholmely procedure: double wedge osteotomy for certain high-arched feet.

Essex-Lopresti procedure: for fractured calcaneus; use of a Steinmann pin or other metal pin to help achieve and hold fracture reduction.

Evans procedure: for severe flatfoot deformity; osteotomy of the calcaneus.

exostectomy: removal of any excess prominences of bone.

Farmer procedure: for hallux varus; soft tissue repair with the use of a skin flap.

Fowler procedure: for metatarsus varus with severe cavus deformity; plantar fascia and muscle release associated with an opening wedge osteotomy of the first cuneiform.

Fried and Green procedure: for paralysis of posterior tibial muscle; transfer of the peroneus longus, or flexor digitorum longus, or flexor hallucis longus, or extensor hallucis longus to posterior tibial tendon.

Frost procedure: for ingrown nail; a skin flap is made over the lateral nail bed, with removal of the nail and bed followed by closure of flap.

Gallis procedure: for malunion calcaneus; subtalar arthrodesis using a tibial bone graft.

Garceau procedure: for clubfeet; anterior tibial tendon transfer.

Garceau-Brahms procedure: for paralytic clubfeet; transection of the motor branches of the plantar nerve.

Gelman procedure: for clubfeet; identical to the McCauley procedure, except that the inferior calcaneonavicular ligament is not incised.

Giannestras procedure: for plantar callosity; proximal shortening of metatarsal.

Gill procedure: for dropfoot; wedge of bone taken from the superoposterior calcaneus with insertion of that block into the posterior tibiotalar joint.

Girdlestone-Taylor procedure: for claw toes; transfer of the long flexors of the involved toe to the extensor hood mechanism.

Grice procedure: for congenital talipes valgus; a soft tissue medial and lateral foot release procedure.

Grice-Green procedure: for talipes valgus; tibial bone graft to subtalar joint; for paralysis of gastrocsoleus; transfer of peroneus longus, peroneus brevis, and posterior tibial tendon.

Hammon procedure: first metatarsal osteotomy and bone graft for a dorsal bunion.

Hark procedure: for congenital talipes valgus; multiple extensor and flexor Z-tendon lengthenings with bony repositioning.

Harris-Beath procedure: for flatfeet; talonavicular and subtalar arthrodesis.

Hauser procedure: for bunion deformity; excision of the medial exostosis and transfer of the adductor tendon from the proximal phalanx to the distal metatarsal.

Hauser procedure: for tight heel cord; division of proximal posterior and distal medial two thirds of the Achilles tendon.

Heifetz procedure: for ingrown nail; excision of affected ingrown side of nail and nail bed.

Herndon-Heyman procedure: for congenital talipes valgus; medial and lateral foot release with tendon lengthening.

Heyman procedure: for clubfeet; soft tissue release for clubfoot, including deltoid ligament.

Hibbs procedure: for claw toes and cavus feet; plantar fascia release with transfer of the extensor digitorum longus to the third cuneiform.

Hoke procedure: triple arthrodesis done with reshaping of the head of the talus.

Hoke procedure: for flatfeet; navicular bone and two medial cuneiforms are fused.

Ingram procedure: for congenital talipes valgus; Z-plasty lengthening of peroneus brevis tendon, medial release, reduction of navicular bone, and anterior tibial tendon transfer.

intermediate phalangectomy: for hammertoe deformity; excision of the middle phalanx.

Japas procedure: for high-arched feet; a combination of plantar fascia release and dorsal wedge osteotomy of the tarsal bones.

Jones procedure: for cock-up deformity of great toe and other problems; transfer of the extensor hallucis longus to the distal first metatarsal; currently done with a distal interphalangeal joint fusion.

Juvara procedure: for a bunion deformity; an oblique osteotomy at the proximal portion of the metatarsal to correct an abnormal transverse and/or sagittal plane deformity.

Keller procedure: for hallux rigidus or bunion; resection of the proximal phalanx of the great toe.

Kendrick procedure: for metatarsus adductus; soft tissue release for all tarsal metatarsal joints.

Kidner procedure: for an accessory navicular bone; removal of the accessory navicular bone with or without transfer of the posterior tibial tendon under the navicular bone.

Kiehn-Earle-DesPrez procedure: for plantar ulcer; closure of ulcer and transfer of extensor digitorum longus to distal metatarsal shaft.

Lambrinudi procedure: a triple arthrodesis done

by resection of the head and inferior portion of the talus.

Lange procedure: for metatarsus varus; simple oblique osteotomy of the second, third, and fourth metatarsals; lateral closing wedge osteotomy of the first metatarsal at the base.

Lapidus procedure: for bunion correction; a closing wedge and fusion at the junction of the first metatarsal and cuneiform bone.

Liebolt: for paralytic equinus foot; a two-stage procedure involving a Hoke triple arthrodesis followed by an ankle fusion.

Lisfranc amputation: amputation through the tarsometatarsal joint.

Lloyd-Roberts procedure: for clubfoot deformity in early childhood; soft tissue release.

Lowman procedure: for flatfeet; transfer of the anterior tibialis with navicular cuneiform fusion.

Ludloff procedure: for hallux valgus; oblique osteotomy of the first metatarsal.

mallerotomy: incision into the ankle by elevation of the lateral malleoli for exploration or as part of a fracture reduction.

matricectomy: for toenail deformity or chronic disease; excision of all or a part of the nail plate (matrix) to eliminate growth of the nail.

Mayo procedure: resection of the distal first metatarsal for bunion deformity.

McBride procedure: excision of the medial exostosis, medial capsular reefing, sesamoidectomy, and transfer of the adductor hallucis tendon into the distal first metatarsal.

McCauley procedure: very extensive medial release of multiple joint capsules, tendon sheaths, abductor hallucis, and, if needed, posterior capsulotomy later.

McElvenny procedure: excision of a plantar nerve neuroma.

McElvenny procedure: for hallux varus; lateral capsular reefing procedure associated with use of the extensor hallucis brevis tendon for repair.

McKeever procedure: for hallux valgus or rigidus; fusion of the first metatarsophalangeal joint.

McReynolds procedure: for fractured calcaneus; open reduction and fixation with staples.

Miller procedure: for severe flatfoot deformity; navicular-cuneiform fusion.

Mitchell procedure: a distal metatarsal osteotomy for bunion deformity; breaking and shifting of metatarsal with excision of exostosis and medial capsular reefing.

neurectomy: excision of a neuroma anywhere in the body; but in the foot, excision of an interdigital neuroma between the second and third or third and fourth toes.

Ober procedure: for paralytic clubfeet; a method of transfer of the posterior tibial tendon to the third cuneiform or metatarsal.

onychotomy: incision into the nail bed.

opening abductory wedge osteotomy (OAWO): for bunion deformity; osteotomy of the first metatarsal base with use of bone graft to open the wedge and bring the first metatarsal closer to the second.

opening wedge osteotomy: for bunion deformity; in orthopaedics, a variety of procedures with or without tendon transfers, with proximal cut in the metatarsal and reduction of the deformity.

Osmone-Clarke procedure: for talipes valgus; soft tissue release of the medial and lateral foot with peroneous brevis tendon transfer.

osteotripsy: for callosities; may be any percutaneous reduction of a bony prominence.

panmetatarsal head resection: usually for severe arthritic deformity, resection of all of the metatarsal heads.

pantalar fusion: for instability of the hindfoot; fusion of the tibiotalar, subtalar, calcaneocuboid, and talonavicular joints.

partial ostectomy: to relieve pressure on the skin; removal of bony prominence.

Peabody procedure: for metatarsus varus; resection of the proximal portion of the second, third, and fourth metatarsals, with osteotomy of the fifth and capsular release of the first metatarsals.

Peabody procedure: for paralysis of gastrocsoleus complex; transfer of anterior tibial tendon to the calcaneus.

phenolization: for nail deformity in which a permanent elimination of a part or entire nail plate is desired. Phenol is applied to the nail matrix after the nail plate is removed in order to destroy any further nail growth.

PIP fusion: operation commonly done for claw toes or hammertoes; removal of the proximal interphalangeal joint and then fusion.

Reverdin-Green procedure: for bunion deformity; an osteotomy of the first metatarsal head.

Rose procedure: for ingrown nail; removal of the ellipse of soft tissue to ingrown portion of nail.

Ruiz-Moro procedure: proximal phalangectomy of the fifth toe for cock-up deformity.

Siffert-Foster-Nachamie procedure: for paralytic clubfeet; triple arthrodesis.

Silver procedure: simple excision of medial exostosis for bunion deformity.

Steindler matricectomy: for nail deformity; removal of a part of the nail matrix to eliminate one border of the nail plate.

Steindler procedure: plantar release of the proximal muscles and fascia of the foot for high-arched feet.

step dowm osteotomy: for abnormally long lesser metatarsal; an osteotomy to shorten the bone.

Stone procedure: for hallux rigidis; resection of the dorsal first metatarsal exostosis.

subtalar arthrodesis: for arthritis and other conditions of the talocalcaneal joint; fusion of the talus to the calcaneus.

subtalar arthroereisis: for severe flatfoot with calcaneal valgus; insertion of an inert spacer into the subtalar joint.

Suppan procedure: for nail deformity; this is a name applied to a variety of procedures to eliminate all or a part of the nail matrix.

syndactylization: soft tissue fusion of two toes in case of clavus or for other reasons.

TAL (tendon Achilles lengthening): a variety of procedures used to lengthen a tight or spastic Achilles tendon.

talectomy: excision of the talus for severe soft tissue contractures.

Thomas procedure: for malunion calcaneus; subtalar arthrodesis using an iliac crest graft.

transmetatarsal amputation: an amputation through the midportion of the metatarsals.

triple arthrodesis: for flail hindfoot and other deformities caused by arthritis. Procedure involves fusion of the calcaneus to the cuboid, navicula to the talus, and talus to the calcaneus.

Turco procedure: for clubfeet; soft tissue release of the posteromedial capsule as well as Achilles tendon lengthening.

V-Y plasty: for claw toes, transection of skin in V-shaped incision with closure in the shape of a Y.

Whitman talectomy procedure: talectomy for calcaneovalgus foot.

Whitman-Thompson procedure: for talipes calcaneus or talipes calcaneovalgus; complete excision of the talus.

Wilson procedure: for bunion deformity; an oblique osteotomy of the first metatarsal neck area.

Winograd procedure: for an ingrown nail; excision of an ingrown portion of toenail, with curettement of the nail bed.

Wolf procedure: for plantar callosity; proximal shortening of the metatarsal.

Young procedure: anterior tibialis transfer for flatfoot.

Z-plasty: for tight heel cord; complete Z-shaped cut requiring suturing of Achilles tendon.

Zadik procedure: for ingrown nail; excision of the entire nail.

11

Physical medicine and rehabilitation: physical therapy and occupational therapy

I. PHYSICAL THERAPY*

Physical medicine and rehabilitation (PM&R) is a medical specialty that is based on the fundamentals of neuromuscular physiology, exercise physiology, and functional anatomy. Typical diagnostic procedures utilized are electromyography and nerve conduction studies.

The *physiatrist* is the physician specialist in PM&R certified by the American Board of Physical Medicine and Rehabilitation after completing a residency and other requirements. In some distinct centers for rehabilitation, a physiatrist is the medical director of the unit. However, some units are organized on a programmatic basis, and have a group of other medical specialists overseeing individual programs; for example, a rheumatologist with the arthritis program, a neurologist with the neuromuscular disease program, and an orthopaedist with the musculoskeletal program.

The *physical therapist* is a health care professional who has completed an entry-level education program accredited by the Commission on Accreditation in Physical Therapy Education. For the advanced clinician, the American Board of Physical Therapy Specialties grants certification to those candidates who have achieved advanced clinical competence and successfully completed a

standardized examination process. Board Certified Specialty areas are: cardiopulmonary physical therapy, neurologic physical therapy, clinical electrophysiologic physical therapy, orthopaedic physical therapy, pediatric physical therapy, and sports physical therapy. The practice of physical therapy is regulated by statute in all 50 states, the District of Columbia, and Puerto Rico. Foreign-trained physical therapists may obtain licenses statutes by providing evidence of educational equivalency and meeting the state's examination requirements.

The remaining members of the rehabilitation team will usually include the occupational therapist, speech therapist, rehab nurse, social worker, and psychologist. Additional members might include a vocational counselor, special educator, prosthetist/orthotist, and numerous medical specialists. Other members of the in-house team include the *Physical Therapist Assistant*, a skilled technical health worker who, under the supervision of a physical therapist, assists in the patient's treatment program. The work of the assistant is regulated either by licensure, certification, or registration in 34 states and Puerto Rico. The assistant may provide the specific elements of a treatment program as delegated by the physical therapist, following the therapist's evaluation, goal, and treatment program development. Some typical activities the assistant might participate in are ambulation training, whirlpool, repetitive exercise programs, teaching safe body mechanics, and activities of

---

*Contributed in part by Patricia Helm-Williams, P.T., M.A., Associate Director, Department of Practice, American Physical Therapy Association, 1111 North Fairfax Street, Alexandria, VA 22314.

daily living. The *physical therapy aide* is an individual who is trained on the job to assist in the physical therapy department, rendering such services as transporting patients, preparing and maintaining treatment areas and equipment, stocking linen, and clerical tasks.

The goal of the rehabilitation team is to enhance each patient's physical capabilities utilizing the team's individual professional skills, expertise, and knowledge to evaluate, plan, and implement treatment interventions tailored to the needs of the patient. In this patient-centered approach, the patient and/or family participates in setting realistic goals to be achieved during the rehabilitation process.

Physical therapist services provide identification, prevention, remediation, and rehabilitation of patients with acute or prolonged physical dysfunction. Such intervention encompasses examination and analysis, therapeutic application of physical and chemical agents, exercises, and education to promote functional independence.

In association with orthopaedic surgery, the rehabilitation team works closely with and is considered an integral part of the orthopaedic rehabilitation program. The physical therapist consults with the orthopaedist and other primary care physicians in the evaluation and treatment of clients with congenital or acquired developmental disabilities, making recommendations for treatment. Services are provided for preoperative and postoperative care of the surgical patient after restorative surgery, trauma, or correction of congenital anomalies. In addition, treatments include the prevention of pulmonary complications after surgery. Strengthening and range of motion exercises are designed for patients with sports-related injuries such as ligamentous tears and bone fractures. Amputees fitted with prostheses are instructed in their use and maintenance. The spinal cord injured patient is given muscle strengthening exercises. In the cases of musculoskeletal injuries, instructions and training in ambulation are taught and may be continued at home, sometimes with the aid of a family member, to whom the principles must also be taught. Physical therapy treatments may include the evaluation and treatment of abnormal

gait patterns resulting from pathologic conditions, such as muscle weakness, paralysis, or biomechanical defects. There are many conditions for which the rehabilitation team is prepared to offer assistance. Patients are referred for rehabilitative services due to neuromusculoskeletal diseases, such as arthritis, stroke, spinal cord injuries, and in the treatment of temporomandibular joint syndrome (TMJ) and chronic pain. The goal is to decrease pain and increase function. This specialty is not only involved in the treatment protocol but in teaching and educating patients in continued rehabilitation.

Physical therapy services

Physical therapists practice in a variety of settings to include acute care hospitals, rehabilitation centers, skilled nursing facilities, convalescent homes, home health, schools, industry, sports clinics, pediatric facilities, or may set up a private practice to provide physical therapy services.

The following is a quick reference to typical services (though not inclusive) that are routinely provided by the physical therapist.

Evaluation-general

Strength
Functional ability
Range of motion
Cognitive level
Coordination
Sensation
Ambulatory status

Evaluation-specific

Manual muscle testing
Cardiopulmonary function
Electroneurophysiologic
Neurodevelopmental
Isokinetic
Limb girth
Gait
Posture
Muscle tone
Wound
Neonatal

Treatment techniques

Therapeutic exercise
  Passive
  Active assistive
  Active
  Resistive (isometric, isotonic, concentric, eccentric, isokinetic)
Specific techniques
  Proprioceptive neuromuscular facilitation (PNF)
  Bobath (neurodevelopmental)
  Rood
  Brunstrom
Muscle reeducation
  Brushing
  Icing
  Tapping
  Quick stretch
  Neurodevelopmental training
Mobility
  Bed (bedbound patient)
  Transfer techniques
  Wheelchair mobility and safety
  Ambulation, parallel bars, walker, crutches, cane, prosthetic, orthotic
Hydrotherapy
  Cold/ice
  Heat (moist)
  Whirlpool (for increasing circulation, decreasing pain, debriding open wounds)
  Therapy pool (for gravity-free exercise and ambulation)
  Paraffin
Physical agents
  Electrodiagnostic test (EMG, nerve conduction velocity studies)
  Electrical stimulation
  Functional electrical stimulation (FES)
  Diathermy
  TENS (Transcutaneous electrical nerve stimulation)
  Ultrasound
  Infrared
  Ultraviolet
Mobilization
  Soft tissue
  Joint
Cardiac care

Cardiac rehabilitation
Cardiac stress testing
Pulmonary
  Bronchial drainage
  Breathing exercises
Pediatric
  Neurodevelopmental
  Scoliosis care (education and exercise, pre- and postoperative care)
  Musculoskeletal
Intermittent Compression (edema control, postmastectomy, etc.)
Traction
  Cervical
  Pelvic
Patient education (an essential element of most treatment plans)

Consultation services

Consultative services are available for clients with special or extraordinary needs that require the recommendations of a multidisciplinary group.

Physical therapy treatments

cervical traction: a means of separating the cervical vertebrae 1 to 2 mm to help relieve painful neck conditions or cervical radiculopathies; may be intermittent or continuous.

contrast baths: alternately exposing affected limb to warm and cool water or specified periods. This is a means of reducing swelling, diminishing pain, and improving joint range of motion.

diathermy: electromagnetic waves with a specific wavelength (shortwave diathermy, microwave diathermy) used as a means of producing heat deep inside tissues.

hot packs: silicone gel, clay, or other material in bags that can be heated to provide superficial heat for tissues.

hydrotherapy treatments: as commonly used today, immersion of affected limbs (sometimes including the trunk) in a tank of water at a specified temperature. The water may be moving (whirlpool), which is one means of debriding tissue. There are also tanks in which a patient may sit (Lo-Boy) and in which he may be almost totally immersed (Hubbard tank). In a pool the buoyancy of water can assist patients with partially paralyzed legs to walk.

infrared treatment: use of "heat lamp," which is an infrared light that heats the superficial tissues, resulting in reflexive deep vessel dilation; used in treating muscle injuries or tight muscles.

intermittent compression: a book or sleeve that is fitted to the leg or arm and alternately pressurized with air and then deflated; this provides a pumping action that is used to reduce disabling edema. It is often prescribed after radical surgery for breast cancer.

paraffin bath: a combination of wax and mineral oil at 126° F used as a means of heating the hands and feet. It may be applied by dip-immersion technique or dip-and-wrap technique.

pelvic traction: application of pelvic belt with caudad pull, which may be continuous or use greater force intermittently; can be done in the hospital or at home.

phonophoresis: technique that uses ultrasound to drive a medication, dissolved or suspended in a coupling fluid, through the skin into underlying tissues.

ultrasound: normally used for its deep-heating effects, which are externally applied through a water-based electric coupling agent but may also be applied on the limb to be treated and the apparatus immersed in water. Athletic injuries, such as contusions, pulled muscles, and tendinitis, are often treated with this modality.

Physical therapy exercises

range of motion (ROM) exercises: designed to maintain or increase the amount of movement in a joint. They may be one of the following.

passive: force is applied to bring about motion in a joint or joints by either a therapist or the patient, without any muscle function in these joints.

active-assistive: exercise performed by the patient but requiring assistance from a therapist, another extremity, or a mechanical device because of muscle weakness or pain.

active: exercise performed by patient without assistance or resistance; the therapist is only an instructor-observer.

DeLorme exercises: originally established on the basis of the 10 repetition maximum (RM), which is the maximal amount of resistance a muscle can lift through full ROM exercises 10 times; the term is frequently interchanged with progressive resistive exercises (PRE), which are designed to build strength and increase endurance through graduated resistance for a prescribed number of repetitions.

isometric exercises: muscle contraction without joint movement in which the resistance may be provided by a fixed object (wall, stabilized bar) or the antagonistic muscle group (flexors versus extensors); a muscle strengthening exercise without causing muscle to work through its range of motion.

isotonic exercises: muscle contraction with movement of the joint through a specified ROM against a fixed amount of resistance.

eccentric lengthening exercises: strengthening exercises in which the external force overcomes the actively contracting muscle, forcing the muscle to lengthen.

isokinetic exercises: strengthening exercises requiring special equipment in which there is an accommodating resistance, resulting in a maximal force against the contracting muscle throughout its full ROM.

aerobic exercises: exercises in which oxygen consumption is inhaled at a rate sufficient for a continuous process of energy production for muscle contraction; the goal is to increase endurance required for long-distance running or after cardiac complications.

anaerobic exercises: exercises in which the expenditure of energy is at a faster rate than that for which the cardiorespiratory mechanism can provide, the goal being to exert the maximal amount of force or energy in a short amount of time, as in a 50-yard dash.

Codman exercises: exercises for a stiff shoulder in which the patient is bent over at the waist (90 degrees) and the hand hangs like a pendulum toward the floor. A weight may be placed in the hand and the arm is then moved through various arcs to increase the ROM in that shoulder.

gait training: the use of parallel bars, crutches, walkers, and canes with specific instructions to the patient. Weight-bearing may be described as non-weight-bearing (NWB), partial weight-bearing (PWB), or full weight-bearing (FWB). Ambulation with crutches is often described as three-point gait, and with walker, four-point gait.

pulley exercises: a rope on pulley system used to increase ROM of a joint or strengthen muscles; resistance can be applied by another limb or by weights.

resistive exercise table: commonly used for lower extremity problems, such as after knee surgery; resistance can be applied by weights ("NK" table in some locales) or by a graded hydraulic system.

Williams flexion exercises: for patients with lower back pain; designed to enhance flexion of the spine, avoid extension of the spine, and strengthen the abdominal muscles.

Physical testing*

Given that the circulation is intact, the major parameters in assessing the function of a limb are range of motion, sensation, and strength. These can be tested directly by the application of forces to the muscle and stimuli to the skin or can be assessed indirectly by electrodiagnostic modalities such as electromyography. In muscle testing, strength is graded by the following scale as assessed directly by the examiner. Range of motion (ROM) is measured with a goniometer, an instrument that measures joint motion in degrees.

Key to manual muscle evaluation†

100% 5 N Normal: Complete ROM against gravity with full resistance

75% 4 G Good: Complete ROM against gravity with some resistance

50% 3 F Fair: Complete ROM against gravity

25% 2 P Poor: Complete ROM with gravity eliminated

10% 1 T Trace: Evidence of contractility

0　0 0 Zero: No evidence of contractility

S　　　　Spasm ⎱ If spasm or contracture ex-
C　　Contracture ⎰ ists, place S or C after the grade of a movement incomplete for this reason

dynamometer: any instrument used to measure strength. One example is a handgrip dynamometer that can be adjusted to test strength in different positions of grasp, recording directly from a pressure gauge.

Cybex: an isokinetic apparatus that can be used to test and record the maximal strength of a muscle as it acts on a joint through a full range of motion. The recording is used to evaluate the progress of a patient's condition during recovery or to confirm the existence and extent of injury. There are several machines available for use in muscle strengthening programs, such as *Orthotron, Kinetron*, and the *Nautilus*.

Sensory testing includes a variety of sensations.

heat and cold testing: self-explanatory.

interferential current: application of two medium frequency alternating currents that interfere with each other. Used for pain control and muscle stimulation.

pinprick test: a gross test to check two variables: (1) the actual ability to feel a pinprick and (2) the ability to determine the difference between sharp and dull.

pressure testing: involves sensation produced by touch to a localized area using an instrument that indicates the pressure needed to produce sensation.

proprioceptive testing: tests the ability to sense the position of a body part with the eyes closed.

tendon reflex examination: graded from 0 to 4 and varies widely in meaning from examiner to examiner; the test is performed by strik-

---

*For more specific information on various tests and examinations, an excellent source is American Orthopaedic Association: Manual of orthopaedic surgery, ed. 6, Chicago, 1985, The Association.

†From Daniels, L., and Worthingham, C: Muscle testing: techniques of manual examination by comparison, ed. 3, Philadelphia, 1972, WB Saunders Co.

ing the tendon briskly and watching muscle reaction.

transcutaneous electrical nerve stimulation (TENS): the introduction of low-voltage, pulsed, direct current into tissue to reduce pain. The units are portable and carried on patient's belt.

two-point discrimination: ability to perceive difference between one or two points of touch at the fingertips or elsewhere; this test of fine sensation is measured in centimeters or millimeters.

vibratory sense examination: tests the patient's ability to feel vibrations with use of a tuning fork.

electromyography (EMG): an electrodiagnostic test conducted on a special machine that evaluates the capability of nerves and muscles to transmit and respond to normal or stimulated electric impulses. The muscle is evaluated by direct insertion of a small needle to which the muscle responds with characteristic contractile activity, which is referred to as "insertional activity." Once the muscle has acclimated to the presence of the needle, individual muscle fiber activity can be seen electrically on an *oscilloscope* and is described by the specific wave patterns. Disorders affecting the nerves, such as a herniated disk, will eventually cause changes in the wave pattern of the muscle. Other disorders commonly evaluated with this study include entrapment syndromes and other neuropathic and muscle disorders. *Conduction time* is the measurement of nerve stimulation applied through the skin, allowing the nerve to transmit impulses. The conduction time is increased in neurologic disorders, such as vitamin B_1 deficiency and carpal tunnel syndrome caused by local nerve pressure.

nerve conduction test: often performed with the EMG, this is a test of the integrity of peripheral nerve(s) that involves placing an electric stimulator over the nerve and measuring the time required for an impulse to travel over a segment of nerve; useful in the diagnosis of nerve entrapment syndrome and polyneuropathies.

II. OCCUPATIONAL THERAPY*

Occupational therapy is the specialty concerned with the rehabilitation of individuals who are limited by physical injury or illness, psychosocial dysfunction, developmental or learning disabilities, poverty or cultural differences, or the aging process. Occupational therapists work to maximize independence, prevent disability, and maintain health through a process of screening, evaluation, treatment, and consultation. Services are provided individually or in groups by two types of practitioners.

The registered occupational therapist (OTR) is a professional who possesses unique skills and credentials, has been educated in a baccalaureate or master's curriculum accredited jointly by the Committee on Allied Health Education, American Medical Association, and the American Occupational Therapy Association (AOTA), and has passed the national certification examination of the American Occupational Therapy Certification Board (AOTCB) and holds current registration with that body. A certified occupational therapy assistant (COTA) has satisfactorily completed an occupational therapy assistant curriculum approved by AOTA, has passed a national certification examination, holds current certification with the AOTCB, and works under the supervision of an OTR. Graduate programs for OTRs prepare the therapist for the role of specialized practitioner, educator, or researcher. Most U.S. jurisdictions regulate Occupational Therapy, the majority through licensure laws.

Specific occupational therapist services

Specific occupational therapist services include but are not limited to the following:

- Education and training in activities of daily living (ADL).

---

*Prepared by Barbara E. Joe, M.A., Quality Assurance Specialist and Carol H. Gwin, Assistant Director, Practice Division, American Occupational Therapy Association, 1383 Piccard Drive, Rockville, MD 20850-4375.

- Administering and interpreting such tests as manual muscle and range of motion.
- Design, fabrication, and application of slings and orthoses
- Developing perceptual-motor skills and sensory integrative functioning.
- Restoration of hand functioning.
- Instruction in work simplification, energy conservation, and use of proper body mechanics during activity for work, leisure, and/or daily living.
- Guidance in the selection and use of adaptive equipment.
- Therapeutic activities to enhance functional performance.
- Prevocational evaluation and training and physical capacity evaluation.
- Consultation concerning adaptation to home or work environments.

Occupational therapy assessment

Services are provided to all age groups in a variety of settings, including hospitals, hand clinics, rehabilitation facilities, sheltered workshops, schools, extended care facilities, private homes, community agency clinics, and industrial settings.

Cases most frequently referred to occupational therapy relating to orthopaedics are: amputation, arthritis, hand trauma, fractures (hip, femur, tibia, ankle, humerus, radius, ulna, wrist), total joint replacement, sports injury, osteoporosis, elbow and shoulder arthroplasty, spinal cord injury, and chronic pain. One-fourth of AOTA's more than 40,000 members work with orthopaedic patients.

Before treatment is given, each potential patient's case is *screened* to determine the need for occupational therapy. This is followed by assessment, which consists of obtaining and interpreting data necessary for treatment, including that needed to plan for and document the evaluation process and treatment results. The occupational therapy evaluation includes assessment of functional abilities and deficits as related to the patient's needs.

Specific evaluations, tests, and devices

Specific evaluations, tests, and devices used in the assessment process include but are not limited to the following:

Baltimore Therapeutic Equipment Work Simulator (BTE): a device used for evaluation and work hardening.

bulb dynamometer: a soft, cylindrical, rubber-filled squeeze bulb that measures gross isometric grasp and pinch, calibrated in pounds per square inch, measuring force in pounds by multiplying the reading by 4.

Crawford small parts dexterity test: of fine eye-hand coordination and manipulation of small hand tools.

Functional capacities assessment: simple rating scale on living skills, indicating progress according to 10 functional levels.

Jamar dynamometer: measures gross isometric grasp in five positions and records in either pounds or kilograms.

Jebsen-Taylor hand function test: consisting of seven subtests to measure major aspects of hand function related to activities of daily living.

LIDO lift and workset: provides rehabilitation and evaluation of physical work-related activities.

Martin Vigorimeter: to test handgrip strength.

Minnesota rate of manipulation test: to measure dexterity from seventh grade to adult level.

O'Connor finger dexterity test: designed to measure fine motor ability.

Pennsylvania bi-manual worksample: measures finger dexterity of both hands, gross movements of both arms, eye-hand coordination, ability to use both hands simultaneously.

ecpinch: three-point lateral and fingertip prehension tested with pinch gauge recorded in pounds or kilograms.

Purdue pegboard: measures gross movements of arm, hand, and fingers and fingertip dexterity.

Smith physical capacities evaluation (Smith PCE): objective test to measure ability of individual to perform selected aspects of occupations.

two-point discrimination: measured with calibrated metric aesthesiometer.

Valpar component work sample series. consisting of 16 work samples designed to measure 17 work behaviors by task analysis, developed for workers with industrial injuries.

VonFrey hair test (Simms-Weinstein monofilament): a series of monofilaments with different ratings to determine amount of sensory loss.

WEST (work evaluation systems technology): evaluating work tolerance of upper extremities and/or total body, including ability to measure lifting capabilities and torque strength of hand.

Occupational therapy treatments

Occupational therapy treatment refers to the use of specific activities or methods to develop, improve, or restore the performance of necessary functions, compensate for dysfunction, or minimize debilitation. The therapist plans for and documents treatment performance. The following are categories of necessary functions treated in occupational therapy for orthopedic problems*:

Activities of daily living/physical daily living skills (ADL/PDLS) are components of everyday activity, including self-care, work, and play/leisure activities. These may also be referred to as life skills or life tasks and consist of the following:

bathing: ability to obtain and use supplies and soap, rinse and dry all body parts, maintain bathing position, transfer to and from bathing position, use adapted bathing equipment such as bath mitt, tub bench, grab bars, scrub brush, etc.

toilet hygiene: ability to obtain and use supplies, clean self, and transfer to and from and maintain toileting position on bedpan, toilet, and/or commode.

dressing: ability to select appropriate clothing, obtain clothing from storage area, dress and undress in sequential fashion, fasten/unfasten clothes and shoes, and don and doff appliances, for example, glasses, prostheses, or orthoses.

---

*Definitions taken from *Occupational Therapy Product Output Reporting System and Uniform Terminology for Reporting Occupational Therapy Services, 1981* and revision in preparation.

grooming: ability to obtain and use supplies to shave, apply and remove cosmetics, wash, comb, style and brush hair, care for nails, care for skin, and apply deodorant.

feeding/eating: ability to set up food, use appropriate regular or adapted utensils and tableware, and bring food or drink from table to mouth.

functional mobility: ability to move from one position or one place to another as in bed mobility, wheelchair mobility, transfers (bed, chair, tub, toilet, car), and functional ambulation with or without adaptive aids, driving, or use of public transportation.

functional communication: ability to use equipment or systems to enhance or provide communication, such as writing equipment, telephones, typewriters, communication boards, call lights, emergency systems, braille writers, augmentative communication systems, and computers.

Work activities include home management tasks such as clothing care, cleaning, meal preparation and cleanup, household maintenance, care of others, and safety procedures. The latter is important in preventing falls in areas such as bathroom, kitchen, and stairs.

Vocational activities consist of vocational exploration, job acquisition, and timely and effective job performance.

Play or leisure involves choosing and engaging in activities for amusement, relaxation, spontaneous enjoyment, or self-expression.

sensorimotor skills: consist of performance patterns of sensory and motor behavior prerequisite to self-care, work, and play and leisure performance, such as:
range of motion (ROM)
gross and fine coordination
muscle control
coordination
dexterity
strength and endurance
sensory awareness, including
    tactile awareness
    stereognosis

kinesthesia
proprioceptive awareness

cognitive skills: necessary mental processes, including orientation, conceptualization/comprehension (concentration, attention span, memory), and cognitive integration (applying diverse knowledge to environmental situations, including ability to generalize and problem solve).

prevention and minimization of debilitation: refers to programs for persons with predisposition to disability, as well as for those who have already incurred a disability, and include the following:

energy conservation: activity restriction, work simplification, time management, or organization of the environment to minimize energy output:

joint protection: procedures to minimize stress on joints, including use of proper body mechanics, avoidance of static or deforming postures, and avoidance of excess weight-bearing.

positioning: placement of body part in alignment to promote optimal functioning.

therapeutic adaptations: design or restructuring of the physical environment to assist self-care, work, and play and leisure performance through selecting, obtaining, fitting, and fabricating equipment, as well as instructing client, family, and staff in its proper use and care, including making minor repairs and modifications for correct fit, position, or use.

Some categories of therapeutic adaptation are:

orthotics, splints, or slings: to relieve pain, maintain joint alignment, protect joint integrity, improve function, or decrease deformity, consisting of

static splints: with no moving parts, designed to maintain joint in desired position.

dynamic splints: to allow for or provide motion by transfer of movement from other body parts or by use of outside forces such as springs, rubber bands, carbon dioxide, or electricity.

functional fracture bracing (using thermoplastics): proximal or distal to fracture, in combination with hinge joint to provide motion and allowing weight-bearing to enhance osteogenesis.

prosthetics: artificial substitutes for missing body parts to augment functional performance, with occupational therapy especially involved in upper extremity prosthetic checkout and training.

assistive/adaptive equipment: additions or devices that assist in performance or in structural or positional changes, such as installing ramps and bars, changing furniture heights, adjusting traffic patterns, and modifying wheelchairs.

Some typical adaptive equipment examples for orthopaedics are reachers, sockdonners, elevated toilet seats, leg-lifter straps, and walker adaptations (platforms and walker bags).

12

Musculoskeletal research

Orthopaedic research is the investigation of and the experimentation on the musculoskeletal system as related to disease and trauma, and its subsequent reconstruction. Research provides a scientific basis for most decisions made in orthopaedic surgery. Of the many achievements made, the greatest advances in recent years have been in the area of prosthetic and orthotic devices, particularly in terms of the positive impact on the quality of life enjoyed by those with fractures of the hip or joints destroyed by disease. Before new technology was developed through research, hundreds of persons suffered major economic and social losses. The treatment of musculoskeletal diseases has been considerably improved, as have fracture healing methods with the use of electricity and magnetic fields, approved by the Food and Drug Administration for general use. Of patients seen by primary physicians across the country, approximately one third have musculoskeletal problems. Therefore there is an increasing need for high-caliber professionals in musculoskeletal research.

This field includes biochemistry, biomechanics, immunology, and prosthetic technology. In the biochemical realm are the studies involving the proteins and special sugars that make up connective tissues. Additionally, minerals are responsible for bone crystallization, nerve conduction, and muscle contraction. Extensive research has been done to study electrical and magnetic forces and fields in different tissues in the normal and diseased states. Biomechanically there are the forces that break bone, stretch tendons, and shear cartilage. These same forces can be studied in healing, deformity, and in the application of surgical and bracing techniques. Immunology is becoming important in understanding the acceptance and rejection of nerve, bone, and tendon grafts. Additionally, immunology is helping in understanding the role of the body's normal defense mechanisms in various bone and soft tissues cancers. Finally, the world of implants has markedly expanded. Not only are materials diversifying, the method of attachment for internal prosthetics has changed rapidly in the past 20 years. The understanding of bone dynamics, wear phenomena, and distribution of forces in internal prosthetics is undergoing a rapid evolution. External prosthetic design is beginning to take on the look of space-age technology with the application of microcomputer devices.

Orthopaedic research consists of biomedical and clinical investigation and requires the commitment and dedication of the orthopaedic research team. This team may consist of the principal investigator, assisted by junior investigators, biochemists, physicists, engineers, physiologists, dentists, veterinarians, laboratory technicians, and many others from the medical and scientific areas. Research endeavors may take months or years, with the ultimate goal to improve the quality of care through the application of biologic and engineering principles to the musculoskeletal system. Interdisciplinary cooperation has been the hallmark of this field of endeavor.

A *research proposal* is an application for a research grant. This proposal is written up by the investigator(s), who submits a protocol outlining the proposed research plan, goals, and potential benefits. In addition the investigator(s) must estimate time, personnel, laboratory space and equipment, and amount of funds required to accomplish the project. Once this information is gathered, the proposal goes before a grants committee reviewing board, which then decides whether it justifies funding. Sometimes a proposal is granted but funds not provided, or only part of a project is funded. Many worthwhile research proposals must await funding before proceeding.

A *research grant* is the name for funds provided to support a specific research project. This support may be given through a large health institution, corporation, pharmaceutic company, private endowment, or government agency. The Orthopaedic Research and Education Foundation (OREF), an independent organization, is currently a principal private supporting mechanism, offering fellowship programs in clinical and laboratory investigations. Another group, the Orthopaedic Research Society (ORS), meets yearly to present papers and exchange ideas with those performing research within the orthopaedic community. The American Academy of Orthopaedic Surgeons Research Advisory Committee (RAC) monitors and advises on administrative requirements for orthopaedic research.

Once research protocols have been investigated and experiments completed, investigators disseminate data on results and benefits obtained through various journals to all clinicians in the field. This chapter presents an overview of research terms.

GENERAL RESEARCH TERMINOLOGY

The following terms are likely to be found in many areas of research, with the exception of biomechanics.

ANOVA: acronym for *an*alysis *o*f *va*riance, a statistical method for detecting significant differences between groups.

assay: assessment of the relative amount of a chemical in solution. Quantity is commonly expressed in terms of parts per million (PPM) or parts per billion (PPB).

cell components: of the many chemicals and parts of a cell, the most commonly described are the following.

centriole
endoplasmic reticulum
filaments
Golgi apparatus
lysosome
microsome
microtubule
mitochondria
nucleolus
nucleus
polyribosomes
ribosome
vessicle

circadian: pertaining to a biologic cycle describing a 24-hour period.

hertz (Hz): a unit of frequency equal to one cycle per second.

in vitro: analysis of reaction taking place outside the body but with attempt to simulate a chemical reaction that takes place within the body.

in vivo: an investigation carried out in tissue within a living body.

microsphere: a small sphere usually made of glass that is injected intravenously for studies of conditions such as blockage of small vessels and muscle injuries.

radioactive tracers: a variety of radioactive compounds commonly used to study the localization of specific elements or compounds. Those most commonly used in orthopaedics include the following:

^{45}Ca (calcium)
^{3}H (equal to tritiated, for example, tritiated thymidine)
^{51}Cr (chromium)
^{35}SO$_4$ (sulfate)
^{67}Ga (gallium)
^{85}S (strontium)

reagent: any substance with specific biologic or chemical action added to the solution of another substance to produce a chemical reaction.

scanning electron miocroscopy (SEM): to examine minute objects, a beam of electrons focused across a specimen produces an enlarged three-dimensional surface contour image of that specimen on a cathode ray tube. A photograph is then obtained.

transmission electron microscopy (TEM): to examine the internal structure of minute objects, a beam of electrons is transmitted through a specimen slice to produce an enlarged two-dimensional picture similar to that produced by a light microscope.

MEASUREMENTS

Most of the measurements used in the current orthopaedic literature are in the metric system, more specifically, the International System of Units. The basic units are the meter for length, kilogram for mass, second for time, and centigrade for temperature. The basic measurements are listed in the box below.

dalton: based on the mass of the C_{12} atom. This unit is used in expressing the weight of molecules, as opposed to molecular weight where the value given is the mass of 6.23×10^{23} molecules of the material. The term dalton is almost equivalent to the term molecular weight.

BONE HEALING AND METABOLISM

Research directed at chemical reactions in living tissue will often overlap with microscopic and electron microscopic techniques. After centuries of technologic refinement in the fields of biochemistry and histology (study of cells), the two fields have developed the ability to see or visually outline molecular structures and confirm by picture what is observed by the biochemist. Many terms listed in this and other sections are part of the investigatory vocabulary of the histologist, electron microscopist, and biochemist.

bone morphogenic protein: protein involved in the stimulation of bone formation.

bone salts: calcium (Ca), phosphate (PO_4), and hydroxyl (OH) ions are the main components of the bone crystal that is directly attached to the collagen molecule. The process by which this attachment occurs is very complicated. Associated terms include the following.

apatite ($Ca_{10}[PO_4]_6[OH]_2$)

alkaline phosphatase

acid phosphatase

brushite

calcium phosphate, dibasic (brushite, $CaHOP_4$ $2H_2O$)

amorphous calcium phosphate ($Ca_9[PO_4]_6$)

calcium pyrophosphate (CaPPi)

calcium phospholipid phosphate

phospholipid

proteolipid

phosphotidyl serine

phosphotidyl inositol

pyrophosphate (PPi, PYP)

calcitonin: a short-chain protein hormone that is involved in bone accretion. The activity of this hormone will reduce the level of serum calcium

Exponent of log base 10	Distance	Stress	Force
10^{-12}		picopascal	
10^{-9}	nanometer	nanopascal	
10^{-6}	micron	micropascal	
10^{-3}	millimeter	millipascal	
10^{-2}	centimeter		
		pascal (1 newton times 1 meter)	newtons (1 gram mass accelerated 1 m/sec)
10^0	meter (39.37 inches)		
10^3	kilometer	kilopascal (KPa)	
10^6		megapascal (MPa)	
10^9		gegapascal (GPa)	
10^{12}		tetrapascal (TPa)	

by its effect on new bone addition at the point where this is taking place.

cement line: the refractile boundary of an osteon, interstitial lamellar system, or border between cartilage and bone. This line marks the completion point of local development or remodeling of bone. Also called a tide mark.

GLA (gamma carboxyglutamic acid): amino acid seen particularly in osteocalcin and chondrocalcin, a protein involved in bone mineral formation.

matrix vesicles: extracellular units that are involved in the initiation of calcium apatite crystal formation.

osteocalcin: vitamin K dependent GlA protein involved in a number of bone formation processes, including the placement of calcium into mature apatite crystals.

parathyroid hormone (PTH): long-chain polypeptide involved in bone crystal removal and elevation of serum calcium; has multiple functions in that it affects the increase of calcium retention by the kidneys and has many other metabolic effects.

phosphoproteins: type of protein generated by bone cells. There are at least three different ones, and their function is unknown.

skeletal growth factor: a bone-derived stimulator of cell division.

somatomedin (insulin-like growth factor I, Sm-C): protein growth factor that is produced in local or distant cells. Stimulates DNA production, cell differentiation, and production of specific cell products.

vitamin D: although a vitamin, it is metabolized by the body and functions as a hormone. Vitamin D is changed chemically by the liver and kidney, aiding in the absorption of calcium by the gut, retention of calcium by the kidney, and removal and replacement process in bone metabolism. Related terms are the following.

1,25-dihydroxycholecalciferol (equivalent of 1,25-dihydroxy vitamin D_3 and 1,25-DHCC)

25-hydroxycholecalciferol (equivalent of 25-HCC)

Wolff's law: the scientific law that states bone will form and remodel in the direction of forces acting on it.

ELECTROBIOLOGY

Recently the application of electric or magnetic fields about fracture sites has been found to stimulate bone formation in the presence of fracture nonunion. The electric stimulation is done by the direct insertion of electrodes into bone using a continuous current. Another method of treatment involves the external application of magnets with the field driven by an external electric current. As a result of years of research, electric or magnetic stimulation is now an approved form of treatment. Terms commonly used in reference to this work are the following:

anode: an electric pole that has a positive charge and attracts negative ions.

capacitor (capacitive coupling): in orthopaedic bone stimulation application, not a true capacitor. Two plates are placed parallel to a resistor and applied to the skin on opposite sides of a nonunion. A high-frequency (60 kHz) current then produces small currents in the deep tissues.

cathode: an electric pole that has a negative charge and attracts cations, which are positively charged ions. In the stimulation of bone formation this is the active pole around which the bone is formed.

magnetic field: the magnetic force field developed as a result of a fluctuating electric current. The field has polarity that is described by north and south poles. In the stimulation of fracture healing the magnetic polarity is directed so that the forces are perpendicular to the site of the fracture.

The magnetic pulses are of two general types. One is a short burst of rapid pulses with repetitions of 15 times a second. This pulse is used mostly in nonunion bone stimulation. The second is a single wider pulse at 72-75 Hz used to stimulate vascular ingrowth such as in avascular necrosis.

stress-generated potentials (SGP): any electrical potential produced by mechanical deformation of tissues, particularly bone cartilage and ligaments.

piezoelectric potentials: a charge that is developed on molecular surface of a material, such as bone collagen and apatite crystals due to bending of that material.

streaming potentials: potentials created near the charged molecular surface created by the passage of charged ions in fluids during the course of deformation.

zeta potential: the relative electric potential produced at the point of the slip plane of passing fluid that contains electrically charged ions. This slip plane is usually 7 Å from the surface.

CARTILAGE AND JOINTS

The surface of bone at the joint is covered with a glistening white to blue-white tissue called hyaline cartilage. This cartilage is composed of living cells that slowly replace themselves, getting nourishment from the circulation in bone and fluid in the joint. For the most part there is no circulation in cartilage. The matrix, material between the cells, is composed of collagen and proteoglycan aggregates. Since much of the research on bone and soft tissues involves collagen, these terms are listed separately.

Proteoglycans are principally found in cartilage. However, they are also found in bony matrix, which is composed almost completely of collagen. Proteoglycans come in many forms, depending on the anatomic location. The basic structure of proteoglycan aggregates is a number of proteoglycan subunits composed of specific mucopolysaccharides attached to the protein core. The subunits are then attached by link protein to hyaluronic-acid chain. The final structure is a molecule that may well have a molecular weight of well over a million. The mucopolysaccharides that make up the side chain of these subunits will vary from one area of the body to the next and will also vary in specific mucopolysaccharide disorders. The various subunits are described with specific chemical compounds.

cathepsin: enzyme that separates proteoglycan from core protein.

chondrocalcin: a protein found in epiphyseal plate cartilage. It is involved in the formation of calcium apatite crystals in the area of hypertrophied cartilage.

core protein: the central protein of the proteoglycan subunit.

glycosaminoglycans (GAG, mucopolysaccha- **rides):** the ammoniated and sulfated sugars that make up the 4 to 60 molecule sugar chains that attach to the core protein.

chondroitin: a sulfated sugar with 40 to 60 repeating units of glucuronic acid (glucuronate) and N-acetylgalactosamine; makes up part of proteoglycan subunit.

chondroitin sulfate A (chondroitin 4 sulfate)
chondroitin sulfate B (chondroitin 6 sulfate)
chondroitin sulfate C (dermatin sulfate)

keratin sulfate: a sulfated sugar with 5 to 20 repeating units of galactose and N-acetylglucosamine; makes up part of proteoglycan subunit.

hyaluronic acid: repeating units of glucuronic acid (glucuronate) and N-acetylglucosamine that make up the core of the proteoglycan aggregate.

glucosamine: any given ammoniated sugar. Also called hexosamine.

hyaluronidase: enzyme that breaks up hyaluronic acid.

link protein: specific 40,000 to 50,000 molecular weight protein that connects proteoglycan subunit to hyaluronic acid chain.

proteoglycan: complex molecule incorporating ammoniated sugars.

proteoglycan aggregate: complex structure of proteoglycan subunits attached by link protein to hyaluronic acid chains (Fig. 12-1).

proteoglycan subunit: proteoglycans attached to core protein.

COLLAGEN

Collagen is a protein material found in all connective tissues of the body. It is also found in plants and is the basic ingredient in gelatin. Collagen is produced by cells and acts as the supporting structure that lends cohesion to a variety of connective tissues. Bone is almost purely a combination of collagen and bone crystals. Some collagen is found in cartilage. The tendons and ligaments are composed mostly of collagen, but it is a slightly different type than the collagen found in bone.

There are three chains of proteins that make up a single fibril. The chains are composed of different amino acid sequences and mixtures and are labeled with Greek letters, for example, alpha, beta, and gamma. Different combinations of these chains

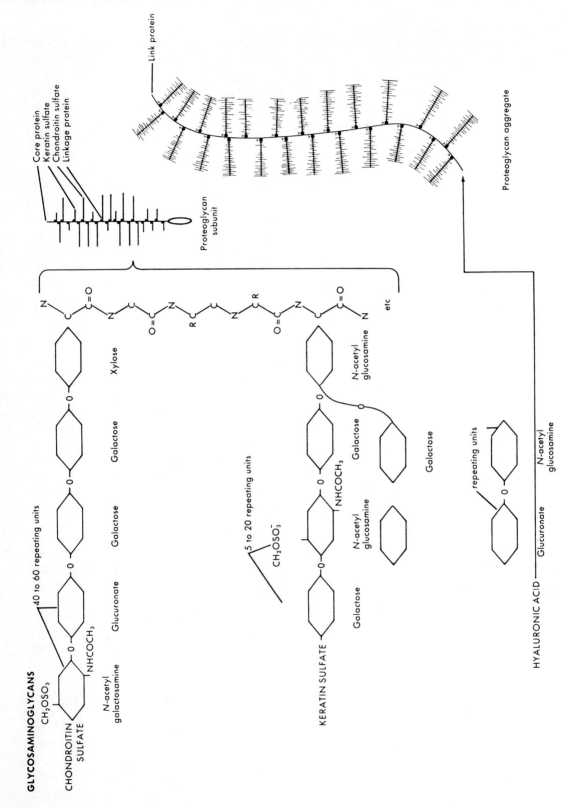

Fig. 12-1. Proteoglycan molecular structure.

then compose the fibrils. Depending on the chain composition, the fibrils are labeled as type I through VI collagen. The following terms are related to collagen metabolism.

collagenase: enzyme that breaks down collagen molecules.

cross-linking: the chemical attachment of molecular chains to make fibrils and fibrils to make collagen fibers. Once these links are interrupted, the molecule is rapidly broken down by collagenase.

fiber: when applied to collagen, denotes the complete collagen fiber that is composed of many collagen fibrils.

fibril: mature collagen with intermolecular cross-links completed.

histidinohydroxymerodesmosine: an important amino acid in cross-linking.

hydroxylysine: amino acid that is hydroxylated after incorporation into protocollagen.

hydroxylysinonor leucine: an amino acid important in cross-linking.

hydroxyproline: amino acid that is hydroxylated after incorporation into protocollagen.

procollagen: collagen that exists as triple helix in single strands with end cystine groups and no cross-linking with other collagen (Fig. 12-2).

protocollagen: 3000A long chain of amino acids predominated with lysine and proline. Alpha 1, 2, and 3 chains have been identified.

tropocollagen: triple helix collagen that has had extra peptides removed, is outside the cell, but has not cross-linked with other collagen strands.

BIOMECHANICS

The terms used in *biomechanics* come more from a physics textbook than from anything normally seen in orthopaedics. The "loads" on bones, muscles, and joints can be studied from the static and dynamic standpoints, looking at forces, work accomplished, and any deformation. The energy absorbed by the system is analyzed with an eye to the deformation and recovery or permanent deformity resulting from the deformation, as in fractures and ruptures. Because much of the tissue is complex, there are peculiarities in its responses that prompt study of elasticity of various structures under the heading of *viscoelasticity*.

The study of motion and the forces that produced the motion is known as *kinesiology*. In human research the interest in the relationship of motion between two parts of the body, such as the leg and thigh, is known as *kinematics*. The gliding of joints is studied in terms of lubrication and viscoelasticity.

Another area of research in biomechanics is the field of design. The shape and material composition of implants are studied from the standpoints of stress, strain, deflection, fatigue, wear, and friction. The body's immunologic response to new implant materials of metals, alloys, ceramics, and plastics has enabled the musculoskeletal system to have thousands of "spare parts," available through use of engineering principles and research. With wider acceptance of implants, the field of biomechanics is drawing an ever-increasing number of nonorthopaedic members to the team.

There is considerable overlap in biomechanical terminology; therefore the frequently used terms are in alphabetic order.

acceleration: change in velocity per unit of time.
   linear acceleration: rate of change of velocity in a straight line (m/sec^2).
   angular acceleration: rate of change of average angular velocity. The instant center is that point about which the rotation occurs (degrees/sec^2).

allowable stress: a stress value that is higher than that of normal loads but is lower than the yield stress of the material. The unit of measure is newtons per square meters (pascals) or pounds per square inch.

angular displacement: change of angular position of a line measured in degrees.

anisotropic material: a material in which the mechanical properties vary depending on the spatial direction of forces.

average angular velocity: angular displacement divided by the time taken for that displacement (degrees/sec).

average velocity: displacement divided by the time taken for that displacement (cm/sec).

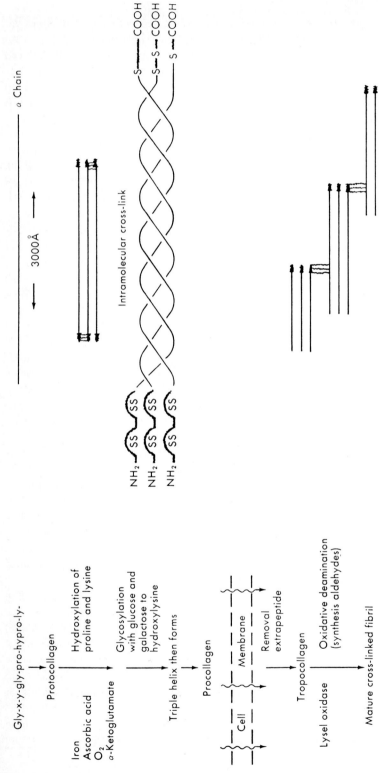

Fig. 12-2. Collagen synthesis.

bending: deformation of a structure in response to a load applied to an unsupported portion of that structure.

bending moment: a quantity at a point in a structure equal to the product of the force applied and the shortest distance from the point to the force direction. The unit of measure is newton meters or foot-pound force.

bending moment diagram: a diagram showing amount of bending moment at various sections of a long structure subjected to bending loads.

biomechanical adaptations: biologically mediated changes in the mechanical properties of tissues (material properties and/or structural changes) in association with the application of mechanical variables to those tissues.

brittle failure: failure by fracture before permanent deformation occurs, for example, breaking glass versus plastic failure seen in the bending of a willow stick.

centroid: a point on which the total area may be centered.

center of gravity (center of mass): point in a body where the body mass is centered.

coefficient of friction: the ratio of tangential force to the normal interbody compressive force required to initiate motion between the two bodies. No units of measure.

compression: the force that tends to push two objects together, the unit of measure is newtons or foot-pound force.

couple: a pair of equal and opposite parallel forces acting on a body and separated by a distance. The moment or torque of a couple is defined as a quantity equal to the product of one of the forces and the perpendicular distance between the forces. The unit of measure for the torque is newton meters or foot-pound force.

coupling: a phenomenon of consistent association of one motion (translation or rotation) about an axis with another motion about a second axis. One motion cannot be produced without the other.

creep: the viscoelastic deformation of a material with time when it is subjected to a constant, suddenly applied load. The deformation-time curve approaches a steady state asymptotically.

degrees of freedom: the number of independent coordinates in a coordinate system required to completely define the position of an object in space.

displacement: change in the position of a particle; compared with a specific point of reference when studying deformation or other motion.

ductile failure: failure of a structure because of excessive plastic deformation, such as pulling on a wire, with stretching and eventual breakage.

ductility: the property of a material to absorb relatively large amounts of plastic deformation energy before deformation. The opposite is brittleness.

dynamic load: a load that varies with time.

elastic behavior: exhibited when deformation caused by a load returns to original position when the load is removed, as in a rubber band.

elastic modulus: an index of the degree to which an object is changed in shape per unit of force applied to it.

elongation: the amount of deformation of a metal that a tensile stress or load will produce, a measure of ductility.

energy: the ability to do work, the amount of work done by a load on a body, measured in newton meters or foot-pound force.

equilibrium: the condition of a body that is not accelerating; the sum of all forces acting on an object is zero. To clarify, an object will remain still or move in the same direction or at the same angular velocity unless there is some external force applied to change it; Newton's law.

fatigue failure: failure by fatigue either with or without permanent deformation, caused by cyclic loading, for example, to bend a paper clip a number of times to point of breaking.

fatigue fracture: a fracture or break in a material caused by repeated applications of loads that are less than the yield strength but greater than the fatigue limit.

fatigue limit: the load a material can endure indefinitely without bending or breaking when subjected to cyclic loading.

fatigue strength (endurance limit): the maximum

load a material can withstand without fracture when subjected to 10 million cyclic loads.

force: any action that tends to change the state of rest or of motion of a body to which it is applied; unit of measure is newtons or pound force.

free-body analysis: a technique for determining the stresses at a point in a structure subjected to external loads.

helical axis of motion: a unique axis in space that completely defines a three-dimensional motion between two rigid bodies, analogous to instantaneous axis of rotation for plane motion.

hysteresis: a phenomenon associated with energy loss exhibited by viscoelastic materials when they are subjected to loading and unloading cycles.

impulse: product of the force and the time interval of application; measured in newton seconds or pound force seconds.

inertia: the property of all material bodies to resist change in the state of rest or motion under the action of applied loads.

instantaneous axis of rotation: when a body moves in a plane, there is a point in the body or some hypothetical extension of it that does not move. An axis perpendicular to the plane of motion and passing through that point is the instantaneous axis (center) of rotation.

isotropic: the properties of a material are the same for forces applied in all directions.

joule: unit of measure; 1 newton times 1 meter (newton meter).

kilopond: a force equal to the gravitational force applied to one kilogram of mass at the earth's surface.

kinematics: division of mechanics (dynamics) that deals with the geometry of the motion of bodies; displacement, acceleration, and velocity, without taking into account the forces that produce the motion.

kinetic energy: the value assigned to the energy of a moving object.

loading: any force applied to an object. In orthopaedics the normal forces acting on bone, joints, tendons, or ligaments, are called *functional loads*, loads that distract are *tensile loads*, and those that compress are *compressile loads*.

mass moment of inertia: the quantitative measure of inertia for change in angular velocity. The unit of measure is kilogram meter squared or pound foot squared.

modulus of elasticity: the ratio of normal stress to normal strain in a material. The unit of measure for the modulus of elasticity (E) is newtons per square meter or pound force per square foot.

moment: quantity necessary to angularly accelerate a mass.

moment of inerta of an area: a measure of the distribution of a material in a certain manner about its centroid. The distribution determines the strength in bending and torsion. The unit of measure is meters or feet to the fourth power.

momentum: product of mass and velocity of a moving body, may be angular or linear. When linear the unit of measure is kilogram meters per second or pound feet per second.

newton: amount of force required to give a 1 kilogram mass an acceleration of 1 meter per second.

normal strain: the quantity described by the quotient of the change of length of a line and its original length.

normal stress: the quantity described by the quotient of distributed force and area when the force is perpendicular to the area.

pascal: one newton per square meter.

plastic behavior: exhibited when deformation caused by a load which does not return to the original position when the load is removed, for example, stretching gum.

plasticity: the property of a material to permanently deform when it is loaded beyond its elastic range.

Poisson ratio: the ratio of transverse to axial strain, generally noted by the Greek letter ν (nu), and no unit of measurement.

polar moment of inertia: a property of a cross-section of a long structure that gives a measure of the distribution of the material about its axis so as to maximize its torsional strength. The unit of measure is meter or foot to the fourth power.

potential energy: energy that may be stored within a structure as a result of deformation or displacement of that structure. The unit of measure is newton meters (joules) or foot pound force.

rigidity: the amount of load required to give a structure one unit of deformation.

shear modulus: the ratio of shear stress to the shear strain in a material. The unit of measure is newtons per square meter (pascals) or pound force per square foot.

shear strain: the change in angle between two lines originally at right angles in a solid (measured in radians).

shear stress: the quantity described by the quotient of force and the area, when the force is applied parallel to the area.

SI units: system of international units such as meter, kilogram, second, and centigrade degree.

statics: the branch of mechanics that deals with the equilibrium of bodies at rest or in motion with zero acceleration.

stiffness: a measure of resistence offered to external loads by a specimen or structure as it deforms.

stiffness coefficient: the property of a structure defined by the ratio of force applied to the deformation produced. It quantifies the resistance that a structure offers to deformation.

strain: the change in unit length or angle in a material subjected to a load.

strain energy: energy stored in a body by virtue of its being deformed under the application of a load, for example, a spring.

strength: the maximal load that a structure can withstand before functional failure occurs (load strength) or the maximal energy that a structure can withstand before functional failure occurs (energy strength).

stress: the force per unit area of a structure and a measurement of the intensity of the force. Stress may be compressile, force directed into the material; tensile, forces away from or distracting the material; or shear, forces parallel to the surface. Units of measure are newtons per square meter or pound force per square foot.

stress-strain diagram: the plot of stress, usually on *y* axis, versus strain, usually on *x* axis. Also called *load deformation curve.*

torr: a measure of pressure, one torr equals 1 mmHg pressure. One standard atmospheric pressure is equivalent to 760 torr.

torque: the force acting about a pivot point described by force times distance from the pivot point.

torsion: a type of load that is applied by a couple of forces that are parallel and directed opposite to each other about the long axis of a structure.

torsional rigidity: the torque per unit of angular deformation. The unit of measure is newton meters per radian or foot-pound force per degree.

toughness: the ability of a material to absorb energy by bending without breaking.

ultimate load: the largest load a structure can sustain without failure. The unit of measure is newtons or pound force if the load is a force; and newton meters or foot-pound force if the load is a torque or moment.

vector: a quantity that has both magnitude and direction.

viscoelasticity: the property of a material to show sensitivity to the rate of loading or deformation.

viscoelastic stability: the type of stability in which the critical load is a function of time as well as the geometric and material properties of the structure.

viscosity: the property of materials to resist loads that produce shear; the ratio of shearing stress to shearing strain rate; the ratio of shearing stress to velocity gradiant. Commonly represented by η (eta) or μ (mu). The unit of measure is newton seconds per square meter, or pound force per square foot, and poise (1 poise = 0.1 newton seconds per square meter).

weight: the force applied by gravitational pull.

work: the product of force multiplied by the displacement through which the force moves.

yield stress: that point of stress on the load deformation curve at which appreciable deformation takes place without any appreciable increase in load. The unit of measure is newtons per square meter or pound force per square foot.

BIOMATERIALS

Historically many different types of materials have been used in attempts to replace bone and joints artificially. Wood, ceramics, and unsophisticated metals were the first materials used, and later metal alloys, including Vitallium and stainless steel, were accepted as having the least wear problems associated with little reaction from the body.

Research into biomaterials is currently directed at long-term use of joint replacement materials. From a bioengineering standpoint, loosening, fatigue failure, and wear are the major problems being investigated. Porous materials that allow bony ingrowth are being researched for the potential development of devices that do not require the use of polymethylmethacrylate "cement" fixation. Biodegradable materials for fracture fixation are also being studied.

metal alloy: a combination of metallic elements with no chemical bonding, but where the combination renders sought-after characteristics of nonreactiveness, durability, and certain biomechanical characteristics. Some standard alloys and some being investigated are the following.
cobalt chrome
Elgiloy
HS25
MP35N
multiphase alloy
nitrided titanium 6-4
stainless steel 316L
titanium
titanium 6-4
Vitallium

bioceramics: ceramic materials composed of glass, glass metals, or metal combinations, resulting in smooth, form-holding products; used mostly in joint replacement. Types are the following.
alumina
low-surface reactive bioglass
nearly inert bioceramics
resorbable bioceramics

Plastic materials have been used for years, with polyethylene receiving the greatest use. Several new plastics are currently under study for increased utilization, such as the following.
Delrin (polyacetyl)
UHMWPE (graphite-fiber reinforced ultrahigh molecular weight polyethylene)

synthetic ligaments: There are two basic types of synthetic ligaments under investigation: those that have cells growing into the fabric, and those that rely entirely on their structure. Some of the materials used are the following:
carbon fiber
coated carbon fiber
Dacron tape
Gor-tex
polypropylene
Proplast
woven bovine collagen
Zenotech

Orthopaedic abbreviations

Many abbreviations are used in orthopaedic terminology that are not used by the general medical profession. The Joint Commission on Accreditation of Health Organizations (JCAHO) has directed that each hospital establish a standard list that is used and known by all specialties. However, the orthopaedic physician facilitates many more to expediently fulfill his needs in a clinical situation. The "physician's shorthand" given here is a compendium for recognition as a reference only.

Care must be taken when using abbreviations. In some cases a single abbreviation may serve for several words. For example, the abbreviation "quad" could refer to quadrilateral (hip), quadriceps (musculature), and quadriplegic (paralysis). Therefore consider the context of the material being read to determine which word is used. References vary widely in the use of capitalization of abbreviations.

CONDITIONS, DISEASES, AND SYNDROMES

ALS: amyotrophic lateral sclerosis; anterolateral sclerosis
ARDS: adult respiratory distress syndrome
AS: arteriosclerosis; aortic stenosis
AVF: arteriovenous fistula
AVM: arteriovenous malformation
CA: carcinoma
CDH: congenitally dysplastic hip; congenitally dislocated hip
CP: cerebral palsy
CREST: *c*aleinosis, *R*aynaud, *e*sophogeal, *s*clerodactyly, *t*elangiectasia
CVA: cerebrovascular accident (stroke)

DISI: dorsiflexed intercalated segment instability
Disl: dislocation
DJD: degenerative joint disease
DVT: deep vein thrombosis
FA: false aneurysm
FB: foreign body
FFC: fixed flexion contracture
Fract or fx: fracture
FUO: fever of undetermined origin
HNP: herniated nucleus pulposus
IDK: internal derangement of the knee
INFH: ischemic necrosis of femoral head
ITT: internal tibial torsion
LCP: Legg-Calvé-Perthes disease
LE: lupus erythematosus
LLD: leg length discrepancy
LOM: limitation of motion
MD: muscular dystrophy
MI: myocardial infarction
MS: multiple sclerosis
OCD: osteochondritis dissecans
PE: pulmonary embolism
PFC: pelvic flexion contracture
PFFD: proximal femoral focal deficiency
PID: pelvic inflammatory disease
PMD: progressive muscular dystrophy
polio: poliomyelitis
PVC: premature ventricular contraction
PVD: peripheral vascular disease
quad atrophy: quadriceps atrophy
RA: rheumatoid arthritis
SCFE: slipped capital femoral epiphysis
SLE: systemic lupus erythematosus
staph: *Staphylococcus* or implies *Staph. aureus* species

strep: *Streptococcus*
sympt or sx: symptoms
TB or TBC: tuberculosis
TIA: transient ischemic attack
THR: total hip replacement
TMJS: temporomandibular joint syndrome
URI: upper respiratory tract infection
UTI: urinary tract infection
VATER: *v*ertebral, *a*nd *t*racheosophogeal, *e*sophogeal, *r*adical
VDDR: vitamin D–dependent rickets
VDRR: vitamin D–resistant rickets
VISI: volar flexed intercalated segment instability

GENERAL ANATOMY

abd: abdomen
ANS: autonomic nervous system
ant: anterior
AV: arteriovenous; atrioventricular
BB to MM: belly button to medial malleolus (examination)
CNS: central nervous system
collat: collateral
CSF: cerebrospinal fluid
CV: cardiovascular
D/3, distal/3: distal third
DP: dorsalis pedis (pulse)
GB: gallbladder
GI: gastrointestinal
GU: genitourinary
HEENT: head, ears, eyes, nose, throat (examination)
inf: inferior
lig: ligament
ligg: ligature; ligament
LLE: left lower extremity
LLL: left lower limb
LLQ: left lower quadrant
LSK: liver, spleen, and kidneys
LUE: left upper extremity
LUL: left upper limb
LUQ: left upper quadrant
M/3, middle/3: middle third
med: medial
mm: muscles; mucous membrane

MM: mucous membrane
NV: neurovascular
P/3, proximal/3: proximal third
PERRLA: pupils equal, round, regular to light accommodation
PNS: peripheral nervous system
post: posterior
px: pneumothorax
quad: quadriceps; quadrilateral; quadriplegic
RLE: right lower extremity
RLL: right lower limb
RLQ: right lower quadrant
RUE: right upper extremity
RUL: right upper limb
RUQ: right upper quadrant
sup: superior

SPECIFIC ANATOMY
Spine and related terms

AAL or ant ax line: anterior axillary line
AC: acromioclavicular (joint)
ASIS: anterosuperior iliac spine
C-1 to C-7: cervical vertebrae
C-spine: cervical spine
cva: costovertebral angle (Do not confuse with CVA—cerebrovascular accident.)
D-spine: dorsal spine*
ICS: intercostal space (ribs)
IS: interspace
L-1 to L-5: lumbar vertebrae
LS: lumbosacral (spine)
L-spine: lumbar spine
MAL: midaxillary line
MCL: midclavicular line
MSL: midsternal line
PAL: posterior axillary line
PSIS: posterosuperior iliac spine
S-1 to S-5: sacral vertebrae
SC: sternoclavicular (joint)
SI: sacroiliac (joint)
T-1 to T-12: thoracic vertebrae
T-spine: thoracic spine*

---

*When reference is made to the dorsal and thoracic spines, they are one and the same. T-spine or D-spine may be used in clinical notes.

Hands

abd poll: abductor pollicis
add poll: adductor pollicis
ADQ: abductor digiti quinti M.
APB: abductor pollicis brevis
APL: abductor pollicis longus
CMC: carpometacarpal
DIP: distal interphalangeal (joint); DIPJ
DP: distal phalanx
DPC: distal palmar crease
ECRB: extensor carpi radialis brevis
ECRL: extensor carpi radialis longus
ECU: extensor carpi ulnaris
EDC: extensor digitorum communis
EDL: extensor digitorum longus
EDQ: extensor digiti quinti
EHL: extensor hallucis longus
EIP: extensor indicis proprius
EPB: extensor pollicis brevis
EPL: extensor pollicis longus
FCR: flexor carpi radialis
FCU: flexor carpi ulnaris
FDL: flexor digitorum longus
FDP: flexor digitorum profundus
FDQB: flexor digiti quinti brevis
FDS: flexor digitorum sublimis
FPB: flexor pollicis brevis
FPL: flexor pollicis longus
IP: interphalangeal (joint)
MCP: metacarpophalangeal (joint)
MP: middle phalanx (or metaphalangeal) joint
ODQ: opponens digiti quinti M.
PB: peroneus brevis
phal: phalanx or phalanges
PIP: proximal interphalangeal (joint); PIPJ
PL: peroneus longus
PP: proximal phalanx
PQ: pronator quadratus
PT: pronator teres
UN: ulnar nerve (finger spreader)

Fingers

1st digit: thumb
2nd digit: index
3rd digit: long
4th digit: ring
5th digit: little

Feet

CAWA: closing abductory wedge osteotomy
DIP: distal interphalangeal (joint); DIPJ
DP: dorsalis pedis pulse
HA: hallux abductus
HD: heloma durum (hard corn)
HM: heloma molle (soft corn)
HT: hammertoe
HV: hallux valgus
IHW: inner heel wedge
IPJ: interphalangeal joint
IPK: intractable plantar keratosis
MHW: medial heel wedge
MPJ: metaphalangeal joint
MPV: metatarsus primus varus
MT bar: metatarsal bar
MTA: metatarsus adductus
MTJ: midtarsal joint
MTP: metatarsophalangeal (joint)
MTV: metatarsus varus
OAWO: opening abductory wedge esteotomy
PIP: proximal interphalangeal (joint); PIPJ
PTP: posterior tibial pulse
PW: plantar wart
STJ: subtalar joint
TEV: talipes equinovarus
TMT: tarsometatarsal

SURGICAL PROCEDURES AND RELATED TERMS

5 in 1: five procedures done during same surgery for ligamentous repair of the knee for rotatory instability
Anes: anesthesia
AO: Arbeitsgemeinschaft fur osteosynthesefragen
Bx: biopsy
CR: closed reduction
CTR: carpal tunnel release
en bloc: in a lump; as a whole
ESIN: elastic stable intramedullary nailing
H: per hypodermic
I&D: incision and drainage

IM: intramuscular; intermuscular; intramedullary (rod)
IV: intravenous
lam: laminectomy
lami: laminotomy
LASER: light amplification by stimulated emission of radiation
lat men: lateral meniscectomy
LP: lumbar puncture
med men: medial meniscectomy
OR: operating room; open reduction
ORIF: open reduction/internal fixation
OW: open wedge (osteotomy)
PLIF: posterolateral interbody fusion
PO, postop: postoperatively
preop: preoperatively
prog: prognosis
PTT: patellar tendon transfer
RR: recovery room
SDR: surgical dressing room
SQ: subcutaneous
STSG: split-thickness skin graft
Sub-Q, SC: subcutaneous (under the skin)
surg: surgical; surgery
TAL: tendon Achilles lengthening
TG: tendon graft
THA: total hip arthroplasty
THR: total hip replacement
TJR: total joint replacement
TT: tendon transfer
TTAP: threaded titanium acetabular prosthesis

Amputation and prosthesis sites

AE: above elbow
AK: above knee
BE: below elbow
BK: below knee

X-RAY EXAMINATIONS

AP: anteroposterior
BMP: bone marrow pressure
CAT (scan): computerized axial tomography
CXR: chest x-ray examination
IVP: intravenous pyelogram
KUB: kidney, ureter, and bladder view of abdomen
lat: lateral

MRI: magnetic resonance imaging
obl: oblique
PA: posteroanterior
R: Roentgen, x-ray examination
RA: radium
RAD: roentgen absorbed dose
REM: roentgen-equivalent-man
SPECT: single photon emission computerized tomography
tomo: tomogram
XIP: x-ray in plaster (examination)
XOP: x-ray out of plaster (examination)

CASTS AND SPLINTS

DBS: Denis Browne splint
FWB: full weight-bearing
HCTU: home cervical traction unit
ICT: intermittent cervical traction
LAC: long-arm cast
LANC: long-arm navicular cast
LAS: long-arm splint
LLC: long-leg cast
LLS: long-leg splint
LLWC: long-leg walking cast
MAST: medical antishock trousers
NWB: non-weight-bearing
PTB: patellar tendon-bearing (cast, orthosis, prosthesis)
PWB: partial weight-bearing
SAC: short-arm cast
SANC: short-arm navicular cast
SAS: short-arm splint
SDD: sterile dry dressing
SLC: short-leg cast
SLS: short-leg splint
tx: traction

EXERCISES AND TESTS (PHYSICAL AND OCCUPATIONAL THERAPY)

A(ROM): active range of motion
AA: active-assistive (range of motion)
ABD: abduction
ADL: activities of daily living
ADD: adduction
AG: antigravity
AGE: angle of greatest extension

AGF: angle of greatest flexion
BME: brief maximal effort
CMS: circulation, muscle sensation
DKB: deep knee bends
DTRs: deep tendon reflexes
ERE: external rotation in extension
ERF: external rotation in flexion
FABER: flexion in abduction and external rotation
FADIR: flexion in adduction and internal rotation
FES: functional electrical stimulation
FF: further flexion
FFC: fixed flexion contracture
IRE: internal rotation in extension
IRF: internal rotation in flexion
MMT: manual muscle testing
OT: occupational therapy
P: passive
PCE (Smith): physical capacities evaluation
PEMF: pulsating electromagnetic fields
PFC: pelvic flexion contracture
PNF: proprioceptive neuromuscular facilitation
PR: pelvic rock
PREs: progressive resistive exercises
PT: physical therapy
RM: repetition maximum
ROM: range of motion
SLR: straight leg raising
TENS: transcutaneous electrical nerve stimulation
TT: tilt table
WC: wheelchair
WEST: work evaluation systems technology
WFE or Wms flex ex: Williams flexion exercises
∥ bars: parallel bars

Reflex tests

AJ: ankle jerks
BJ: biceps jerks
EJ: elbow jerks
KJ: knee jerks
TJ: triceps jerks

Physical therapy treatments

CB: contrast baths
EMG: electromyography
HP: hot packs
HT: Hubbard tank

IR: infrared (light)
MWD: microwave diathermy
NCV: nerve conduction velocity
PB: paraffin baths
SWD: shortwave diathermy
US: ultrasound
UV: ultraviolet (light)
WPB: whirlpool bath

MISCELLANEOUS

abd: abdominal (pad)
ADL: activities of daily living
adm: admission
ASAP: as soon as possible
BP: blood pressure
c̄: with; cum
C: centigrade
Cath: catheter
CC: chief complaint
c/o: complaint of
decub: decubitus position; lying down
DIE: died in emergency room
disch: discharge
DL: danger list
DOA: date of admission; dead on arrival
DOE: date of examination
Dx or diag: diagnosis
ECG: electrocardiograph(gram); EKG
EDC: estimated date of confinement
EEG: electroencephalograph(gram)
EOM: extraocular movement
expir: expiration
F: Fahrenheit
FH: family history
H&P: history and physical (examination)
HPI: history of present illness
Hx: history
L&W: living and well
mx: management
NB: note well
OD: oculus dexter (right eye); overdose
OPD: outpatient department
Ortho: orthopaedics
OS: oculus sinister (left eye). Also abbreviated OL.
OU: both eyes
p̄: after

P&A: percussion and auscultation
PE, Px: physical examination
PH: past history
PI: present illness
PMHx: past medical history
PRN: whenever necessary
prog: prognosis
pt: patient
PTA: prior to admission
R/O: rule out
ROS, SR: review of systems
RRE: round, regular, and equal
RTC: return to clinic
RV: return visit
s̄: without
SH: social history
SL: serious list
SOS: if necessary
stat: immediately
TPR: temperature, pulse, respiration
TPN: total parenteral nutrition (IM, IV, etc.)
VSL: very serious list
WD, WN: well developed, well nourished
WNL: within normal limits
x̄: except
⊖ **or ō:** negative
+ or ⊕: positive
Δ: difference, deltoid muscle
↑ **or >:** increase, greater than
↓ **or <:** decrease; less than
♂: male
♀: female
1°: primary
2°: secondary
3°: tertiary

PRESCRIPTIONS (℞)
Forms

amp: ampule
aq, aqu: aqueous; water solution
ASA: aspirin
caps: capsules
cpd: compound
ETOH: alcohol
fl: fluid

med: medicine
prep: preparation
quant: quantity
℞: (Latin) to take; recipe
sol, soln: solution
tabs: tablets

Amounts

dr, ʒ: dram (4 ml)
g, gm: gram (15 grain)
gr: grain (60 milligram)
gtt: drop (0.05 ml)*
kg: kilogram (1,000 gram)
mg: milligram (1/60 grain)
oz, ℥: ounce (8 dram, 30 ml)
qt: quart (32 oz, 0.946 liter)
s̤s̤: ½ (e.g., gtt s̤s̤ = ½ drop)
wt: weight

Directions

Sig: let it be labeled; directions

When:
ac: before meals
ad lib: as desired
ASAP: as soon as possible
c̄c: with meals
dc, D/C: discontinue
hs: at bedtime
p̄: after
pc: after meals
pp: after meals (postprandial)
sos: repeat once if need exists
stat: immediately
sum: take
ut dict: as directed

How often:
bid: twice a day (ii)
prn, PRN: as often as necessary; ad lib
q: every
qam: every morning

*Units of measure are usually not capitalized.

qd, od: every day
qh: every hour
q3h: every 3 hours
qid: four times a day (iiii)
qn: every night
qod: every other day
qpm: every afternoon or evening
qs or QS: as much as suffices; quantity sufficient
quotid, in d: daily
tid: three times a day (iii)

Where:
IM: intramuscular (injection)
IV: intravenous (injection)
NPO: nothing per oral (by mouth)
po: per oral
pr: per rectum
Sub-Q: subcutaneous

NOTE: Laboratory abbreviations remain within that chapter.

APPENDIX B

Anatomic positions and directions

In orthopaedics, anatomic positions and directions are frequently used to provide an accurate description of specific anatomic locations. These basic directions may be compared to looking at a map to determine the longitude and latitude of an area. Humans are three-dimensional subjects with points of reference made in the orthograde (upright) position. The surface locations and anatomic planes are described as follows.

SURFACE LOCATION

The location of a structure is described in reference to a standing person facing the examiner with outstretched hands in a palms-up position. The basic directional terms are:

anterior (ventral): forward or front surface.

posterior (dorsal): back surface.

lateral: sides, away from midline.

medial: middle, toward the midline.

superior: upper area, above, toward the head.

inferior: lower area, below, toward the tail end.

These reference points may be combined to give a more precise location to a specific region on a surface or in structures deep within the body, for example, the exposed hip in a surgical procedure. When these terms are compounded and hyphen omitted, the combining forms may be:

anteromedial	posterosuperior
anterosuperior	anteroposterior
posteromedial	posterolateral
anterolateral	superolateral
dorsolateral	

ANATOMIC PLANES

The term *plane* comes from the Latin word, planus, meaning a flat, level surface. There are three directions of planes, all in reference to a standing person facing the examiner: vertical anterior to posterior (sagittal), vertical side to side (coronal or longitudinal), and horizontal (transverse).

anteroposterior planes

median (midsagittal) plane: vertical plane directly through the midline of the body, transecting the nose, navel and spine, and dividing body into left and right halves.

median or sagittal plane: any of the anteroposterior planes through the midaxis, dividing body in half; the term sometimes implies the median plane only. If the word sagittal is used to denote the median plane, then other sagittal planes are called parasagittal planes.

vertical side to side planes

coronal (frontal plane) a plane parallel with long axis of body at right angles to median sagittal plane going through coronal sutures of the skull (approximately center of body) and dividing body into front and back parts.

longitudinal: lengthwise and parallel with long axis of body or part; any of the vertical side to side planes. Coronal and longitudinal planes have been used interchangeably to describe each other. In this case, the context of

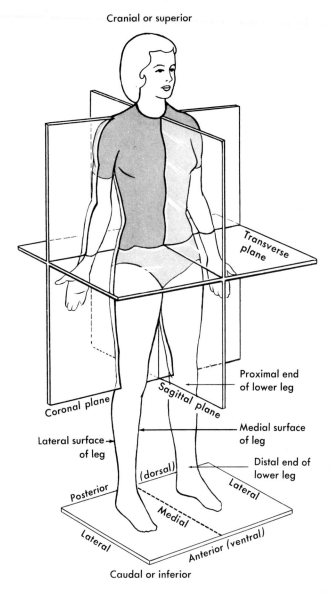

Fig. 1. Anterior view of human figure demonstrating meaning of terms used in describing the body. (From Anthony CP and Kolthoff N: Textbook of anatomy and physiology, ed 9, St Louis, 1975, The CV Mosby Co.)

the sentence will indicate the reference point of the plane.

horizontal (transverse) plane: any of the horizontal planes across the body at right angles to coronal and sagittal planes parallel to baseline.

SPECIFIC LOCATIONS

When describing limb anatomy, the nomenclature is very specific. The four appendages are correctly referred to as the upper and lower limbs, two forelimbs, and two hindlimbs. The *thigh* indicates that portion above the knee and the *shank* the portion between the knee and ankle. The *calf* is the posterior aspect and the *shin* the anterior aspect of the leg. The sole (bottom) of the foot is called the *plantar surface,* and the top is the *dorsal surface.* The *brachium* refers to that portion of the arm above the elbow and below the shoulder. The *antebrachium* refers to the portion of the arm below the elbow but above the wrist. The *ventral side* of the hand is the palm or *volar surface,* with the opposite side being the *dorsum* or *dorsal surface.* The forearm is similarly divided into volar and dorsal aspects.

JOINT MOTIONS*

Ranges of joint motion refer to the extent of movement within a given joint. Joint motion may be active, passive, or active assistive. The major joint areas involve the shoulder (glenoid), elbow (cubitus), hip (coxa), and knee (genu).

All the hinge joints have motion described in terms of *flexion* and *extension.* Except for the ankle, the 0-degree position occurs when the limb is held out straight, and the degree of flexion is then stated in terms of degrees from the 0-degree extended position. The knee and elbow will occasionally extend beyond the 0-degree limit, and this motion is expressed in degrees of *hyperextension.* The wrist has approximately 90 degrees of extension and 90 degrees of flexion (dorsiflexion and palmar flexion). Other measured motions include:

circumduction: a maneuver or movement of a ball-and-socket joint in a circular motion; for example, the shoulder can circumduct 180 degrees with six movements possible.

flexion: to bend from the joint as in flexion movements of the spine at the waist (anterior or lateral). In the foot or hand is expressed as:

dorsiflexion: the toe-up motion of the ankle expressed in degrees from the 0-degree position of the foot at rest on the ground in standing position.

valgus: the distal part is away from the midline,

*Further information about the assessment and recording of joint motions is obtainable from American Academy of Orthopaedic Surgeons: Joint motion—method of measuring and recording. Chicago, 1965, The Academy.

plantar flexion: the toe-down motion of the foot at the ankle expressed in degrees from 0-degree position of the foot at rest on the ground in standing position.

palmar flexion: of the wrist with palm up in flexion

extension: in the limbs is to extend distally away from body, or bending back posteriorly as in the spine.

pronation: palm-down position of hand with elbow at a 90-degree angle, brought about by the motion of the radius around the ulna (posterior rotation). In the foot, the plantar surface is turned down.

supination: palm-up position of the hand with elbow flexed at a 90-degree angle, brought about by motion of the radius around the ulna (anterior rotation). In the foot, the plantar surface is turned inward.

ulnar deviation: of the hand at the wrist such that the hand is directed in an ulnar direction; measured in degrees from 0 with hand in midline.

radial deviation: of the hand at the wrist such that the hand is directed radially; measured in degrees from 0 with hand in midline.

abduction: movement away from midline of body in frontal plane; applied to hip, shoulder, fingers, thumb, and foot. The midline reference point is a central line in the body for proximal joints and the central part of a limb for distal joints.

adduction: movement toward the midline in frontal plane as in abduction. On verbal transcription in clinical notes the person dictating will sometimes say "a-b-duction" or "a-d-duction" to clarify distinction between *ab*duction and *add*uction.

anteversion: in reference to the neck of humerus or femur, is an anterior rotation.

eversion: when applied to the heel, describes the degree of motion of the heel pushed outward with ankle in neutral position; when applied to the foot, describes the combined motions of dorsiflexion, pronation, and abduction.

inversion: when applied to the heel, describes the degree of motion of the heel pushed inward with ankle in neutral position; when applied to the foot, describes the combined motions of plantar flexion, supination, and adduction.

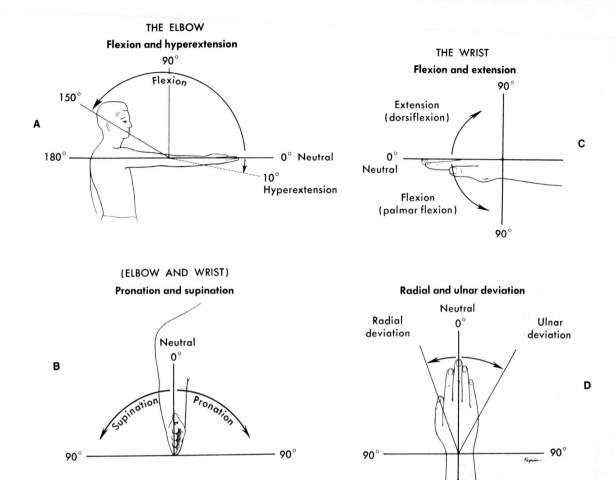

THE ELBOW

Flexion and hyperextension

THE WRIST

Flexion and extension

(ELBOW AND WRIST)

Pronation and supination

Radial and ulnar deviation

Fig. 2. A, Elbow. *Flexion:* 0 to 150 degrees. *Extension:* 150 degrees to 0 (from angle of greatest flexion to 0 position). *Hyperextension:* measured in degrees beyond the 0 starting point. This motion is not present in all individuals; when it is, it may vary from 5 to 15 degrees. **B,** Elbow and wrist. *Pronation:* 0 to 80 or 90 degrees. *Supination:* 0 to 80 or 90 degrees. *Total forearm motion:* 160 to 180 degrees. **C,** Wrist. *Flexion* (palmar flexion): 0 to about 80 degrees. *Extension* (dorsiflexion): 0 to about 70 degrees, **D,** Wrist. *Radial deviation:* 0 to 20 degrees. *Ulnar deviation:* 0 to 30 degrees. (From American Academy of Orthopaedic Surgeons: Joint motion—method of measuring and recording, Chicago, 1965, The Academy.)

retroversion: in reference to the neck of femur or humerus, is a posterior rotation.

apposition: contact of two adjacent parts; bringing together as in a finger movement, the thumb to index finger.

opposition: applied mostly to the thumb but also to little finger; describes the motion required to bring about opposition, or the setting opposite,

of thumb against little finger (pulp surfaces). For the thumb, opposition is the combined action of abduction, rotation, and flexion.

external rotation: in frontal plane is away from midline.

internal rotation: in a frontal plane is toward the midline.

valgus: the distal part is away from the midline,

THE HIP

Rotation in extension   **In flexion**

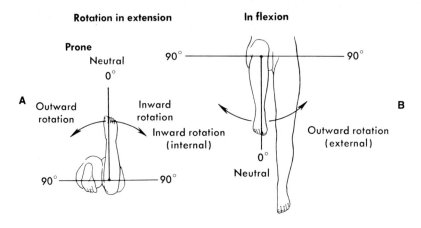

Prone

A

B

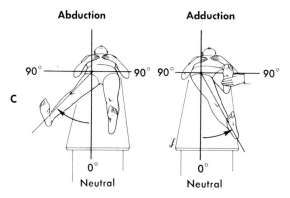

Abduction   **Adduction**

C

Fig. 3. The hip. **A,** *Inward rotation:* measured by rotating leg outward. *Outward rotation:* measured by rotating leg inward. **B,** *Inward rotation (internal):* measured by rotating leg away from midline of trunk with thigh as the axis of rotation, thus producing inward rotation of the hip. *Outward rotation (external):* measured by rotating leg toward midline of trunk with thigh as the axis of rotation, thus producing outward rotation of the hip. **C,** *Abduction:* outward motion of the extremity is measured in degrees from 0 starting position. *Adduction:* to measure examiner should elevate opposite extremity a few degrees to allow leg to pass under it. (From American Academy of Orthopaedic Surgeons: Joint motion—method of measuring and recording, Chicago, 1965, The Academy.)

for example, genu valgus (knock-kneed).

varus: the distal part is toward the midline, for example, genu varus (bowlegged).

ANATOMIC DIRECTIONS AND CONFIGURATIONS

The following are other associated terms referring to directions of anatomy or physical signs.

a, an: no, not.

ab: away from.

ad: toward.

Age: angle of greatest extension.

AGF: angle of greatest flexion.

alignment: linear position of one part of an extremity compared with another; to bring into a straight line.

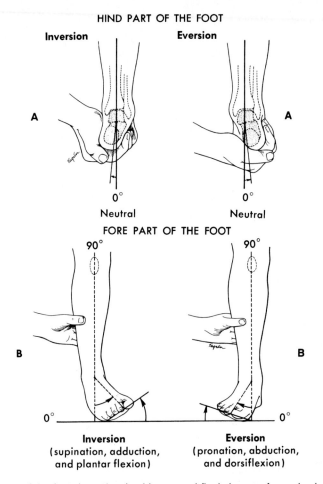

HIND PART OF THE FOOT

Inversion   **Eversion**

A   A

0°   0°

Neutral   Neutral

FORE PART OF THE FOOT

90°   90°

B   B

0°   0°

Inversion   **Eversion**
(supination, adduction,   (pronation, abduction,
and plantar flexion)   and dorsiflexion)

Fig. 4. A, Hind part of the foot. *Inversion:* heel is grasped firmly in cup of examiner's hand. Passive motion is estimated in degrees, or percentages of motion, by turning heel inward. *Eversion:* motion is estimated by turning heel outward. **B,** Fore part of the foot. *Active inversion:* foot is directed medial. This motion includes supination, adduction, and some degree of plantar flexion; can be estimated in degrees or expressed in percentages as compared with the opposite foot. *Active eversion:* sole of foot is turned to face laterally. This motion includes pronation, abduction, and dorsiflexion. (From American Academy of Orthopaedic Surgeons: Joint motion—method of measuring and recording, Chicago, 1965, The Academy.)

ambi: on both sides.

ambidextrous: using both right and left hands effectively.

amph-, amphi-: both ways, all around, both sides.

an-, ana-: up, increase, throughout, again.

angulation: sharp bend of a structure to form an angle.

ante-: forward, before.

antecedent: to precede, or go before.

anterior: front view, ventral side, face surface, superior.

antero-: before, in front of.

apex: top, tip, point of activity, summit, vertex (refers to C-2).

apical: pertaining to apex.

apo-: away from.

asymmetric: lacking symmetry; uneven, as one limb to another.

axis: line of symmetry, rotation, or revolution; pivot dividing line; also second vertebra.

basilar: base of a part.

bilateral: both sides.

cat-, cata-: down, through, concealed.

caudal, caudad: tail, inferior to or bottom point of reference, away from head.

centri-: center.

cephalic: head end, cranial end, uppermost point of reference.

circumference: around, outer circular boundary.

co-, com-, con-: together, with.

concave: rounded, depressed surface.

contralateral: opposite side.

convex: rounded, elevated surface.

craniad: toward the head.

curvilinear: curved away from straight line.

de-: away, from, down.

deep: depth from surface.

delta: triangle (deltoid).

dexter: right.

dia-: between, through, across, apart.

diffuse: widely distributed.

THE THUMB

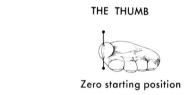

Zero starting position

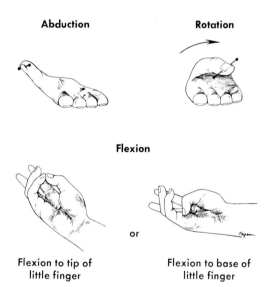

Abduction

Rotation

Flexion

or

Flexion to tip of little finger

Flexion to base of little finger

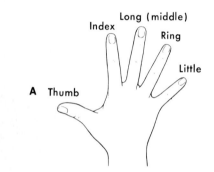

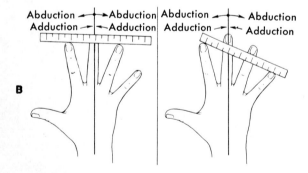

Fig. 5. **A,** Nomenclature of fingers. To avoid mistakes fingers and thumb are referred to by name rather than by number. **B,** Finger spread in abduction and adduction can be measured in centimeters or inches from the tip of index finger to tip of little finger. Individual fingers spread from tip to tip of indicated fingers. (From American Academy of Orthopaedic Surgeons: Joint motion—method of measuring and recording, Chicago, 1965, The Academy.)

Fig. 6. Thumb opposition. The motion is a composite of three elements: (1) abduction, (2) rotation, and (3) flexion. This motion is considered complete when tip, or pulp, of thumb touches tip of fifth finger or, according to some surgeons, when tip of thumb touches base of the fifth finger. (From American Academy of Orthopaedic Surgeons: Joint motion—method of measuring and recording, Chicago, 1965, The Academy.)

dis-: apart from.

distal: away from, furthest point of reference.

dorsal: back or posterior aspect.

ec-: out, out from.

ectopic: located away from normal position; out of place.

em-, en-: in, within.

endo-: within, in.

epi-: on, above, over.

eso-: in, inward, inside.

ex-, exo-: out, outside.

external: outside, describing walls, cavities, or hollow viscera.

extra-: beyond, outside, without.

facet: flat surface.

fore: in front of, before.

hyper-: over, above, excessive.

hypo-: under, below, deficient.

in-, ino-: into, in.

inferior: below point of reference, underneath.

infra: below or under.

in situ: in its natural place or position.

inter-: between.

intercalary: middle.

internal: inside; describing walls, cavities or hollow viscera.

interstitial: spaces within a structure.

intra-: within.

intro-: into, beginning.

ipsilateral: same side.

juxta: close to.

juxtaposition: apposition.

lat, latero-, lateral: sides, right and left; away from median plane, outer surface.

latus: broad.

levo: left.

linear: elongated, straight line.

longitudinal: lengthwise, parallel to the long axis of the body or an organ. (coronal or frontal planes).

medi-, medial: middle or median plane, toward midline, inner surface, link making halves.

megalo-: large.

meso-: large.

met-, meta-: beyond, from one place to another, point of change.

oblique: slanted, inclined.

palmar: side of hand suface, face up.

para-, par-: beyond, beside.

parallel: equal in lines or surface; in the same direction.

patent: open, unobstructed, apparent, evident.

peri-, peripheral: immediately around, sphere.

perpendicular: exactly upright; being at right angles to a given line or plane.

pivot: to turn as in a circular motion.

plantar: sole, bottom of the foot.

posterior, postero-, post-: after, behind, tail end, back, inferior to surface.

prone: face down (lying face down).

proximal: close to nearest point of reference.

re-: back, again.

recurvatum: bending backward; a flexure or hyperextension.

residual: left behind.

retrad: backward, toward back part.

retro-, retrograde: going backward, behind.

rotation: turning in a circular motion.

sinister: left.

sub-: under.

summit: top.

super-, supra-: above.

superficial: near the surface.

superior, supero-: uppermost side, above point of reference, toward head (cephalic).

supine: lying on back, face up.

sym-, syn-: together.

symmetric: exhibiting symmetry, even alike.

terminal: end.

trans-, transverse: across.

ultra: beyond.

unilateral: one side.

ventral: belly side (abdomen), anterior, front, face up.

vertex: top, summit.

vertical: perpendicular to the plane of the horizon (vertex).

volar: underneath suface, palm or sole.

Bibliography

General

American Academy of Orthopaedic Surgeons, Heck CV, editor: Fifty years of progress (1922–1983), Chicago, 1983, The Academy.

American Medical Association. Manual of style, ed 8, Baltimore, 1989, Williams and Wilkins.

American Orthopaedic Association, Brashear, HR, editor: Manual of Orthopaedic Surgery, ed 6, 1987, The Association.

American Orthopaedic Association. History of Orthopaedics. In Manual of Orthopaedic Surgery, 1986, pp 1-8.

Cozen L: Office orthopaedics, ed 4, Springfield, Ill, 1975, Charles C Thomas, Publishers.

Cyriax J: Textbook of orthopaedic medicine: diagnosis of soft tissue lesions, ed 8, Philadelphia, vol 1, 1984, Baillier Tindall.

Dorland's illustrated medical dictionary, ed 26, Philadelphia, 1981, WB Saunders Co.

Glanz WD et al.: Mosby's medical and nursing dictionary, ed 2, St. Louis, 1986, The CV Mosby Co.

Hilt NE and Cogburn SB: Manual of orthopaedics. St. Louis, 1977, The CV Mosby Co.

Stedman's medical dictionary. ed 25, Baltimore 1984, Williams and Wilkins.

Thomas CL, editor: Taber's cyclopedic medical dictionary illustrated, ed 13, Philadelphia, 1979, FA Davis Co.

Webster's new collegiate dictionary, Springfield, Mass, 1977, G&C Merriam Co.

Fractures

DePalma AF: The management of fractures and dislocations: an atlas. ed 3, vols 1-2, Philadelphia, 1981, WB Saunders Co.

Klafs CE and Arnheim DD: Modern principles of athletic training, ed 5, St Louis, 1981, The CV Mosby Co.

Kulund DN: The injured athlete, Philadelphia, 1982, JB Lippincott Co.

Owen R, Goodfellow J, and Bullough P: Scientific foundations of orthopaedics and traumatology, London, 1980, William Heinmann Medical Books, Ltd.

Peterson L: Sports injuries. Chicago, 1986, Yearbook Medical Publishing.

Rockwood CA, Green D: Fractures in adults, Philadelphia, 1984, JB Lippincott Co.

Rockwood CA, Wilkins KE, King RE: Fractures in children, Philadelphia, 1984, JB Lippincott Co.

Schultz RJ: The language of fractures, Huntington, NY, 1976, RE Krieger Publishing Co.

Seligson D and Pope M: Concepts in external fixation. New York, 1982, Grune & Stratton.

Diseases

Aegerter E and Kirkpatrick JA: Orthopaedic diseases: physiology, pathology, radiology, ed 4, Philadelphia, 1975, WB Saunders Co.

Albright JA and Brand RA: Scientific basis of orthopaedics, New York, 1979, Appleton-Century-Crofts.

American Academy of Orthopaedic Surgeons and the International Society for the Study of the Lumbar Spine: Glossary on spinal terminology, document 675-680, Chicago, 1980, The Academy.

Bogumill GP and Schwamm HA: Orthopaedic pathology: a synopsis with clinical and radiographic correlation, Philadelphia, 1984, WB Saunders Co.

Fitzgerald RH et al.: Orthopedic knowledge update, American Academy of Orthopedic Surgeons, 1987.

Gartland JJ: Fundamentals of orthopaedics, ed 4, Philadelphia, 1987, WB Saunders Co.

X-ray and scanning techniques

Greulich WW and Pyle SI: Atlas of the development of the hand and wrist, ed 2, Stanford, Calif, 1959, Stanford University Press.

Tanner JM, et al: Assessment of skeletal maturity and prediction of adult height (TW2) method, ed 2, London, 1983, Academic Press.

Todd TW: Atlas of skeletal maturity, St Louis, 1937, The CV Mosby Co.

Test sign and maneuvers

Hoppenfeld S: Physical examination of the spine and extremities. New York, 1976, Appleton-Century-Crofts.

Polly HF, Hunder GG: Physical examination of the joints, ed 2, Philadelphia, 1978, WB Saunders Co.

Trumbly CM: Physical disabilities, ed 2, Baltimore, 1983, Williams & Wilkins.

Laboratory evaluations

Kjeldsberg CR, Knight JA: Body fluids, ed 2, American Society of Clinical Pathologists, 1987.

Casts, splints, and dressings

American Academy of Orthopaedic Surgeons: Emergency transportation of the sick and injured, ed 3, Chicago, 1981, The Academy.

Schmeisser GA: A clinical manual of orthopedic traction techniques, Philadelphia, 1963, WB Saunders Co.

Schneider RF: Handbook for the orthopaedic assistant, ed 2, St Louis, 1976, The CV Mosby Co.

Simon RR, Koenigsknecht SJ: Emergency orthopedics: The extremities, ed 2, Norwalk, Conn, 1987, Appleton & Lang.

Prosthetics and orthotics

American Academy of Orthopaedic Surgeons: Atlas of limb prosthetics, Chicago, 1984, The Academy.

Bunch WH and Keagy RD: Principles of orthotic treatment, St. Louis, 1976, The CV Mosby Co.

Redford JB: Orthotics etcetera, ed 3, Baltimore, 1986, Williams and Wilkins.

Anatomy and surgery

American Orthopaedic Association: Manual of orthopaedic surgery, Chicago, 1979, The Association.

Burchardt H: The biology of bone graft repair, Clin Orthop (Philadelphia) 174:28, 1983.

Crenshaw AH: Campbell's Operative Orthopaedics, ed 7, St Louis, 1987, The CV Mosby Co.

Friedlaender GE: Immune responses to osteochondral allografts: current knowledge and future directions, Clin Orthop (Philadelphia) 174:58, 1983.

Haimovici H: Vascular surgery: principles and techniques, New York, 1984, Appleton-Century-Crofts.

Moore KL: Clinically oriented anatomy, ed 2, Baltimore, 1985, Williams and Wilkins.

Rutherford RB, editor: Vascular surgery, ed 2, Philadelphia, 1984, WB Saunders Co.

Tomford WW and Friedlaender GE: Bone banking procedures, Clin Orthop (Philadelphia) 174:15, 1983.

Weiland AJ: Current concepts review: vascularized free bone transplants, J Bone Joint Surg (Boston) 63A:166, 1981.

Hand

Lichtman DM: The wrist and its disorders, Philadelphia, 1988, WB Saunders Co.

Foot

Jahss MH: Disorders of the foot, vols I and II, Philadelphia, 1982, WB Saunders Co.

Mann RA: Surgery of the foot, ed 5, St Louis, 1986, The CV Mosby Co.

Physical therapy (PT)

American Occupational Therapy Association Commission on Practice Uniform Reporting System Task Force: Uniform terminology system for reporting occupational therapy services, Rockville, Md., 1979, The Association.

Kamenetz HL: Dictionary of rehabilitation medicine, New York, 1983, Springer Publishing Company.

Research

Brighton CT, Black J, and Pollack S: Electrical properties of bone and cartilage, New York, 1979, Grune & Stratton.

Frankel V: Orthopedic biomechanics, Philadelphia, 1970, Lea & Febiger.

SUGGESTED READINGS
Orthopaedics Journals and tapes

ACTA Chirurgiae Orthopaedicae et Traumatologiae Cechoslovaca (Praha)

ACTA Orthopaedica Belgice (Bruxelles)

Aktuelle Probleme in Chirurgie und Orthopadie (Bern)

Advances in Ortho Surg 1985 (Baltimore)

American Journal of Sports Medicine (Columbus, GA)

Archives of Orthopaedic and Traumatic Surgery (Berlin)

Archivio Putti di Chirurgia Degli Organi di Movimento (Firenze)

Arthritis & Rheumatism (Atlanta)

Arthroscopy (New York)

Audio Digest Foundation (Ortho Tapes) (Chicago)

Beitrage zur Orthopadie und Traumatologie (Berlin)

Bone (New York)

Bone and Mineral (Amsterdam)

Bulletin of the Hospital for Joint Diseases Orthopaedic Institute (New York)

Chirurgia Narzadow Ruchu I Ortopedia Polska (Warszara)

Chirurgia Degli Organi di Movimento (Bologna)

Clinical Orthopaedics and Related Research (Philadelphia)

Clinics in Sports Medicine (Philadelphia)

Continuing Education in Ortho Surg (Recert) (AAOS) (Chicago)

Foot and Ankle (Baltimore)

Hand Clinics (Philadelphia)

Instructional Course Lectures (Chicago)

International Orthopaedics (Berlin)

Italian Journal of Orthopaedics and Traumatology (Bologna)

Journal of Arthroplasty (New York)

Journal of Bone and Joint Surgery. American Volume (Boston)

Journal of Bone and Joint Surgery. British Volume (London)

Journal of Bone and Mineral Research (New York)

Journal of Hand Surgery (St. Louis)

Journal of Orthopaedic Research (New York)

Journal of Orthopaedic Trauma (New York)

Journal of Pediatric Orthopedics (New York)

Journal of Orthopaedics and Sports Physical Therapy (Baltimore)

Journal of Sports Medicine & Physical Fitness (Rome)

Magyar Traumatologia, Orthopaedia es Helyreallito Sebeszet (Budapest)

Nippon Seikeigeka Gakkai Zasshi. Journal of the Japanese Orthopaedic Association (Tokyo)

Orthopaedic Audio-synopsis (AAOS) (Chicago)

Orthopaedic Clinical Update Monograph (AAOS) (Chicago)

Orthopade (Berlin)

Orthopedic Clinics of North America (Philadelphia)

Orthopaedic Nursing (Pitman, NJ)

Orthopaedic Review (Lawrenceville, NJ)

Orthopaedic Survey (Chicago)

Orthopedics (Thorofare, NJ)

Ortopediia Travmatologiia I Protezirovanie (Kharkov)

Revue de Chirurgie Orthopedique et Reparatrice de 1 Appareil Moteur (Paris)

Skeletal Radiology (Berlin)

Spine (Hagerstown MD)

Yearbook of Orthopaedic Trauma & Surgery (Chicago)

Yearbook of Sports Medicine (Chicago)

Zeitschrift fur Orthopadie und Ihre Grenzgebiete (Stuttgart)

Osteopathic medicine

Journal of the American Osteopathic Association (Chicago)

Index

Parapodium orthosis, 123
Parathyroid hormone, 244
Paratonia, 89
Paratrooper fracture, 12
Paravertebral muscle spasm, 53
Paraxial hemimelia, 62
Paresis, 48
Paresthesia, 48
Parham band, 140
Parkinson disease, 48
Paronychia, 206, 211, 225
Parosteal chondrosarcoma, 29
Parosteal osteosarcoma, 28
Parrot-beak meniscus tears, 60, 61
Pars interarticularis, 171
Parsonage-Turner syndrome, 49
Partial adactylia, 62
Partial aphalangia, 62
Partial dislocation, 20
Partial hand amputation, 115
Partial hemimelia, 62
Partial meniscectomy, 190
Partial ostectomy, 230
Partial patellectomy, 191
Partial thromboplastin time, 97
  activated, 96
Partridge band, 140
Parvin maneuver, 83
Pascal, 250
Passive range of motion exercises, 235
Patch angioplasty, 158
Patella, 183, 184
  bipartite, 61
  dislocatiotns of, 21
  high-riding, 61
  subluxation of, 21
    chronic, surgery for, 190
  subluxing, 61
  surgery of, 190-191
Patella alta, 61
Patella baja, 61
Patellar fracture, 11
Patellar pad, 124
Patellar retraction test, 87
Patellar shaving, 191
Patellar tendon bearing orthosis, 122
Patellar tendon weight-bearing cast,
  105
Patellectomy, 191
Patello-femoral angle, lateral, 73
Patency, 156
Patent, 267
Pathologic dislocation, 20

Pathologic fracture, 12
Patrick test, 81, 82
Pauciarticular, 40
Paulos procedure (knee), 190
Pauwels angle, 73
Pauwels fracture classification system,
  17
Pauwels osteotomy, 135, 181
Pauwels-Y osteotomy, 135, 181
Pavlik harness, 123
Payr sign, 85
PCA total hip replacement, 145
PCA unconstrained devices, 146
PCA unicompartmental devices, 145
PCE, Smith, 238
PE, 42
Peabody procedure (foot), 230
Pearson attachment, 109, 111
Pectus caranatum, 67
Pectus excavatum, 67
Pedicle, 171
Pedicle bone grafts, 213
Pedicle flap, 213
Pedicle graft, 137, 193, 213
Peg graft, 138
Pegboard, Purdue, 238
Pellagra, 48
Pellegrini-Steida disease, 38
Pelvic band for above-knee prosthesis,
  118
Pelvic femoral angle, 73
Pelvic girdle, 177
Pelvic rock test, 82
Pelvic sling, 110
Pelvic traction, 110-111, 235
Pelvis
  anatomy of, 177-179
  blood vessels of, 187
  fractures of, classification of, 14, 19
  and hips, 177-182
  and proximal femur, fractures of, 10-
    11
  Otto , 21
  surgery of 180-182
surgical approaches to, 195
Pemberton osteotomy, 134, 181
Pennsylvania bi-manual worksample,
  238
Per primam, 201
Percutaneous transluminal angioplasty,
  157
Perforating arteries, 188
peri-, 267

Periarticular fibrositis, 37
Periarticular fracture, 6
Perilunate dislocation, 20
Perineal loops, 128
Periosteal fibroma, 37
Periosteal osteosarcoma, 28
Periosteotomy, 133
Periosteum, 132
Periostitis, 31
Periostomy, 133
Peripheral, 267
Peripheral nervous system, 46
Peripheral neuropathy, 48
Peritoneum, 178
Peroneal artery, 188
Peroneal muscles, 221
Peroneal nerves, 188
Peroneal spastic flatfoot, 225-226
Peroneus brevis muscle, 221
Peroneus longus muscle, 221
Peroneus tertius muscle, 221
Perry procedure (knee), 191
Perthes disease, 30, 32
Pertrochanteric fracture, 11
Pes, 226
Pes anserinus muscle, 185
Pes calcaneocavus, 226
Pes calcaneovalgus, 226
Pes calcaneus, 226
Pes cavovalgus, 226
Pes cavovarus, 226
Pes cavus, 226
Pes equinovalgus, 226
Pes equinovarus, 226
Pes planovalgus, 226
Pes planus, 226
  lanus, surgical procedures for, 227
Pes valgus, congenital convex, 224
Petaling edges of cast, 106
Petechiae, 66, 67
Petit mal epilepsy, 47
Petrie spica cast, 105
-pexy, 201
PFFD, 60
PGP nail, 140
pH, 100
Phalan maneuver, 84
Phalan test, 84
Phalangectomy, 215
  intermediate, 229
Phalanx, 208, 221, 223
Phalen-Miller opponensplasty, 214
Phantom pain, 201

Sagittal stress test, 87
Saha procedure (shoulder), 163
St. George-Buckholz ankle prostheses, 146
St. George fully constrained devices, 145
St. George sledge unicompartmental devices, 145
Salicylates, 96
Saline dressing, 108
Salmonella bone infection, 51
Salter fracture, 7
Salter osteotomy, 134, 181
Salter-Harris fracture, 7, 8
Salter sling, 123
Saltiel orthosis, 122
Salts, bone, 243
Salzer resurfacing procedure, 144
Sanfilippo syndrome, 36
Sanguinous, 67
Saphenous nerve, 188
Saphenous vein, 188
Saponification, 67
Sarbó sign, 89
Sarcoid, Boeck, 31
Sarcoma
    epithelioid, 29
    osteogenic, 28
    reticulum cell, 29
Sargent procedure (knee), 190
Sarmiento osteotomy, 135, 181
Sarmiento procedure (pelvis/hip), 182
Sarmiento total hip replacement, 144
Sartorius muscle, 179
Saucerization, 201
SBO, 55
Scaglietti hip reduction, 181
Scalene block 194
Scalenus muscle, 172
Scales and ratings, 90-91
Scanning electron microscopy, 242
Scanning techniques, x-ray films and, 69-77
Scanogram, 71
Scanography, 71
Scans, 75-76
Scaphoid, 221
Scaphoid fractures, classification of, 15
Scaphoid pads, 129
Scapula, 159
    surgery of, 161
Scapulectomy, 163

Scarborough total hip replacement, 144
Schanz hip osteotomy, 181
Schatzker fracture classification system, 18
Schede hip osteotomy, 181
Scheie syndrome, 36
Scheuermann disease, 26, 29, 32, 55
Schlein elbow prosthesis, 147
Schlesinger sign, 85
Schmorl nodes, 55
Schneider arthrodesis, 149, 182
Schneider nail, 140
Schneider rod, 140
Schreiber maneuver, 89
Schrock procedure (shoulder), 163
Schultze-Chvostek sign, 90
Schwann tumor, 37
Schwannoma, 49
Sciatic nerve, 179, 180, 188
Sciatic notch, greater, 178
Sciatic plexus, 178-179
Sciatica, 54, 57, 58
Scleroderma, 45
    focal, 45
    limited, 45
Sclerosing hyperostosis, diffuse idiopathic, 40
Sclerosing osteomyelitis, chronic, of Garre, 28
Sclerosis
    lateral, amyotrophic, 46
    Mönckeberg, 45
    multiple, 47
Sclerotomal pain, 57
Scoliorachitis, 54
Scoliosis, 54
    types of, 53, 54-55
Scoliosis cast, 104
Scotchcast, 104
Scott procedure (shoulder), 163
Scottish Rite orthosis, 123
Scout film, 71
Screen, type and, 97-98
Screws for internal fixation, 139-140
Scudari procedure (knee), 191
SD, 115
Seattle orthosis, 122
Sebaceous, 67
Secondary closure, 199, 201
Secondary fracture, 7
Secondary union, 13
Sed. rate, 94
Seddon arthrodesis, 212

Sedimentation rate, 94
Segmental fracture, 6, 7
Segmental graft, 138
Segmentation, failure of, of vertebra, 59
Segond fracture, 11
Segs., 99
Seinsheimer fracture classification system, 18
Seizure, 64
Self-bearing ceramic total hip replacement, 145
Selig procedure (pelvis/hip), 182
SEM, 242
Semicircular fixation devices, 141
Semiconstrained elbow devices, 147
Semiconstrained knee prostheses, 146
Semi-Fowler position, 111
Semilunar cartilages, 188
Semimembranosus muscle, 185
Semitendinosus muscle, 185
Senegas approach to hips, 195
Senile osteoporosis, 49, 50
Sensitivity, culture and, 95
Sensorimotor skills, 239-240
Sensory testing, 236-237
Sepsis, 67, 201
Septa, 206
Septic, 201
Septic thrombophlebitis, 42
Septicemia, 67
Sequelae, 67
Sequestration of disk, 58
Sequestrectomy, 133
Sequestrum, 28
Serendipity view, 71
Serial casts, 106
Serologic test for syphilis, 95
Serology, abbreviations for, 100
Seropurulent, 67
Serosanguineous, 67
Serous, 67-68
Serum alkaline phosphatase, 93
Serum calcium, 96
Serum chemistries, abbreviations for, 99-100
Serum gamma glutamyl transpeptidase, 96
Serum globulin, immune, 99
Serum GT, 96
Serum lead level, 96
Serum protein electrophoresis, 97
Sesamoids, 132, 209, 223